Tsunami of Diseases

Headed Our Way

Know Your Food

Before Time Runs Out

By
Dr. Sahadeva dasa

B.com., FCA., AICWA., PhD
Chartered Accountant

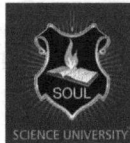

SOUL
SCIENCE UNIVERSITY

Soul Science University Press
www.cowism.com

A Food Manifesto For The Future

Readers interested in the subject matter of this
book are invited to correspond with the publisher at:
SoulScienceUniversity@gmail.com   +91 98490 95990
or visit DrDasa.com

First Edition: January 2013

Soul Science University Press expresses its gratitude to the
Bhaktivedanta Book Trust International (BBT), for the use of quotes by
His Divine Grace A.C.Bhaktivedanta Swami Prabhupada.

ISBN 97893-82947-01-1

Published by:
Dr. Sahadeva dasa for Soul Science University Press

Cover Design by:
Sailesh Ijmulwar, Waar Creatives, Hyderabad

Printed by:
Rainbow Print Pack, Hyderabad

To order a copy write to chandra@rgbooks.co.in
or buy online: Amazon.com, Rgbooks.co.in

Dedicated to....

His Divine Grace A.C.Bhaktivedanta Swami Prabhupada

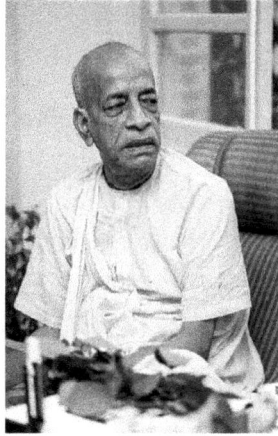

"The maximum duration of life for human beings in Kali-yuga will become fifty years.... the bodies of all creatures will be greatly reduced in size...cows will be like goats...most plants and herbs will be tiny, and all trees will appear like dwarf sami trees...and all human beings will have become like asses..."
(Srimad Bhagavatam 12.2.11-16)

By The Same Author

Oil-Final Countdown To A Global Crisis And Its Solutions

End of Modern Civilization And Alternative Future

To Kill Cow Means To End Human Civilization

Cow And Humanity - Made For Each Other

Cows Are Cool - Love 'Em!

Capitalism Communism And Cowism - A New Economics

For The 21st Century

Noble Cow - Munching Grass, Looking Curious And Just

Hanging Around

Let's Be Friends - A Curious, Calm Cow

Wondrous Glories of Vraja

We Feel Just Like You Do

(More information on availability on DrDasa.com)

Contents

Preface

.

Food is our common ground, a universal experience. If you're
happy, you eat. If you're sad, you eat. You lose a job, you
eat. You get a job, you eat. Therefore the bread is rightly called 'the
staff of life'.

Civilization as it is known today could not have evolved, nor
can it survive, without an adequate food supply.

It's amazing how pervasive food is. Every second commercial is
for food. Every second TV episode takes place around a meal. In the
city, you can't go ten feet without seeing or smelling a restaurant.
There are 20 feet high hamburgers up on billboards.

But there is trouble with our food today. Traditional societies
had good food but we just have good table manners. Our progress
is unfortunately destroying this important aspect of our existence.
There is even a saying that if you're going to America, bring your
own food.

We have taken food for granted. Its a mistake for which we are
paying dearly. Food doesn't grow on supermarket shelves.

A disease tsunami is sweeping the world. Humanity is dying out.
This is the result of our deep ignorance about our food.

When you have your health you have everything. Most people
who are sick and dying would trade all their possessions to feel
better and live longer. When they toast each other, no matter what
the language, it's usually some variant of, "to your good health."
There's nothing more important.

If you don't have good health, the other things like food, housing, transportation, education and recreation don't mean much.

Its time to realize that so long as you have 'healthy' food in your mouth, you have solved all questions for the time being.

We live in a culture of profit-seeking leeches that are only too happy to sell us compromised foods and line their pockets with the profits gained from pillaging our health. When are we going to stop them?

What is it going to take for us to demand accountability from the people who produce our food and those government agencies that supposedly protect the health of the public?

When will we pull our heads out of the sand and see the reality we face?

Sahadeva dasa

Dr. Sahadeva dasa
1st January 2013
Secunderabad, India

Section-I

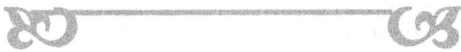

Food

A Sacred Gift
Of Life

Food - A Sacred Gift

Food is any nourishing substance that is eaten, drunk, or otherwise taken into the body to sustain life, provide energy, promote growth etc. It is usually of plant or animal origin, and contains essential nutrients, such as carbohydrates, fats, proteins, vitamins, or minerals. The substance is ingested by an organism and assimilated by the organism's cells.

Today, most of the food energy consumed by the world population is supplied by the food industry, which is operated by multinational corporations that use intensive farming and industrial agriculture to maximize system output.

Food - A Sacred Gift, A Blessing From Beyond

Ask any child where their food comes from, and the chances are he or she will say the supermarket.

And most adults don't know a lot more about how food ends up on their plate either.

In our concrete, day-to-day experience it seldom comes to our awareness that our food is a gift, a blessing from beyond. This is so because all food originates from reproducing plant life – life that God created. It takes water, air and sunlight for plants to grow, elements that are also created and regulated by God. The animals that become our food are dependent on this same plant life, air, water, and sunlight.

The divine source of our food is hidden from us by modes of production, packaging and distribution. The food we eat is manufactured in factories, bakeries and dairies or comes to us in trimmed bunches of produce without blemish.

Also, the divine source of our food is hidden from us by a consumer attitude of entitlement. It doesn't matter to us where food comes from because we deserve it; food is our right. Food is something we buy with our hard-earned money.

Food comes to us as a natural result of our hard work. To say food is a gift is to denigrate the efforts of our hard work and that of people in the food industry who labor in the fields, factories and retail sector to provide our food. We do not see food as a gift. Given the framework of the Western worldview and socioeconomic system, which places high currency on "individual rights," saying "food is a right" seems so politically correct.

In our economy it is by attributing rights to people that we acknowledge they are valued as human beings. In our economy the highest human values are enshrined as rights. We claim food as a right, and in our best charity we attribute that right to everyone.

Traditional societies had a much more spiritual understanding of food than we have in today's culture, where the Darwinian evolutionary ideas cloud our understanding.

Moreover, we live in a mortal economy, where food has been treated as a weapon, as a commodity. The truth is that food is a gift from the Creator, a blessing so that we may all live.

Every once in a while, something happens and the reality of a higher control bursts into our awareness. The trappings of our society and economy are stripped away. Then we see our daily food for what it is, a sacred gift of life.

Commodification Of Our Eating

Scanning and dropping packages in a Walmart basket is rarely occasioned with reflection upon one's place in the universe. The commodification of our eating has eliminated the empathy between consumers and consumed. Chemically nurtured and internationally distributed monocropping has robbed farmers of their connection with the rhythms of the soil and their relationship with the divine nature. Mass-produced and nutritionally bankrupt diets have broken the social ties of traditional cuisine. And the subjugation of meal-time to our commutes has eliminated the occasion to reflect upon and feel gratitude for this great gift of life.

In traditional societies, they treated this gift with respect due such a life-giving substance. Farmers considered Earth to be mother and farming to be a sacred act of worship. They sang and prayed for the rain and acknowledged their place in the cycles of nature. Animals were not treated as bags of flesh but their sacrifice was respected and their spirits revered.

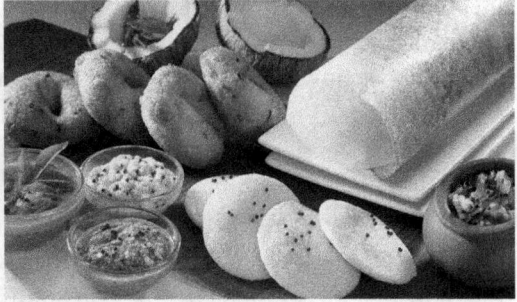

Cooking was sanctified and communities defined themselves in terms of their diets. Ceremonies and rituals were observed to bind people together through food. And the final act of eating was sanctified as prayers were spoken and bread was broken and friends and families fed their living with a sense of gratitude.

As these relationships and connections began to be displaced by commerce and greed, the sacred was squeezed out of our food system from the outside in.

"The shared meal elevates eating from a mechanical process of fueling the body to a ritual of family and community, from the mere animal biology to an act of culture."
~ Michael Pollan

2.

Food Prayers

Humankind's First Act of Worship

P rayer is how human beings relate to God, nature, and their place in the Divine order of things. Prayer is the principal channel we use in our search for the ultimate meaning of life and the fulfillment thereof.

Expressing thanks for food is humankind's first act of worship. In every culture there are sacred beliefs or divine commandments that require honoring the giver of life - God or the Divine principle - through acknowledging the sacred gift of food.

All civilizations and all religions through all ages associated food with God or gods; all primitives associate food with a supernatural power or spirits. All recognize the earth's bounty (crops and food) as a reflection of Divine goodness.

A grace is the thanks-to-God utterance before or after a meal. Food has always been recognized as the unmerited gift from God. Grace is the Divine reality underlying all religion and faith--that is, God's loving generosity.

Whether that expression of thanks (gratia) for the gift of food is voiced in a tribal ritualized saying or uttered silently or sung eloquently, a person's intrinsic spiritual nature imposes a

"... the way we eat represents our most profound engagement with the natural world. Daily, our eating turns nature into culture, transforming the body of the world into our bodies and minds."
~ Michael Pollan

recognition that the very food before him or her is sacred and comes to him or her from the beyond. In fact, our very table is sacred as the saying goes, "One eats in holiness and the table becomes an altar."

Expressing Mankind's Profound Debt To God

The Supreme Lord commands prayers of thanks for food. According to Adrian Butash, there are many ways to analyze and classify food prayers: by country, by culture, by language, by religion, by God, by food, by sacred imagery--to name a few.

In the ancient esoteric Jewish sect Essene, the members attributed highest sanctity to food. They never ate anything cooked by others, to the point of preferring to starve instead. Before their meals, they bathed themselves in cold water and after this purification, they assembled in a special building as though into a holy precinct. When they were quietly seated, the baker served out the loaves of bread in order, and the cook served only one bowlful of one dish to each man. Before the meal the priest said a prayer and no one was permitted to taste the food before the prayer. Afterwards they lay aside the garments which they had worn for the meal, since they were sacred garments.

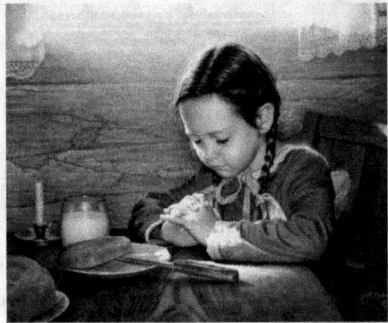

In India's Vedic system, food cannot be eaten unless it is first offered to God. It then becomes prasadam, the mercy of God.

In religions of the Far East, food and associated prayers play a central role. The modern Chinese expedient gratia before the banquet meal, Duo xie, duo xie (a thousand thanks, a thousand thanks), is merely the cultural evolution of worship chanted to the many food gods of Chinese antiquity. In cultural circles, the grace is - Ren Yi Shi Wei Tian' which translates as 'people perceive food to be almost like God.'

Shinto is the old native religion of Japan that reveres ancestors and nature spirits. Amaterasu is the most eminent of the Shinto deities. She is the beneficent sun goddess who taught mankind the cultivation of food. Inari is the grain god. Norito prayers petition the gods for good harvests. The Setsubun ceremony celebrates the start of a new season of seeds and planting. These rites, expressing thanks for the bounty of the earth, are popular even today.

The Bible has several citations: "And thou shall eat and be satisfied, and bless the Lord your God" (Deut. 8:10). Then there is The Lord's Prayer, "Give us today our daily bread" (Mat 6:11). These famous words are recorded in what is known as the "model prayer" that Jesus gave to his disciples instructing them how to pray.

"Bread" in the Bible and in the Middle East represented life itself, as grains used in bread making were the staple food. When people say this prayer, they are acknowledging that all sustenance comes from God, and that we are dependent upon him to give it to us every day.

A verse from the Koran instructs Muslims on the sacred origins of food and the requirement of food prayers: "Eat of your Lord's provision, and give thanks to Him" (34:15).

Buddhism's history is rich with reverence for food and thankfulness for its nourishment. Buddhists have used prayers of blessing and offering in everything from the cultivation of crops to the dedication of each plate of food to the betterment of humanity.

According to them, food can be truly blessed only when the one giving thanks has lived a life of service to both the universe that has given the food and those who suffer and are without food. Buddhism commands thankfulness for food by its "vow to live a life which is worthy to receive it."

Native American Indian tribes share a common reverence for the earth and all that is given from its bounty. Animals, harvests and water must be accepted with thankfulness in rituals and prayers. Respect for the food gift is often expressed by asking a plant or

The world's quest for happiness operates within a context of reverence for God through an inimitable link to food. In this uncertain age when ethnic differences divide people, we should strive to embrace our common humanity that is expressed so succinctly in food prayers. These prayers talk to us with the wisdom of the ages and teach us that we are all one family, all part of one mystical soul. Food prayers throughout history may be seen as evidence of our profound sense of awe in the face of The Infinite. ~ Adrian Butash

animal that must be used for food for its forgiveness in taking its life and explaining why its death was necessary. In Native American thought, human beings are dependent upon the earth, not master over it.

People go to church and say, "God, give us our daily bread." Actually, if He did not give it to us, we would not be able to live. That is a fact. The Vedas also say that the one Supreme Personality supplies all the necessities of every other living creature. God is supplying food for everyone. We human beings have our economic problem, but what economic problem is there in societies other than human society? The bird society has no economic problem. The species of life, and out of that, human society is very, very small. So they have created problems -- what to eat, where to sleep, how to mate, how to defend. These are a problem to us, but the majority of creatures -- the aquatics, the fish, the plants, the insects, the birds, the beasts, and the many millions upon millions of other living creatures -- do not have such a problem. They are also living creatures. Don't think that they are different from us. It is not true that we human beings are the only living creatures and that all others are dead. No. And who is providing their food and shelter? It is God. The plants and animals are not going to the office. They are not going to the university to get technological education to earn money. So how are they eating? God is supplying. The elephant eats hundreds of pounds of food. Who is supplying? Are you making arrangements for the elephant? There are millions of elephants. Who is supplying?

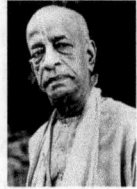

So the process of acknowledging that God is supplying is better than thinking, "God is dead. Why should we go to church and pray to God for bread?" In the Bhagavad-gita it is said, "Four kinds of people come to Krishna: the distressed, those who are in need of money, the wise, and the inquisitive." One who is inquisitive, one who is wise, one who is distressed, and one who is in need of money -- these four classes of men approach God. "My dear God, I am very hungry. Give me my daily bread." That's nice.

~ Srila Prabhupada (Science of Self Realization)

3.

You Are How You Eat

Eating With Awareness And Gratitude

You are what you eat. That is only half the truth. According to the nutritional scientist, Deborah Kesten, what you eat is as important as how you eat. And eating with that awareness may enhance your health and certainly enhance your whole quality of life. She is the author of "The Healing Secrets of Food."

According to her, it's important to appreciate the food we have got and eat it with gratitude. One's demeanor can greatly alter how the body processes food. For example, in the 1960s, cardiologist Meyer Friedman fed a high-fat, high-cholesterol, butter-laden "killer meal" to two groups of men: loud, aggressive Type A personalities and a mellower Type B group.

The doctor found the Type B group metabolized the fatty meal more effectively than the "hard-driving, competitive and impatient" Type A group. This experiment urged the people to slow down and appreciate food, considering it a blessing of life. Such a mindset is conducive to better digestion and assimilation.

According to the Ksema-kutuhala, a Vedic cookbook from the 2nd century A.D., a pleasant atmosphere and a good mood are as important to proper digestion as the quality of the food.

Look upon your food as God's mercy. Food has to be cooked, served and eaten in a spirit of joyful reverence.

In many experiments, it was observed that food smelled and tasted better to the test subjects when they were in a proper mindset. It is not enough, however, to be relaxed, mellow and spiritual and then gulp down mounds of greasy pizza and sugary snacks and gallons of soda.

Different kinds of cancer are increasing; high blood pressure, diabetes and congestive heart failure are on the rise. For this, the blame goes not only to 'what' we are eating, but also on 'how' we are eating.

After the ceremony, we went back to someone's home for a celebration. There the boy gave a bar mitzvah speech like I'd never heard before. He said: "I want to thank the One and the Only, All in One and One in All." This thirteen-year-old boy really impressed me with his lofty, mystical articulations. He and his fellow ashram dwellers were very spiritual people. After the speech, everyone was invited to have some food-all strictly vegetarian. Everyone was barefoot, having left their shoes at the door. The meal was a buffet, so after the guests got their food, they sat down cross-legged on the floor and ate.

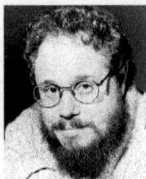

I had three of my kids with me and we helped ourselves and sat down on the floor like everyone else. At that point, my son Nuri, then five years old, looked at me, and exclaimed, appalled, "Daddy, you won't believe it. They didn't say a blessing before they ate."

His shock was cute, and he may have missed it, but the irony struck me as sad. I have met self-acclaimed, highly spiritual people, who have the consciousness to be vegetarians, and the humility to take off their shoes and even sit on the floor. But when it came to consuming their food, they just stuff themselves. They do not even pause and meditate for a moment, to appreciate the food as a Divine gift. On the other hand, my kids, who I can guarantee it are spiritually unsophisticated, would never think of popping a crumb into their mouths without first acknowledging God as the source of the food.

For a thirteen-year-old to talk about "the One in the All and the All in the One" is impressive. But how does one take this high level of philosophical content and turn it into an everyday consciousness? How do we bring it into the office, bring it into the kitchen, bring it into the living room, bring it into the bedroom?

Rabbi David Aaron (Excerpts from "Seeing God)

4.

Feeding the Body, Nourishing the Soul

The Yoga of Cooking and Eating

Cooking is generally thought as something you do to feed yourself and your family. However cooking, if done with the right consciousness, can be a way to reconnect with the divine.

Whether or not that reconnect actually takes place depends on one's consciousness. Our consciousness during our cooking should be that we are "cooking for the pleasure of God and that we want to share our food with others."

Knowing that we're cooking for someone else can help remove some of the selfishness we harbor in our hearts and can increase the quality of selflessness. Since the process of yoga is meant to purify the heart and mind and reconnect with the Supreme, cooking with the right consciousness can be transformed into a yoga practice.

This entails that the cook isn't allowed to taste the food while the cooking is taking place. As soon as one hears this, the immediate response is that of complete surprise. How is it possible to cook without tasting what we are doing? It takes practice and a recipe should be followed. Since the food is being cooked for the pleasure of God, God should be the first individual to taste it. It gets even more difficult, as the cook isn't even supposed to be thinking of eating or enjoying the food while cooking.

As bizarre as all this might be sounding, this is the method of cooking adopted by those who adhere to the Bhakti or devotional path within Vedic tradition. One way to express our love for people we care for is to cook for them. So a similar way to cultivate our love for God is to cook delicious preparations with a mood of love and devotion to God.

Gadadhara Pandita Dasa, a follower of Vedic tradition, explains it by the example of a mother. Most people will agree that the best meals are often prepared by a loving mother.

Why a mom enjoys cooking for her children? She gets pleasure from watching them eat what she's cooked.

The food she's prepared is imbued with her feelings of motherly love and care. Her consciousness has entered the food and is being transferred to me. That transference of consciousness creates a powerful bond. So, even though she may or may not use the perfect amount of turmeric, hing or cumin, the most important ingredient is bhakti, or love.

Consciousness affecting material things may seem a bit farfetched, but we witness this effect taking place with works of art and music, and how they're embedded with the consciousness of the particular artists.

When we listen to or examine a work of art or music, the artist's mood also becomes apparent and many times we can be emotionally impacted by that mood. Similarly, cooked food is no less a work of art than traditional art or music and is invested with the emotions and consciousness of the cook.

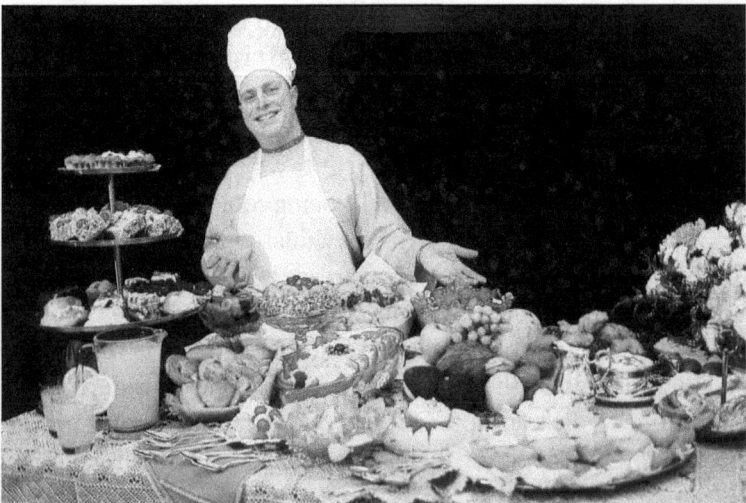

When we eat, we're not only eating the food and it's ingredients, but we're also eating the consciousness of the cook. A very important question we can ask ourselves before our next meal is, "Whose consciousness am I eating?"

It is one of the most important and least understood activities of life that the feelings that go into the preparation of food affect everyone who partakes of it. This activity should be unhurried, peaceful and happy because the energy that flows into that food impacts the energy of the receiver.

That is why the advanced spiritual teachers of the East never eat food prepared by anyone other than their own disciples. If the person preparing the food is spiritually advanced., an active charge of happiness, purity and peace will pour forth into the food from him, and this pours forth into any one who partakes of it.

To be healthy, we need to prepare our own food, for ourselves and our families. We can return to good eating practices one mouth at a time, one meal at a time, by preparing our own food and preparing it properly.

Food decorating the super market shelves is devoid of any feelings other than that of pure greed and exploitation. Because people are eating such foods, they are turning into desensitized robots. These days no one reacts if a man is killed in broad daylight.

"That anyone should need to write a book advising people to "eat food" could be taken as a measure of our alienation and confusion. Or we can choose to see it in a more positive light and count ourselves fortunate indeed that there is once again real food for us to eat."
~ Michael Pollan, In Defense of Food: An Eater's Manifesto

5.

Foods

Civilized Vs. Uncivilized

Civilization is synonymous in every sense with the growth of agriculture. Cultivating crops forms the basis of civilization. The existence in the belief of the power of the fruits or grains has provided the world with many rituals, beliefs and festivals. The festival calendars of antiquity are based on agriculture. Our modern calendar descends from ancient agricultural calendars.

The cultivation of plants for food, as opposed to the use of plants as they grow naturally in the environment, marked the evolution of humanity from a user of food to a producer of food.

All civilizations have depended on agriculture for subsistence. Growing food on farms results in a surplus of food, particularly when people use intensive agricultural techniques such as irrigation and crop rotation.

Grain surpluses have been especially important because they can be stored for a long time. A surplus of food permits some people to do things besides produce food for a living: early civilizations included artisans, priests and priestesses, and other people with specialized careers. A surplus of food results in a division of labor and a more diverse range of human activity, a defining trait of civilizations.

Meat Comes Under Uncivilized Category

According to Webster's definition, the world civilized means to bring out of a primitive state; to be marked by refinement in taste and manners; to become cultured. According to this definition, killing of billions of animals in most despicable conditions, in spite of availability of so much food can hardly be considered civilized.

George Bernard Shaw rightly put it, "While we ourselves are the living graves of murdered beasts, how can we expect any ideal conditions on this earth?" Also Einstein was right in saying, "Vegetarian food leaves a deep impression on our nature. If the whole world adopts vegetarianism, it can change the destiny of humankind."

Uncivilized races living in the jungle and being unqualified to produce food by agriculture may eat animals, but a perfect human society advanced in knowledge must learn how to produce first-class food simply by agriculture and dairy.

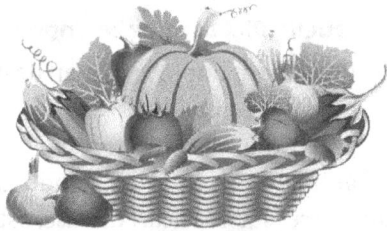

Already, as an emerging social trend, the eating of meat is being looked on as uncivilized. As part of the shift away from meat toward fruit, vegetables, and grains, people are becoming more distanced from the production of the meat they eat and less willing to eat as wide a variety of meats.

Classification of Foods

The Bhagavad-gita (17.8-10) divides foods into three classes: those of the quality of goodness, those of the quality of passion, and those of the quality of ignorance. The most healthful are the foods of goodness. "Foods of the quality of goodness [milk products, grains, fruits, and vegetables] increase the duration of life; purify one's existence; and give strength, health, happiness, and satisfaction. Such foods are sweet, juicy, fatty, and palatable."

Foods that are too bitter, sour, salty, pungent, dry or hot, are of the quality of passion and cause distress. But foods of the quality of ignorance, such as meat, fish, and fowl, described as "putrid,

"Tell me what you eat and I will tell you what you are."
~ Anthelme Brillat-Savarin, 1826

decomposed, and unclean," produce only pain, disease, and bad karma.

In other words, what you eat affects the quality of your life. There is much needless suffering in the world today, because most people have no other criterion for choosing food than price, and sensual desire. The purpose of food, however, is not only to survive, but also to purify the mind and consciousness. As it is said, we should eat to live and not live to eat.

Cruelty Diet Leading To Unprecedented Health Hazards

Plant foods improve human health, while animal 'foods' damage it. The most comprehensive study to date regarding the relationship between diet and human health found that the consumption of animal-derived 'food' products was linked with "diseases of affluence" such as heart disease, osteoporosis, diabetes, and cancer. T. Colin Campbell's landmark research in The China Project found

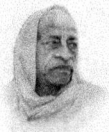

"Actually, giving up meat-eating is not a question of Krishna consciousness but of civilized human life. God has given human society so many things to eat--nice fruits, vegetables, grain, and first-class milk. From milk one can prepare hundreds of nutritious foods, but no one knows the art. Instead, people maintain big slaughterhouses and eat meat. They are not even civilized. When man is uncivilized, he kills poor animals and eats them.

Civilized men know the art of preparing nutritious foods from milk. For instance, on our New Vrndavana farm in West Virginia, we make hundreds of first-class preparations from milk. Whenever visitors come, they are astonished that from milk such nice foods can be prepared.

The blood of the cow is very nutritious, but civilized men utilize it in the form of milk. Milk is nothing but cow's blood transformed. You can make milk into so many things--yogurt, curd, ghee (clarified butter), and so on--and by combining these milk products with grains, fruits, and vegetables, you can make hundreds of preparations.

This is civilized life--not directly killing an animal and eating its flesh. The innocent cow is simply eating grass given by God and supplying milk, which you can live on. Do you think cutting the cow's throat and eating its flesh is civilized?"

— Srila Prabhupada (Science of Self-Realization, Chapter 1)

a pure vegetarian diet to be healthiest. Dr. Campbell estimates that "80 to 90% of all cancers, cardiovascular diseases, and other degenerative illness can be prevented, at least until very old age - simply by adopting a plant-based diet.

The meat, poultry, dairy and egg industries employ technological short cuts— as drugs, hormones, and other chemicals — to maximize production. Under these conditions, virulent pathogens that are resistant to antibiotics are emerging. These new 'supergerms,' whose evolution is traceable directly to the overuse of antibiotics in factory farming, have the potential to cause yet unknown human suffering and deaths.

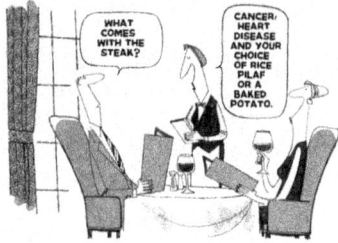

Peculiar new diseases have been amplified by aberrant agribusiness practices. For example, "Mad Cow Disease" (bovine spongiform encephalopathy or BSE), a fatal dementia affecting cattle, spread throughout Britain when dead cows were fed to living cows. When people ate cows with "Mad Cow Disease," they got Creutzfeldt-Jakob Disease (CJD), a fatal dementia that afflicts humans. Another farm animal disease beginning to jeopardize human health is avian influenza.

Millions of people are infected, and thousands die every year from contaminated animal 'food' products. Despite repeated warnings from consumer advocates, the meat inspection systems everywhere remains grossly inadequate, and consumers are now being told to "expect" animal products to be tainted.

Meanwhile, the agribusiness industry, rather than advising consumers to curtail their intake of animal products, has devised extreme measures (irradiation, antibiotics, etc.) to help consumers circumvent the hazards of animal products and maintain their gross over-consumption of meat and processed dairy.

> "Were the walls of our meat industry to become transparent, literally or even figuratively, we would not long continue to raise, kill, and eat animals the way we do."
> ~ Michael Pollan,

6.

Society Needs To Connect To Its Food Source

Before the onset of industrial revolution, all traditional societies were very connected to their food sources, and individual wealth was measured in terms of livestock and land owned.

Contrast this way of life with the way of life in the 21st century. When the United States was founded in 1776, about 90 percent of the population was involved in agriculture and producing food. By the time Abraham Lincoln became president in 1860, the percentage had dropped to about 50%. Today, many years after the industrial revolution, that number is less than 1%.

Most of our society is no longer connected to our food sources, and very few people would even understand the concept that we are dependent upon higher forces of nature to supply our food, our "daily bread." With a Darwinian evolutionary understanding of science and technology, our culture has come to depend on a very few wealthy companies to control the bulk of our food system.

The result of this concentrated power among such a small percentage of our population has been disastrous. The mass-produced foods are toxic and devoid of nutrients. Our poor health, both among the human population as well as the livestock population, has resulted in a very prosperous pharmaceutical industry. We no longer depend upon God for our 'daily bread,' but

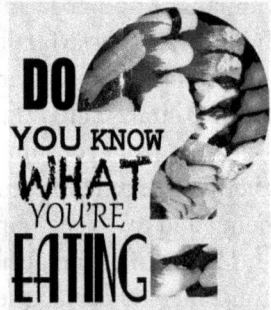

on Mosanto and Cargill. Most of us are not even aware of what the problem is, let alone what the solutions are.

Our eating has been secularized. It has been robbed of its poetry and beaten into the staccato uniformity of packaged snacks. We have insisted upon efficiency as the only criterion of our culinary aesthetic. As a direct result, our prey suffer needlessly, our planet is wilting under the pressures of our demands, our neighbors are strangers, we are unhealthy, and our place in the order of things is lost behind the incessant pace of our living.

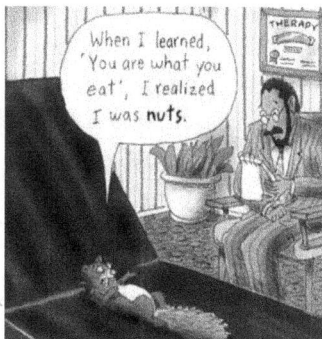

We are in desperate need of reconnecting our eating with the sacred. This needn't mean a complete return to the perspectives and practices of the past. It does necessarily mean a reevaluation of the fundamental principles by which we relate to our eating. Also, it definitely means to be aware of and to reconnect to our food source.

"Imagine if we had a food system that actually produced wholesome food. Imagine if it produced that food in a way that restored the land. Imagine if we could eat every meal knowing these few simple things: What it is we're eating. Where it came from. How it found its way to our table. And what it really cost. If that was the reality, then every meal would have the potential to be a perfect meal. We would not need to go hunting for our connection to our food and the web of life that produces it. We would no longer need any reminding that we eat by the grace of nature, not industry, and that what we're eating is never anything more or less than the body of the world. I don't want to have to forage every meal. Most people don't want to learn to garden or hunt. But we can change the way we make and get our food so that it becomes food again—something that feeds our bodies and our souls. Imagine it: Every meal would connect us to the joy of living and the wonder of nature. Every meal would be like saying grace."

~ Michael Pollan, The Omnivore's Dilemma: A Natural History of Four Meals

Spaghetti Trees

In 1957, the BBC television programme "Panorama" ran a famous hoax, showing Italians harvesting spaghetti from trees. A large number of people contacted the BBC wanting to know how to cultivate their own spaghetti trees!

This programme, narrated by distinguished broadcaster Richard Dimbleby, featured a family carrying out their annual spaghetti harvest.

Just a few companies control the whole world's food supply. Not all of them are humanitarian organizations:

Nestlé is the world's largest food and beverage company.

PepsiCo is the largest U.S.-based food and beverage company.

Unilever is an Anglo-Dutch company that owns many of the world's consumer product brands in foods and beverages.

Kraft is apparently the world's second largest food company, following its acquisition of Cadbury in 2010.

DuPont and Monsanto Company are the leading producers of pesticide, seeds, and other farming products.

Both Archer Daniels Midland and Cargill process grain into animal feed and a diverse group of products. ADM also provides agricultural storage and transportation services, while Cargill also operates a finance wing.

Bunge Limited is a global soybean exporter and is also involved in food processing, grain trading, and fertilizer.

Dole Food Company is the world's largest fruit company. Chiquita Brands International, another U.S.-based fruit company, is the leading distributor of bananas in the United States. Sunkist Growers, Incorporated is a U.S.-based grower's cooperative.

JBS S.A. is the world's largest processor and marketer of chicken, beef, and pork. Smithfield Foods is the world's largest pork processor and hog producer.

Sysco Corporation, mainly catering to North America, is one of the world's largest food distributors.

General Mills is the world's sixth biggest food manufacturing company.

Grupo Bimbo is one of the most important baking companies in brand and trademark positioning, sales, and production volume around the world.

It showed women carefully plucking strands of spaghetti from a tree and laying them in the sun to dry.

But some viewers failed to see the funny side of the broadcast. Others, however, were so intrigued they wanted to find out where they could purchase their very own spaghetti bush.

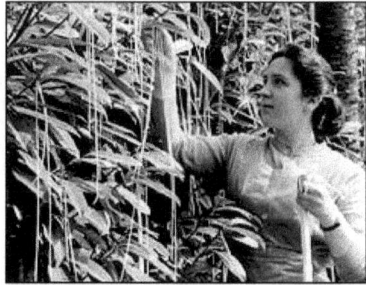

Mr Dimbleby explained how each year the end of March is a very anxious time for Spaghetti harvesters all over Europe as severe frost can impair the flavour of the spaghetti.

He also explained how each strand of spaghetti always grows to the same length thanks to years of hard work by generations of growers.

Spaghetti Trees! This is an example of how much we are disconnected from our food source today. Another example can be the meat vending machines which are gaining popularity everywhere.

People are just forgetting that steak comes from a cow and a pork chop comes from a pig. Also they are forgetting that meat products cost something more than money: a life. At the very least, the blood on a 'real' butcher's apron used to remind them of that.

Several years ago I took my daughter and her friend to our allotments. As we left I dug up a couple of bunches of my prized organic carrots and offered one of them to my daughter's friend.

With a look of absolute disgust the young girl said, "My mommy doesn't get food from the dirt! She goes to Tescos!"

Still, at least she knew what a carrot was.

~Jennifer Hill, Bristol

Section-II

Food

A Sacred Gift

Abused And Defiled

Turned Into A Deadly Curse

"If you're concerned about your health, you should probably avoid products that make health claims. Why? Because a health claim on a food product is a strong indication it's not really food, and food is what you want to eat" ~ *Michael Pollan*

7.

Food

A Victim Of Excessive Human Interference And Meddling

In the preceding chapters we have discussed the old adage - you are what you eat - because every food you eat and every beverage you consume are creating you.

This is so because the foods and beverages you consume are broken down by your body into vitamins, minerals, enzymes, amino acids, fatty acids, and simple sugars, all of which your body then uses as raw materials to create new liver cells, skin cells, brain cells, bone cells, or whatever your body needs to replenish at that time.

But what if you eat foods that your digestive tract cannot break down into the building blocks it needs? Or what if the foods and beverages you consumed had very little nutritional value and therefore very few building blocks for healthy cells and tissue? Worse yet, what if these foods and beverages were also laden with synthetic chemicals which your body had to work harder to eliminate but which did not provide the energy your body needs to do that? Even worse still, what if you exposed your body to synthetic chemicals in such vast quantities that it had to struggle to keep you disease-free?

This is what we mean by excessive human interference and meddling in the divine gift of life - food.

Traditional Food Processing

Mankind has always processed his food; food processing is an activity that is uniquely human. One type of food processing is cooking.

Traditional food processing had two functions: to make food more digestible and to preserve food during times of scarcity. In the past, this processing was carried out by farmers, cooks and artisans. This type of processing resulted in delicious foods and kept the profits on the farm and in the farming communities where it belonged—food processing should be a local cottage industry.

Most importantly, traditional processing enhances or increases the nutrient value of our foods. For example, making of yoghurt and similar products from fresh milk makes the nutrients in the milk still more available and more digestible.

Industrial Food Processing

Unfortunately, in modern times we have abandoned local artisanal processing in favor of factory and industrial processing, which destroys the nutrients in food and makes our food more difficult to digest.

Furthermore, industrial processing depends upon products that have a negative impact on our health, such as sugar, white flour, processed and hydrogenated oils, additives, synthetic vitamins and an extrusion processing of grains. These are the tools of the food processing industry.

Another big problem with foods of the modern civilization is their so called refinement or purification. We have to eat them as the nature intended us to do. Experiments revealed that animals fed on a diet composed of purified proteins, purified starches, purified fats and inorganic salts, although they may live on these for a time, do not grow and in a short time develop various pathological conditions as a result of such "diet." If whey, or fruit juice, or vegetables are then added to the diet, the symptoms improve and the animals thrive better.

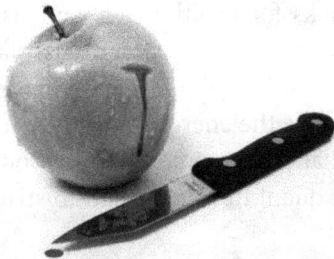

Except for the organic fresh fruits and vegetables we eat, practically everything we have on our table has had something done to it. Our milk is pasteurized, homogenized, condensed, evaporated, heated; Our sugar is the crystallized, refined and bleached sap of cane that has had all the minerals and vitamins removed from it.

Our cereals are cracked, rolled, hammered, frittered, curled, flaked, ironed, roasted, twice roasted, boiled, and in other ways rendered useless. Wheat is milled, its minerals and vitamins removed, the flour is bleached and chemicalized. Its most important food elements are removed in the milling process.

Our dried fruits are heated in drying, bleached with sulphur dioxide, stored for long periods of time and, finally, stewed and mixed with white sugar before being eaten.

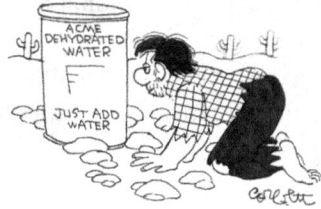

The refining, preserving and cooking processes to which our foods are subjected destroy extraordinarily delicate and tender vital food factors. The refining and cooking processes rob foods of so much of their values that we add salt, sugar, spices, pepper and various other condiments and seasonings to make them palatable. Without the additions of such things they are dull, flat, insipid. Nature has placed delicate flavors and aromas in her foods that appeal to the senses of taste and smell.

Factory Food Preparation—Is Your Food Made by Caring Hands?

Artificial flavors and preservatives are made by chemical companies in factories; they are not being made by the loving hands of a cook. All the artificial ingredients added to the food help the rich get richer and the general public get sicker. The industry has completely processed the life out of the food and then as a concession to the public, thrown in a handful of artificial nutrients. Can you imagine what kind of feeling, what kind of radiation comes from that factory food?

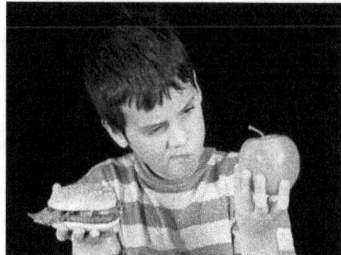

It would be better that an individual did not eat at all than to eat food that has been 'prepared under a feeling of anger, apathy, resentment, depression, or any outward pressure.'

Think of the vibration that in all this food that is made in factories. Nourishing foods starts with the way we farm—the farmer who farms with wisdom and love for the land, the dairyman who farms with love for his animals, the cheese maker who makes cheese with the love of her craft, the baker who bakes with the love of the final product, the beverage maker who makes the type of delicious and nutritious beverage that should be produced in every town and village. Traditional processing puts not only good nutrition, but the vibration of love into our food.

The situation is really very critical. We have to return to good eating practices if we have to preserve our race.

"So what exactly would an ecological detective set loose in an American supermarket discover, were he to trace the items in his shopping cart all the way back to the soil? The notion began to occupy me a few years ago, after I realized that the straightforward question 'What should I eat?' could no longer be answered without first addressing two other even more straightforward questions: 'What am I eating? And where in the world did it come from?' Not very long ago an eater didn't need a journalist to answer these questions. The fact that today one so often does suggests a pretty good start on a working definition of industrial food: Any food whose provenance is so complex or obscure that it requires expert help to ascertain."

~Michael Pollan, The Omnivore's Dilemma: A Natural History of Four Meals

8.

Diminishing Nutrition

And Denaturing of Foods

B y denatured foods we mean foods that have been so altered and impaired in the processes of manufacturing, bleaching, canning, cooking, preserving, pickling, etc., that they are no longer as well fitted to meet the needs of the body as they were in the state nature prepared them.

Such denatured and chemically altered foods are acid forming and yet, the vitamin faddist will tell us only that it is lacking vitamin C or D. Our vitamin knowledge, where it is permitted to obscure all else, usually blinds the so-called dietitians to some of the most important facts and principles of food science.

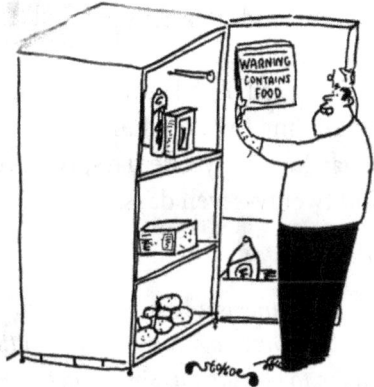

A nation whose diet is made up almost wholly of such 'foodless' foods cannot possibly be well nourished. Why go to great lengths and much trouble to build

> *"Government regulation is an imperfect substitute for the accountability, and trust, built into a market in which food producers meet the gaze of eaters and vice versa."*
> ~ John Robbins

up our soils and then take everything out of the foods that the 'improved' soils have put into them?

Over eighty years ago, Dr. Magendie of Paris, starved one full pen of dogs to death by feeding them a diet of white flour and water, while another pen thrived on whole wheat flour and water. He fed another pen of dogs all the beef tea they could consume, and gave the dogs of another pen only water. The beef tea fed dogs all starved to death. The water fed dogs had lost considerable weight and would have starved also if the experiment had been continued; however, they were alive after those fed on beef tea were all dead. They were fed and all recovered.

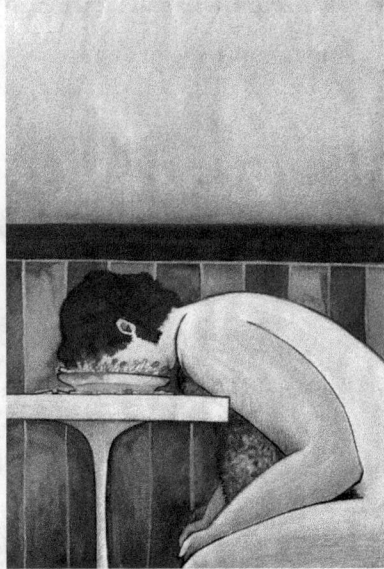

Dogs fed on oil, gum or sugar died in four to five weeks. Dogs fed on fine (white) flour bread lived but fifty days. A goose fed on sugar in twenty-one days; two fed on starch died in twenty-four and twenty-seven days.

> "Eating is an agricultural act,' as Wendell Berry famously said. It is also an ecological act, and a political act, too. Though much has been done to obscure this simple fact, how and what we eat determines to a great extent the use we make of the world - and what is to become of it. To eat with a fuller consciousness of all that is at stake might sound like a burden, but in practice few things in life can afford quite as much satisfaction. By comparison, the pleasures of eating industrially, which is to say eating in ignorance, are fleeting. Many people today seem perfectly content eating at the end of an industrial food chain, without a thought in the world."
>
> ~Michael Pollan, The Omnivore's Dilemma: A Natural History of Four Meals

Learn To Distinguish Between Real Foods And Fake Foods

One of the paths to vibrant health is to choose healthy foods that are rich in as many natural vitamins and minerals as possible, while avoiding processed foods.

That means consistently choosing to eat real foods over fake foods. Real food is what our great-grandparents ate, and it was what we should be eating. Don't eat something your great-grandmother wouldn't recognize as food.

What are real foods? Real food is food that comes from a clean, living source like a plant. Real food ages, and unless fermented for specific results, should be eaten while fresh. Real food has its natural flavors, colors and texture intact. It is minimally processed before it reaches your kitchen, and no chemicals have been added to change its natural state.

Healthy foods can not be stored for a very long time. In contrast, processed foods have a very long shelf life.

The main goal of switching to traditional and healthy foods is to avoid as many toxic chemicals, additives, colors, and preservatives as possible. By themselves, these chemicals may be generally recognized as safe (GRAF) by the FDA, but no studies have ever been done on the effects that combinations of these chemicals have on human health. And we are not so sure about the FDA's commitment to keeping us safe either.

It appears that the general headaches, joint pains, stomach ailments, fatigue, and other "non-specific" health issues that many people experience are related to the chemicals found in our food supply. Many people who substitute real foods for processed, chemical laden foods, stop having these non-specific symptoms.

Modern commerce has robbed these foods of their body-building material while retaining the hunger satisfying energy factors. For example, in the production of refined white flour approximately eighty per cent or four-fifths of the phosphorus and calcium content

"For a product to carry a health claim on its package, it must first have a package, so right off the bat it's more likely to be processed rather than a whole food."
~Michael Pollan, Food Rules: An Eater's Manual

are usually removed, together with the vitamins and minerals provided in the embryo or germ. The evidence indicates that a very important factor in the lowering of reproductive efficiency of womanhood is directly related to the removal of vitamin E in the processing of wheat.

The germ of wheat is our most readily available source of that vitamin. Its role as a nutritive factor for the pituitary gland in the base of the brain, which largely controls growth and organ function, apparently is important in determining the production of mental types. Similarly the removal of vitamin B with the embryo of the wheat, together with its oxidation after processing, results in depletion of body-building activators.

9.

Soil Depletion

Plant, Animal And Human Health Deterioration

Soil and organic matter in the soil may be considered our most important national resource. Plant and animal health and subsequently human health depends on healthy soil. Unfortunately our current farm practices have enormously reduced the supply originally present in the soil and we must expect a permanently lower level of agricultural efficiency if we do not take corrective steps urgently. An adequate supply of organic matter in the soil is vital to the survival of life on the planet.

One of the factors responsible for the global health crisis today is soil deterioration. In the Museum of Natural History (New York), is an exhibit showing the effects of soil deficiency on plant life.

These plants, all of the same kind, were reared in soils lacking some element. The exhibit has to be seen to be fully appreciated. The plants range in size from about three inches to about eighteen inches in height. Their color ranges from pale yellow to dark green. The leaves of some are broad, of others narrow. Some of the leaves are kinky. All of the plants except one is defective both in size, color and features and all except that one were raised in soil lacking some food element. For example, one was raised in a soil lacking iron, (the plant has "anemia"), another in a soil lacking potassium, another in a soil lacking nitrogen, etc.

Deficient soil means deficient food that grows on it. Humans and animals who consume such food also naturally become nutrient deficient. If essential food elements are lacking in their foods, they, like the plants in the experiments, fail and die. Ride along the highway with an experienced farmer and he will point out fertile soil and poor soil, by the vegetation growing thereon; sickly and stunted children (as well as the obese ones) are the result of poor soil.

Global Soil Change : As Serious As Climate Change

Earth's climate and biodiversity aren't the only things being dramatically affected by humans—the world's soils are also shifting beneath our feet.

'Global soil change' due to human activities is a major component of what some experts say should be recognized as a new period of geologic time: the human-made age. This new era will be defined by the pervasiveness of human environmental impacts, including changes to Earth's soils and surface geology.

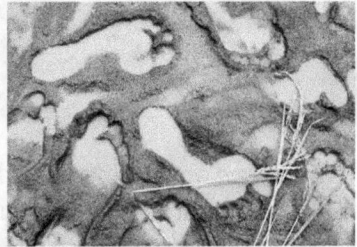

Daniel Richter of Duke University, in his report published in the December 2007 issue of the journal of Soil Science, warns that Earth's soils already show a reduced capacity to support biodiversity and agricultural production. As the amount of depleted and damaged soils increases, global cycles of water, carbon, nitrogen, and other materials are also being affected.

In another paper, Jan Zalaseiwicz of the University of Leicester in England and colleagues argue that the fossil and geologic record of our time will leave distinct signatures that will be apparent far into the future.

Overworked Earth

Today about 50 percent of the world's soils are subject to direct management by humans. Global soil change is also occurring in more remote areas due to the spread of contaminants and alterations in climate. Worldwide, soils are being transformed by human activities in ways that we poorly understand, with possibly dire implications.

The report warns that properties and processes in the soil are more dynamic and susceptible to change than previously thought.

Only recently it has been documented that many aspects of soil chemistry and composition are highly responsive to human activities.

Report also warns that severe soil degradation is increasing globally at a rate of 12.4 million to 24.7 million acres (5 million to 10 million hectares) annually.

Soil Degradation And Climate Change - A Relationship

Soil degradation plays much a larger role in climate change than was previously suspected. That's because organic matter in soils store vast amounts of carbon—more than is present in the atmosphere and in all land vegetation combined.

According to the noted geologist Bruce Wilkinson of Syracuse University, heavily cultivated and degraded soils lose their carbon-storing ability as exposed organic matter breaks down.

Over the past half century or so, global soils have lost approximately a hundred billion tons of carbon [in the form of carbon dioxide] to the atmosphere through such exposure. Humans are now the predominant geological force operating on the planet.

Rates of sedimentation and erosion caused by human activities—mainly industrial agriculture—are ten times higher those attributable to natural processes. On agricultural land, soil is being lost ten times faster than it is being replaced. Humans are rapidly consuming the global soil reservoir. In light of the wasting grains to produce meat and biofuels, this is obviously a very serious change.

Empty Foods, Hollow Lives

We've all heard and read it countless times - "the best way to maintain health is to eat a balanced diet including lots of fruit and vegetables". Of course, this is absolutely correct, so long as those fruits and vegetables are not grown on the mineral-depleted soils that necessitate todays ever-increasing range of chemical 'fertilizers'.

As long ago as in 1920s, the British and US Governments were warned by nutritional experts that the soils on which most crops

"...our modern civilization returns exceedingly little of what it borrows." ~Martin Renner"

were grown were so deficient in mineral content that the foods grown on them contained less than 10% of the vitamins and minerals they should normally have. The intention of these reports was to highlight the problem so that remedial action could be taken to remineralise the soils, leading once again to naturally healthy fruits and vegetables.

But in last one century, no remedial action has been taken and the problem has been intensified by modern intensive farming methods. The fruits and vegetables not only have little or no vitamin and mineral content, but they are routinely sprayed with such a broad selection of chemicals that they are actually poisonous.

How Can Plants Grow Without Vitamins And Minerals?

They can! Even when the soil is burnt out, farmers can still grow good looking fruits and vegetables. Most plants require only three nutrients to grow, namely nitrogen, phosphorus and water. In the presence of these nutrients, virtually all plants will grow into what appear to be healthy, nutritious adult specimens.

However, if the minerals found in their natural habitat are not present, such plants and their relevant fruits and vegetables will be nutritionally "empty".

As a result of this, these plants are less able to defend themselves against natural predators and are susceptible to insect attack and damage from viruses / bacteria. In order to control this, insecticides, antifungals, antibiotics, pesticides and dozens of other categories of chemicals have been designed to limit the damage done to plants by their natural enemies.

Unfortunately, many of these chemicals have not been properly tested to assess their effects on either plant or human health, and virtually none have been tested in combination to assess their

What is lent by earth has been used by countless generations of plants and animals now dead and will be required by countless others in the future. In the case of an element such as phosphorus, so limited is the supply that if it were not constantly being returned to the soil, a single century would be sufficient to produce a disastrous reduction in the amount of life.

~Sears

combined effects. The result is that most fruits, vegetables and other plant-based foods are so contaminated with a huge variety of chemicals, and so deficient in nutrient content that they actually do more harm than good.

Soil Replenishment And Survival of Civilization

The history of preceding civilizations and cultures indicate the imbalances that have developed when minerals have been permanently transferred from the soil. There are only a few localities in the world where great civilizations have continued to exist through long periods and these have very distinct characteristics.

It required only a few centuries, and in some profligated systems a few decades to produce so serious a mineral depletion of the soil that progressive plant and animal deterioration resulted. In such instances, regular and adequate replenishment was not taking place.

In nature's program, minerals are loaned temporarily to the plants and animals and their return to the soil is essential. In the case of a forest system, this replenishment is made by its plant and animal life automatically. But in case of agriculture, we have to make a conscious effort to do it. A few intelligent civilizations have done it but the balance of the cultures have largely failed at this point.

Another procedure for the replenishing of the depleted soils is by the annual overflow of great river systems which float enrichment from the highlands to the lower plains. This is illustrated by the history of the rivers like the Ganges or the Nile which have carried their generous blanket of fertilizing humus and rich soil over their long course and thus made it possible for the plains to sustain a very dense population. Where human beings have deforested vast mountainsides at the sources of these great waterways, the whole situation has reversed.

For example in China, its two great rivers, the Yangtze and the Yellow River have their source in the isolated vastness of the Himalayas in Tibet and through the centuries have provided the replenishment needed for supporting the vast population of the plains. Because of this natural replenishment, the Chinese have been exceedingly efficient in returning to the soil the minerals borrowed by the plant and animal life. Their efficiency as agriculturists has exceeded that of the residents of many other parts of the world.

But this is no longer so. Under the pressure of industrial progress, more and more of the highlands have been denuded. The forests have been ruthlessly cut down. Vast areas that nature had taken millenniums to forest have been denuded and the soil has been washed away in a few decades. These mountainsides have become a great menace instead of a great storehouse of plant food material for the plains.

The heavy rains now find little impediment and rush madly toward the plains, carrying with them not the rich vegetable matter of the previous era, but clay and rocks. This material is not good. Instead of replenishing the soil, it covers the plains with a layer of silt many feet deep, making it impossible to utilize the fertile soil underneath.

We have only to look over the departed civilizations of historic times to see the wreckage and devastation caused by these processes. The rise and fall in succession of such cultures as those of Greece, Rome, North Africa, Spain, and many districts of Europe, have followed the pattern which we are now pursuing with great pride, under the illusion of progress.

The complacency with which the masses of the people as well as the politicians view our trend is not unlike the drifting of a merry party in the rapids over a great water fall. There seems to be no sense of impending doom.

It is apparent that the present and past one or two generations have taken more than their share of the minerals and have done so without duly returning them back. Thus they have handicapped, to a serious extent, the succeeding generations. It is not easy to replenish the minerals in the soil and it practically takes many centuries to accumulate another layer of topsoil.

This constitutes one of the serious dilemmas. A program that does not include maintaining this balance between population and soil productivity must inevitably lead to disastrous degeneration. Over-population means strife and wars.

The history of many civilizations has recorded a progressive rise while civilizations were using the accumulated nutrition in the topsoil, and a progressive decline when these civilizations were destroying these essential sources of life. Their cycle of rise and fall is strikingly duplicated in our present industrial culture.

Alarming Rise In Dust Storms

Another very destructive force is the wind. When surfaces are denuded either at high or low altitudes the wind starts carving up the soil and starts blowing it across the country. These are known as dust storms.

Research shows that dust storms are increasing in certain parts of the world, including China and Africa. In parts of North Africa, annual dust production has increased tenfold in the last 50 years. According to Andrew Goudie, a professor of geography at Oxford University, in Mauritania alone there were just two dust storms a year in the early 1960s, but there are about 80 a year today. Levels of Saharan dust coming off the east coast of Africa in June 2007 were five times those observed in June 2006.

The huge amounts of dust blowing across the Earth may have serious consequences for the environment. Dust storms are transporting prodigious quantities of material for very long distances. Dust storms have also been shown to increase the spread of disease across the globe as they are now combining with airborne pollutants emitted by human activities.

Also, the virus spores in the ground are blown into the atmosphere by the storms with the minute particles. Their increasing frequency could affect the levels of carbon dioxide in the atmosphere, thus directly affecting temperatures and rainfall.

Using satellite imagery, scientists are able to monitor dust storms. Modern agricultural practices, deforestation, drought, winds and increased grazing etc. contribute to dust production.

The cross-boundary nature of dust makes it a truly global issue and one that is not receiving the attention it deserves.

Desertification - Green Earth Turning Into Sand

Desertification is the degradation of land in arid areas, resulting primarily from human activities and influenced by climatic variations. A major impact of desertification is biodiversity loss and loss of productive capacity.

Examples can be cited from various parts of the world. In Africa, if current trends of soil degradation continue, the continent might

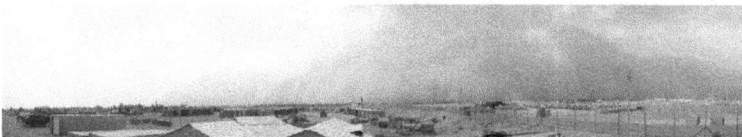

be able to feed just 25% of its population by 2025, according to UNU's Ghana-based Institute for Natural Resources in Africa.

It is a common misconception that droughts by themselves cause desertification. While drought is a contributing factor, the root causes are all related to man's overexploitation of the environment. There is no geological evidence that deserts expanded significantly before the advent of industrialization.

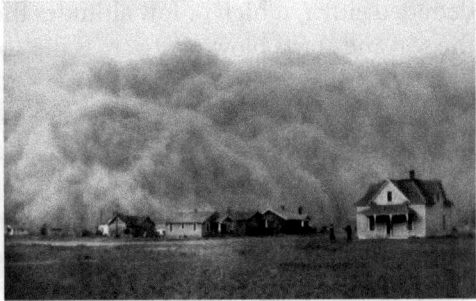

The heavy losses of territory to advancing deserts in China and Nigeria, the most populous countries in Asia and Africa respectively, illustrate the trends for scores of other countries. China is not only losing productive land to deserts, but it is doing so at an accelerating rate. From 1950 to 1975 China lost an average of 1,560 square kilometers of land to desert each year. By 2000, nearly 3625 square kilometers were going to desert annually.

A U.S. Embassy report entitled "Desert Mergers and Acquisitions" describes satellite images that show two deserts in north-central China expanding and merging to form a single, larger desert overlapping inner Mongolia and Gansu provinces. To the west in Xinjiang Province, two even larger deserts—the Taklimakan and Kumtag—are also heading for a merger. Further east, the Gobi Desert has marched to within 150 miles (241 kilometers) of Beijing, alarming China's leaders. Similar phenomenon is taking place in dozens of countries around the World.

> "When you're cooking with food as alive as this -- these gorgeous and semigorgeous fruits and leaves and grains -- you're in no danger of mistaking it for a commodity, or a fuel, or a collection of chemical nutrients. No, in the eye of the cook or the gardener ... this food reveals itself for what it is: no mere thing but a web of relationships among a great many living beings, some of them human, some not, but each of them dependent on each other, and all of them ultimately rooted in soil and nourished by sunlight."
>
> ~Michael Pollan

10.

Not Your Life Or My Life

But Shelf Life

Shelf life is the length of time that food and drinks and many other perishable items are given before they are considered unsuitable for sale, use, or consumption. In many countries, a best before, use by or freshness date is required on packaged perishable foods.

Packaged foods can undergo important changes, even while the material is being processed or while stored on the shelves. The determinations of the loss of vitamins and other nutrients in packaged foods was reported as early as 1938 by the Agricultural Experimental Station of Oklahoma Agricultural and Mechanical College. The report revealed that a material loss occurs in two weeks' time and a very serious loss in one to two months time in certain stock rations.

Unfortunately, the primary focus of today's food production and processing is shelf life and not the wholesomeness or nutritional preservation of the foods. Shelf life basically means the stripping foods of their valuable contents so much that even worms and microorganisms would not care to touch them.

Beautifully decorated shelves are meant for everything but food. Shelf life imprints are indeed yet another way to distinguish what one should or should not eat

Why would you want to put anything in your body that has been sitting on a shelf? Consider this - would you ever consider, even remotely, the concept of milking a cow and placing the fresh milk on a shelf and drinking it several days later? How about several months or even years later? Of course, you wouldn't even think about it.

So, how about if you took that very same milk and did something to it so as to prevent it from naturally degrading and basically rotting, so that you could actually drink it months or years later without having to worry about its adverse impact on health.

This is what the shelf life does to the food. The food thus stored may not contain toxic levels of bacteria but also it does not contain anything nutritious or good for your body in any way, shape or form. How about eating a piece of cardboard?

It's easy and common sense. If it's fresh, whole, real, could be eaten as it is, it's food and you can safely eat it. If it's refined, processed, altered, hydrogenated, boxed, wrapped in plastic and hermetically sealed, well, leave it that way and don't inflict it upon your healthy body!

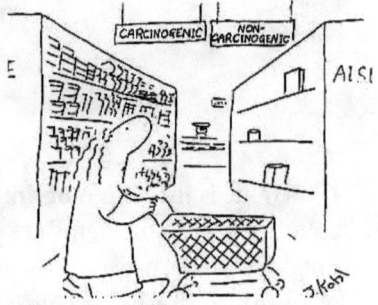

Issues Associated With Sell By / Use By Dates

There is tremendous confusion over actual shelf life of food. Each country has its own standards which they keep changing frequently. According to former UK minister Hilary Benn, the use by date and

> *"Much of our food system depends on our not knowing much about it, beyond the price disclosed by the checkout scanner; cheapness and ignorance are mutually reinforcing. And it's a short way from not knowing who's at the other end of your food chain to not caring–to the carelessness of both producers and consumers that characterizes our economy today. Of course, the global economy couldn't very well function without this wall of ignorance and the indifference it breeds. This is why the American food industry and its international counterparts fight to keep their products from telling even the simplest stories–"dolphin safe," "humanely slaughtered," etc.–about how they were produced. The more knowledge people have about the way their food is produced, the more likely it is that their values–and not just "value"–will inform their purchasing decisions."*
>
> *~Michael Pollan, The Omnivore's Dilemma: A Natural History of Four Meals*

sell by dates are old technologies that are outdated and should be replaced by other solutions or disposed of altogether.

This confusion is resulting in phenomenal wastage of precious food. According to the UK Waste & Resources Action Programme (WRAP), the Western countries waste a whopping 33% of their food production. A major contribution to this wastage is made by the supermarkets who throw away food according to sell by date even if it is in perfectly good condition. With a billion people starving in the Third World, supermarkets in UK alone are throwing away food worth £12bn every year.

But is the food within sell by date safe enough for human consumption? According to the WHO and CDC, every year in the USA there are 76 million foodborne illnesses, leading to 325,000 hospitalizations and 5,000 deaths.

You Can't Judge A Product By Its Label

You need to differentiate fact from fiction when it comes to all the "healthy" labels out there. Spanning everything from "heart healthy" to "boost your child's immunity," these classic marketing ploys are just part and parcel for the food industry. And yet these companies wouldn't get away with the games if their claims didn't reflect conventional wisdom on some level.

The industry's marketing tactics simply manipulate already strained, twisted messages about health and nutrition. The consumer is left to wonder what's truth, half truth and bold-face scheme. Unfortunately, it's never safe to judge a product by its label. In fact, if it needs a label at all, it's already subject to questioning. The safest assumption is this: there's always more to the story.

"What is most troubling, and sad, about industrial eating is how thoroughly it obscures all these relationships and connections. To go from the chicken (Gallus gallus) to the Chicken McNugget is to leave this world in a journey of forgetting that could hardly be more costly, not only in terms of the animal's pain but in our pleasure, too. But forgetting, or not knowing in the first place, is what the industrial food chain is all about, the principal reason it is so opaque, for if we could see what lies on the far side of the increasingly high walls of our industrial agriculture, we would surely change the way we eat." ~ John Robbins

Section-III

Humanity
Dying Out

A Disease Tsunami Is
Sweeping The World

"What an extraordinary achievement for a civilization: to have developed the one diet that reliably makes its people sick!"
~ Michael Pollan

11.

A 'Disease Tsunami' Is Sweeping The World : UN

David Bloom, a health economist with Harvard University, is leading a UN sponsored study on global health. According to him, Chronic illness like heart disease and cancer will cost the world an estimated $US35 trillion over 25 years unless concerted action is taken to combat the "tsunami" of such diseases now taking hold in developing countries.

He warns that the world is confronted by a "perfect storm" of diseases which are already gripping the wealthy countries and are also emerging in the more populous developing world. The preliminary results of analysis for the United Nations indicate the world faces a "staggering burden" unless it acts to quell the often preventable non-communicable diseases.

According to him, in the year 2010, newly diagnosed cancer cases cost the world about $US300 billion in treatment and output forgone by those with the disease. The bill for those with chronic obstructive pulmonary diseases such as bronchitis was about $US400billion.

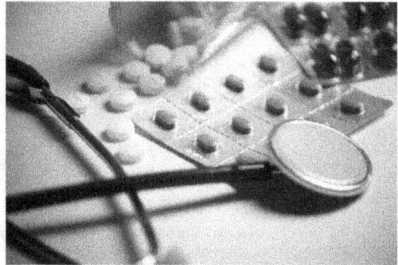

Professor Bloom's earlier report to the World Economic Forum led UN to take the unprecedented step of calling on world leaders to agree to a public health declaration to focus global attention on fighting non-communicable diseases, 80 per cent of which afflict developing countries and are growing rapidly in China and India.

UN has appealed to the world's finance ministers to accept this health warning and realize the economic impact the diseases like diabetes and high blood pressure are having. UN feels that action will be costly but inaction is likely to be far more costly.

> *The sheer novelty and glamor of the Western diet, with its seventeen thousand new food products every year and the marketing power - thirty-two billion dollars a year - used to sell us those products, has overwhelmed the force of tradition and left us where we now find ourselves: relying on science and journalism and government and marketing to help us decide what to eat."*
>
> ~ *Michael Pollan, In Defense of Food: An Eater's Manifesto*

12.

Progress

From Infectious To Man Made Diseases

Industrialisation has spawned its own health problems. In pre-industrial society there were diseases caused by viruses and bacteria. In modern society, in addition to viral and bacterial diseases, there are hundreds of lifestyle diseases - cancer, stroke, diabetes, hypertension, obesity, multiple organ failures etc. Science has miserably failed as far as containment of diseases is concerned.

With the progress of modern science, the general health of masses has only degraded. Of late, several dangerous strains of viruses have surfaced and thanks to global interconnectivity, in matter of days millions can get infected in case of a global outbreak.

Lifestyle Diseases of New Age

Lifestyle diseases (also called diseases of civilization) refer to ailments which have emerged from modern industrialized life style and diet in last few decades. These include Cancer, Hypertension, Obesity, Heart Disease, Diabetes, Alzheimers, Parkinsons, Osteoporosis, Osteoarthritis, Cirrhosis, Nephritis, Stroke, Asthma, Depression etc.

Lifestyle diseases are a result of an inappropriate relationship of people with their environment. The onset of these lifestyle diseases is insidious, they take years to develop, and once encountered do not lend themselves easily to cure.

The increase in the incidence of the above-mentioned diseases is associated with supposed improvements in people's lives. People's lives have got better yet they've become more susceptible to some of the most devastating diseases known to man. Main culprit has been the deterioration in nutrition levels of food.

Sudden vs. Slow Death

Earlier death was caused by sudden onset conditions. Sudden onset conditions are more easily handled by medicine.

In 1900, the top three causes of death in the Western countries were pneumonia/influenza, tuberculosis, and diarrhea/enteritis. Back then communicable diseases accounted for about 60 percent of all deaths. In 1900, lifestyle diseases like heart disease and cancer were ranked number 6 and 8 respectively.

Since the 1940's, most deaths in these countries have resulted from heart disease, cancer, and other lifestyle diseases. And, by the late 1990's, lifestyle diseases accounted for more than 60 percent of all deaths.

Epidemiological Transition - From Infectious To Man Made Diseases

This change from infectious diseases to chronic and life style diseases is known as the 'epidemiological transition'. This was first described in 1971 by Abdel Omran, a professor at the University of North Carolina. Writing in a Quarterly, he drew a map of disease through human history in which he charted this gradual replacement of infectious with chronic, degenerative and man-made diseases.

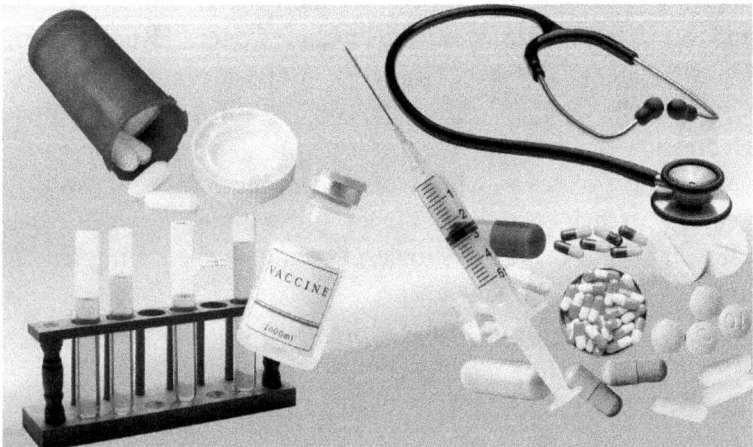

In 2005, about 58 million people died of life-style diseases around the world. By 2020, it's projected that lifestyle diseases will be responsible for seven out of every 10 deaths in the world. In Mexico, for example, three-quarters of all deaths are already in this category.

Emergence of Silent Killers

The World Health Organization has warned that more than 270 million people are susceptible of falling victim to lifestyles diseases. Majority of these people are thought to come from the developing countries.

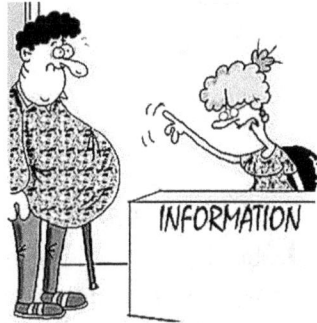

Professor Paul Zimmet, a director of the International Diabetes Institute in Australia says that the world appears to be more preoccupied with AIDS and more recently bird flu, but

"Cardiac day patients? Up the corridor, left at x-ray, right at critical care, straight up the stairs to the fourth floor, fork left at pathology, bear right at neurology and it's dead opposite the mortuary."

far bigger killers are being ignored. It's a time bomb.

The world is just not spending enough money or paying enough attention to deal with this crisis.

"Escherichia colia O157:H7 is a relatively new strain of the common intestinal bacteria (no one had seen it before 1980) that thrives in feedlot cattle, 40 percent of which carry it in their gut. Ingesting as few as ten of these microbes can cause a fatal infection; they produce a toxin that destroys human kidneys."

~Michael Pollan, The Omnivore's Dilemma: A Natural History of Four Meals

13.

Developing Countries

Dual Burden of Diseases

For the first time in history, poor countries are now facing a dual burden of infectious and chronic diseases. While third world governments are funding cash and devising plans to prevent a possible flu pandemic, little is being done to tackle these big killers such as cancer, diabetes and respiratory and heart disease.

India has planned to import equipments worth $215 Billion to diagnose and treat lifestyle diseases in next 5 years. Renowned cardiologist Dr R.R. Kasliwal says that lifestyle diseases pose a greater threat to ordinary Indians than HIV/AIDS.

In the yesteryears, life style diseases were diseases of the affluent and uncommon in the developing world. Gone are those days and now they are an important threat to developing economies, draining a good chunk of their scanty health budget.

Third World Catching Up With The Diseases Of The Rich

These diseases often hit people at the peak of their economic productivity. Developing countries are adopting the least healthy habits of the west. This is particularly true of urban and wealthier classes. Today, already half of new cancer cases occur in developing countries.

Elsewhere the problem is often obesity. On a shopping street in Manila or Johannesburg or Hyderabad, you will find people as fat as those you'd see in a Midwestern American mall. That wasn't the case 10 years ago. But now, many formerly poor people can afford to gorge on calories, often in new fast-food restaurants.

Highest Outbreak of New Diseases In 1980s

Researchers from the Zoological Society of London, the Wildlife Trust and Columbia University have analyzed databases of disease outbreaks and found 335 cases of emerging diseases between 1940 and 2004. Of these, 60.3% were infections which also affected animals, and 71.8% were known to have triggered disease in humans after spreading from animals.

Major outbreaks of disease have become more common around the globe in the past 40 years, according to the largest ever investigation into emerging infections. Diseases such as Ebola and Sars, which originally spread from animals, are an increasing threat to human health, and many infections have now become resistant to antibiotics.

The international team of scientists have warned that tropical regions are likely to become a future hotspot for new diseases, and called for early warning systems to be set up in countries to spot outbreaks before they become unmanageable.

More diseases emerged in the 1980s than any other decade, according to the study.

Digital Age Diseases

A study by the Indian Council for Research on International Economic Relations says that although India's IT boom has brought spiralling corporate profits and higher incomes for employees, it has also led to a surge in workplace stress and lifestyle diseases. Former health minister, Anbumani Ramadoss says, "IT is the fastest-growing industry in our country, but it is most vulnerable to lifestyle diseases. Its future growth could be stunted if we don't address the problem now."

India's rapid economic growth could be slowed by a sharp rise in the prevalence of heart disease, stroke and diabetes, and the successful information technology industry is likely to be the hardest hit. Lifestyle diseases are estimated to have wiped $9bn off the country's national income in 2005, but the cost could reach more than $100bn over the next 10 years if corrective action is not taken soon.

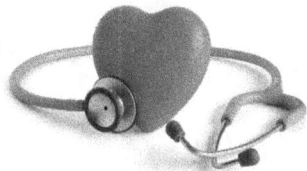

Long working hours, night shifts and a sedentary lifestyle make people employed at such companies prone to heart disease and diabetes. There have also been growing reports of depression and family breakdown in the industry.

Infosys Technologies, India's second-largest software exporter, has a 24-hour hotline for employees suffering from depression to contact psychiatrists. A company director says "We must have prevented at least 30 deaths from suicide because of this hotline in one year." In Bangalore the psychiatrists say their Saturdays are reserved for marriage counselling for the IT sector.

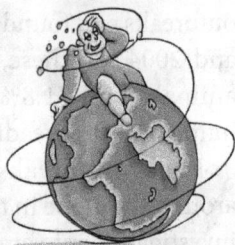

"...There's a lot of money in the Western diet. The more you process any food, the more profitable it becomes. The healthcare industry makes more money treating chronic diseases (which account for three quarters of the $2 trillion plus we spend each year on health care in this country) than preventing them. "

~ *John Robbins*

14.

Globesity

An Obesity Explosion

Obesity is a medical condition in which excess body fat has accumulated to the extent that it may have an adverse effect on health, leading to reduced life expectancy and/or increased health problems. Obesity increases the likelihood of various diseases, particularly heart disease, type 2 diabetes, certain types of cancer, high blood pressure, high blood cholesterol, and osteoarthritis.

For thousands of years obesity was rarely seen. It was not until the 20th century that it became common, so much so that in 1997 the World Health Organization (WHO) formally recognized obesity as a global epidemic.

As of 2005 the WHO estimates that at least 400 million adults (9.8%) are obese, with higher rates among women than men.

As of 2008, The World Health Organization claimed that 1.5 billion adults, 20 and older, were overweight and of these over 200 million men and nearly 300 million women were obese.

Once considered a problem only of high-income countries, obesity rates are rising worldwide. These increases have been felt most dramatically in urban settings. The only remaining region of the world where obesity is not common is sub-Saharan Africa.

Obesity is a leading cause of death worldwide today, with increasing prevalence in adults and children, and authorities view it as one of the most serious public health problems of the 21st century.

Obesity rates have tripled in developing countries over the past 20 years. At the other end of the malnutrition scale, it is one of today's most blatantly visible – yet most neglected – public health problems.

Paradoxically coexisting with undernutrition, an escalating global epidemic of overweight and obesity – "globesity" – is taking over the world. It is a complex condition, one with serious social and psychological dimensions.

Fat Dead - A Deadly Problem

People are getting fatter and fatter. So fat, that mortuaries are having a difficult time accommodating all the dead weight. According to a Reuters report published on August 6, 2007, pathologists are calling for new 'heavy-duty' autopsy facilities to cope with obese corpses that are difficult to move and dangerously heavy for standard-size trolleys and lifting hoists.

The bodies presented "major logistical problems" and "significant occupational health and safety issues," according to a separate study, which found the number of obese and morbidly obese bodies had doubled in the past 20 years.

Professor Roger Byard, a pathologist at the University of Adelaide says, "Specially designed mortuaries would soon be required if the

---

"According to the surgeon general, obesity today is officially an epidemic; it is arguably the most pressing public health problem we face, costing the health care system an estimated $90 billion a year. Three of every five Americans are overweight; one of every five is obese. The disease formerly known as adult-onset diabetes has had to be renamed Type II diabetes since it now occurs so frequently in children. A recent study in the Journal of the American Medical Association predicts that a child born in 2000 has a one-in-three chance of developing diabetes. (An African American child's chances are two in five.) Because of diabetes and all the other health problems that accompany obesity, today's children may turn out to be the first generation of Americans whose life expectancy will actually be shorter than that of their parents. The problem is not limited to America: The United Nations reported that in 2000 the number of people suffering from bad nutrition (empty calories) --a billion--had officially surpassed the number suffering from malnutrition--800 million."

~ Michael Pollan, The Omnivore's Dilemma: A Natural History of Four Meals

---

nation failed to curb its fat epidemic, providing larger storage and dissection rooms, and more robust equipment."

"Failure to provide these might compromise the post-mortem evaluation of markedly obese individuals, in addition to potentially jeopardizing the health of mortuary staff," he adds.

Obesity Can Begin In 9-month-olds Too!

Obesity epidemic has not spared infants also. A new study has revealed that obesity can begin in babies as young as nine months old.

Researcher Brian Moss, at Wayne State University in Detroit says, "With the consistent evidence that the percent of overweight children has steadily increased over the past decade, we weren't surprised by the prevalence rates we found in our study, but we were surprised the trend began at such a young age."

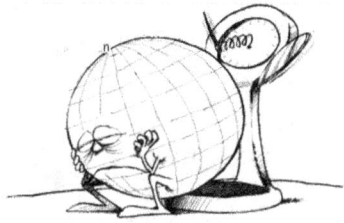

The researchers analysed the Early Childhood Longitudinal Study-Birth Cohort data collected on 16,400 American children born in 2001. Of these, 8,900 were nine-months-old and 7,500 were two-years-old.

Rapid weight gain in childhood can lead to development of insulin resistance and metabolic syndrome.

Fat Feet - Growing Shoe Size

Around the world, there has been a phenomenal increase in demand for bigger shoes. According to a report by The Daily Mail, thirty years ago the standard shoe size for men across Britain was size 7. Five years ago it was an 8. Now it's a 9. And 12, the largest typically in stock at stores, now outsells size 7. Scientists say the obesity epidemic is at play.

Average female shoe size has increased to a size six over the last 10 years, and demand for size nines has triggered an 80 percent increase in stocks at the stores.

The change is attributed to women's feet becoming broader rather than longer due to an increase in average body weight.

Big-footed females are ashamed of stepping out in their shoes but shoemakers have begun to adapt fashionable show designs for larger feet, with celebrities Nicole Kidman, Michelle Obama and Paris Hilton sporting larger footwear on the red carpet.

3 Year Old Girls Worry About Being Fat!

Girls as young as three worry about their body image, according to a new study published in the British Journal of Developmental Psychology

Psychology professor Stacey Tantleff-Dunn and doctoral student Sharon Hayes, University of Central Florida, found that nearly half of the 3 to 6-year-old girls worried about being fat even before they start school.

Experts observed that about one-third would go the extent of changing a physical attribute, such as their weight or hair colour.

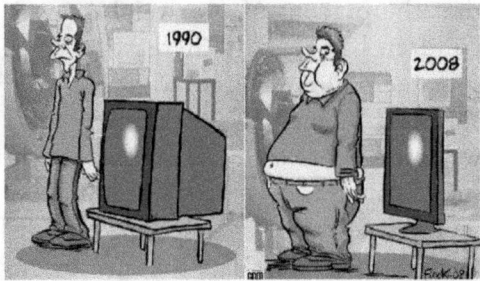

Study says that watching a movie starring a stereotypically thin and beautiful princess may influence young girls' behaviour or self-esteem. Researchers urged parents to take their young girls to see animated movies since they were unlikely to influence how they perceive their bodies.

Professor Tantleff-Dunn says, "We need to help our children challenge the images of beauty, particularly thinness, that they see and idolize and encourage them to question how much appearance should be part of their self-worth. We should help them build a positive self-image with an appreciation for many different types of body attributes."

> *"While the surgeon general is raising alarms over the epidemic of obesity, the president is signing farm bills designed to keep the river of cheap corn flowing, guaranteeing that the cheapest calories in the supermarket will continue to be the unhealthiest."*
> *~Michael Pollan, The Omnivore's Dilemma: A Natural History of Four Meals*

Epidemic of Under-nutrition

On the other end of the nutritional scale lies under-nutrition. Malnutrition has triggered two global epidemics - epidemic of under-nutrition and an epidemic of obesity. One leads to underweight and the other, to overweight.

Under-nutrition causes stunted growth and wasting (being extremely thin) in nearly 300 million children. Nearly 4 million children die each year from nutritional risks, including underweight, and vitamin and mineral deficiency, particularly of vitamin A, iron, iodine and zinc.

WHO's Director of Nutrition for Health and Development, Francesco Branca says, at the same time 43 million children under age five are overweight.

Often we have in the same countries, at the same time, the presence of under-nutrition and overweight.

Underweight in women and children is responsible for more premature deaths and disability than any other preventable risk factor - more than unsafe sex, more than tobacco use and more than overweight.

15.

Diabetes

Scourge of A Sweet Death

Diabetes mellitus, often simply referred to as diabetes, is a group of metabolic diseases in which a person has high blood sugar, either because the body does not produce enough insulin, or because cells do not respond to the insulin that is produced. This high blood sugar produces the classical symptoms of polyuria (frequent urination), polydipsia (increased thirst) and polyphagia (increased hunger).

There are three main types of diabetes:

Type 1 diabetes: results from the body's failure to produce insulin, and presently requires the person to inject insulin.

Type 2 diabetes: results from insulin resistance, a condition in which cells fail to use insulin properly, sometimes combined with an absolute insulin deficiency.

Gestational diabetes: is when pregnant women, who have never had diabetes before, have a high blood glucose level during pregnancy. It may precede development of type 2 diabetes.

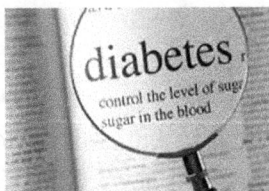

Global Diabetes Epidemic Balloons To 350 Million

The number of adults with diabetes worldwide has more than doubled since 1980 to 347 million, a far larger number than previously thought.

Around 3.8 million deaths every year are attributable to complications of diabetes; six deaths every minute. This is roughly the same number as those dying from HIV/AIDS.

The top 10 countries, in numbers of sufferers, are India, China, USA, Indonesia, Japan, Pakistan, Russia, Brazil Italy and Bangladesh.

Overall, direct health care costs of diabetes range from 2.5% to 15% of annual health care budgets, depending on local diabetes prevalence and the sophistication of the treatment available.

The costs of lost production may be as much as five times the direct health care cost, according to estimates derived from 25 Latin American countries.

In a study published in the Lancet journal, it was found that of the 347 million people with diabetes, 138 million live in China and India and another 36 million in the United States and Russia.

The most common type of diabetes, Type 2, is strongly associated with obesity and a diet of processed foods.

People with diabetes have inadequate blood sugar control, which can lead to serious complications like

"I agree, buying in bulk does save you money, but I don't think that applies to insulin."

heart disease and stroke, damage to the kidneys or nerves, and to blindness.

Experts say high blood glucose and diabetes cause around 3 million deaths globally each year, a number that will continue to rise as the number of people affected increases.

As a result, diabetes is a booming market for drugmakers like Novo Nordisk, Sanofi, Eli Lilly, Merck and Takeda.

Dozens of diabetes treatments, both pills and injections, are on the market. Global sales of the medicines totaled $35 billion last year and could rise to as much as $48 billion by 2015, according to drug research firm IMS Health.

For this Lancet study, the largest of its kind for diabetes, researchers analyzed fasting plasma glucose (FPG) data from 2.7 million participants aged 25 and over across the world, and then used advanced statistical methods to estimate prevalence.

They found that between 1980 and 2008, the number of adults with the disease rose from 153 million to 347 million.

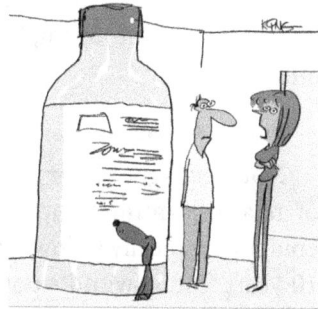

The proportion of adults with diabetes rose to 9.8 percent of men and 9.2 percent of women in 2008, compared with 8.3 percent of men and 7.5 percent of women in 1980.

Diabetes has taken off most dramatically in Pacific Island nations, which now have the highest diabetes levels in the world, the study found. In the Marshall Islands, a third of all women and a quarter of all men have diabetes.

Among wealthy countries, the rise in diabetes was highest in North America and relatively small in Western Europe. Diabetes and glucose levels were highest in United States, Greenland, Malta, New Zealand and Spain, and lowest in the Netherlands, Austria and France.

India - A Case Study

Not long ago, public health officials considered this a disease of relatively minor importance. That has changed. A diabetes epidemic typically follows an obesity epidemic with a lag of about 10 years. India, with its population of 1.1 billion, has upwards of 100 million diabetics and that figure is growing every year. China is in similar situation. An extreme case is the Pacific island of Nauru, where half a century ago diabetes was unknown. Now 40 per cent of adults have it.

Diabetes is very much a disease of the cities. It is rife in India's boomtown like Hyderabad. Make the slow, laborious drive out of the clogged-up city into the neighbouring villages, and the much thinner rural population is less likely to be diabetic.

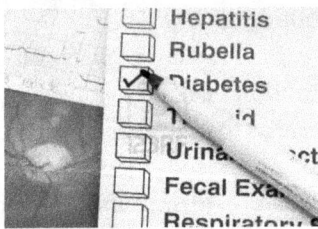

The problem is only partly the traditional Hyderabad biryani dish, made with meat, rice and lots of oil or ghee. Rich Indians now get a far larger proportion of their energy from fat than poor Indians do. A national survey found that by 2000, 12 per cent of urban Indians over the age of 20 already had diabetes.

It's not just that people in poor countries are adopting unhealthy habits. Once ill, they are much less likely than those in rich countries to see a doctor and receive treatment. A survey in Egypt published in 2000, for instance, showed that one in three people with very severe hypertension didn't even know they had the condition. Even if they knew, they struggled to find doctors. In Uganda, there is only one doctor of any kind for every 20,000 people, compared with one for 500 in the UK.

Diabetes Treatment - Runaway Budgets

India spent $32bn on diabetes care in 2010.

A study on the financial burden of diabetes on the common man in the country has found that 60% of diabetics - irrespective of their socio-economic status - pay for the expenditure incurred for treatment and management of the disease from their personal savings.

The study, "The Socio-economics of diabetes from a Developing Country" conducted by the Diabetes Research Centre in Chennai, says the next common method of payment was by selling, mortgaging immovable assets or taking loans with interest rates as high as 39%.

The situation is especially grim for those patients whose monthly income is Rs.10,000 or less. Around 60% of them borrow, mortgage or sell their property just to keep their blood sugar level under control. On an average, a diabetic in India spends Rs 25,931 annually on diagnosis and treatment of the ailment, and its attendant complications.

World Diabetes Day is on 14 November and all over the planet events are taking place to draw attention to this crisis.

Already it kills more people than HIV/Aids and the prognosis is grim. Diabetes causes myriad medical complications: heart disease, blindness, kidney failure, loss of limbs and death.

16.

Chronic Kidney Disease

Wasting Away Populations

As seen in previous chapters, contemporary societies are in the midst of an epidemic of chronic non-communicable diseases and that includes chronic kidney disease (CKD).

Chronic kidney disease is a world wide health problem. According to World Health organization (WHO) Global Burden of Disease project, diseases of the kidney and urinary tract contribute to global burden with approximately 850,000 deaths every year. This is 12th leading cause of death and 17th cause of disability.

This global prevalence, however, may be grossly underestimated for a number of reasons. Patients with chronic kidney disease are at high risk for cardiovascular disease and cerebro vascular disease, and they are more likely to die of cardiovascular disease than to develop end-stage renal failure.

Chronic kidney disease is another important disease related to diabetes mellitus and hypertension. As more and more individuals become diabetic, the prevalence of chronic kidney disease due to diabetic nephropathy also increases. Uncontrolled hypertension also contributes to the burden of chronic kidney disease.

Three simple tests can detect CKD: blood pressure, urine albumin and serum creatinine. The world observes World Kidney Day on March 10.

USA - An Update

The number of individuals initiating renal replacement therapy in the United States population has grown exponentially over the past two decades. Cases of end-stage renal disease (ESRD) attributed to diabetes accounted for most of this increase. It has now been officially recognized as an epidemic.

According to Centre For Disease Control and Prevention (CDC) 2010 figures, currently 26 million American adults (more than 10 percent of the population) have chronic kidney disease and millions of others are at increased risk. Surveys in Australia, Europe, and Japan describe the prevalence of CKD to be 6–16% of their respective populations. (El Nahas AM, Bello AK, 2005, Chronic kidney disease: the global challenge)

Mystery Kidney Disease in Central America

A mysterious epidemic is sweeping Central America – it's the second biggest cause of death among men in El Salvador, and in Nicaragua it's a bigger killer of men than HIV and diabetes combined.

But the epidemic extends far beyond Nicaragua. It's prevalent along the Pacific coast of Central America – across six countries.

"It is important that the chronic kidney disease (CKD) afflicting thousands of rural workers in Central America be recognized as what it is – a major epidemic with a tremendous population impact," says Victor Penchaszadeh, a clinical epidemiologist at Columbia University in the US. He is also a consultant to the Pan-American Health Organization on chronic diseases in Latin America.

El Salvador's health minister recently called on the international community for help. She said the epidemic is "wasting away our populations."

India - Grim Situation

India's diabetes epidemic has triggered surging demand for dialysis as the disease destroys kidneys, leaving them with only months to live without treatment.

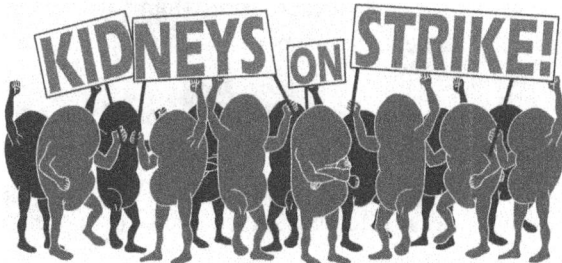

According to Fresenius Medical Care AG, the world's biggest provider of kidney dialysis, sales of blood-filtering products in India have grown more than 30 percent annually since 2006. Apollo Hospitals Enterprise Ltd. and Fortis Healthcare India Ltd., the country's biggest private-hospital operators, are opening dialysis centers nationwide as the number of Indians with diabetes is predicted to reach 101 million by 2030.

The Indian market for kidney-care products and services grew to $152 million in 2008 from $97 million in 2007. New machines are coming up in every nook and corner of the country. Every major health-care provider wants a share of this market.

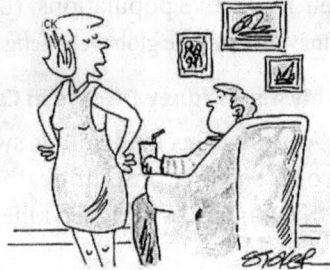

"WELL?! DON'T YOU NOTICE ANYTHING DIFFERENT? I GOT A NEW KIDNEY!"

The number of people lining up at hospitals to get dialysis, a procedure in which waste is removed from the blood, is increasing almost 30 percent each year. The global dialysis market was valued at $69 billion in 2010.

More than 90 percent of the people who develop chronic kidney failure each year in India die within months because of a lack of treatment, doctors from the All India Institute of Medical Sciences and the health ministry in New Delhi said in a 2009 study. Only a very small percentage of patients can afford the treatment.

Death Sentence

A year of dialysis and medication for a patient with chronic kidney disease in India can range from 60,000 rupees at a subsidized provider to more than 700,000 rupees for the home-based treatment.

While that's less than the cost of more than $30,000 in the U.S., the price is still a barrier for most patients in India, where a majority of people live on less than $2 a day.

Kidney transplants aren't an option for most people, either. Only 3,500 kidneys are transplanted each year. Now there is alarming rise in chronic kidney diseases among children. Slowly progressive, chronic kidney disease often goes unnoticed in children until the kidneys have been severely affected.

17.

Heart Disease

A Global Disease Requiring A Global Response

Cardiovascular disease or heart disease are a class of diseases that involve the heart or blood vessels (arteries and veins). Cardiovascular disease is the leading cause of death globally and is projected to remain so. It has no geographic, gender or socio-economic boundaries.

Every year, heart disease and stroke causes as many deaths as HIV/AIDS, tuberculosis, malaria and diabetes plus all forms of cancer and chronic respiratory disease combined.

The percentage of premature deaths from cardiovascular disease range from 4% in high-income countries to 42% in low-income countries.

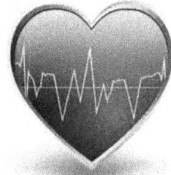

An estimated 17.3 million people died from cardiovascular diseases in 2008. By 2030, almost 23.6 million people will die from cardiovascular diseases. In recent years, cardiovascular risk in women has been increasing and has killed more women than breast cancer.

The heart is arguably the organ that suffers most from increasing economic globalisation. Increasing industrialisation and urbanisation, while raising living standards for many, is also accompanied by a stressed lifestyle, hypertension and host of other unhealthy habits which ultimately take their toll on the person's heart.

In nearly all regions of the world, heart failure is both common and on the rise. In Hong Kong there has been a 10% annual increase in hospital admissions over the past five years (unpublished data). In Africa, at least 3–7% of all hospital admissions are caused by heart failure. In South America cardiovascular disease is now the leading cause of death, and the prevalence rate of heart failure is about 4% in those older than 65 years. Similar prevalence rates were found in the Arab population.

One out of every four Americans has cardiovascular disease, that converts to about 57 million Americans. Heart disease and stroke account for almost 6 million hospitalizations each year and cause disability for almost 10 million Americans age 65 years and older. Almost 1 million Americans die of cardiovascular diseases each year, which adds up to 42% of all deaths. CVD costs the nation $274 billion each year, including health expenditures and lost productivity. The 1999 cost is estimated to be $286.5 billion, and the burden continues to grow as the population ages.

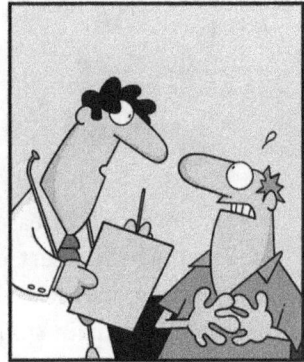

"It's normal for a man your age to have chest pains when he drips hot, melted pizza cheese on his shirt."

10% of the Indian population has cardiac problems with around four per cent of the rural population being afflicted with Coronary Artery Disease (CAD), considered a disease of the developed world.

By 2016, it is estimated that 68 million people in the country will be afflicted by the CAD problem.

With the magnitude of the problem being very high in the next 10 years, it would mean 80 per cent of the global burden of CAD and cancer will be borne by India and lower middle income countries. CAD has also been recognised as a global epidemic.

A trend has emerged, particularly in the early 2000s, in which numerous studies have revealed a link between fast food and an increase in heart disease. These studies include those conducted by the Ryan Mackey Memorial Research Institute, Harvard University and the Sydney Center for Cardiovascular Health. Many major fast food chains, particularly McDonald's, have protested the methods used in these studies and have responded with 'healthier' menu options.

18.

Global Cancer Epidemic

A 'Crisis in Slow Motion'

Cancer, known medically as a malignant neoplasm, is a large group of different diseases, all involving unregulated cell growth. In cancer, cells divide and grow uncontrollably, forming malignant tumors, and invade nearby parts of the body. The cancer may also spread to more distant parts of the body through the lymphatic system or bloodstream.

Every month 600,000 people die of cancer in the World which is more than AIDS, tuberculosis, and malaria combined.

In response to this situation and the epidemic of other non-communicable diseases, the United Nations (UN) authorised a High-Level Meeting (HLM) in September 2011 to address the prevention and control of these diseases. The outcomes document generated by the HLM - known as a Political Declaration - is only the second of its kind to address a health issue on a global scale, the first being the outcomes document from the 2001 UN General Assembly Special Session on HIV/AIDS.

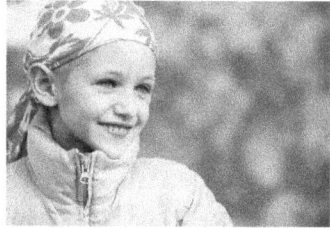

> *"As long as one egg looks pretty much like another, all the chickens like chicken, and beef beef, the substitution of quantity for quality will go unnoticed by most consumers, but it is becoming increasingly apparent to anyone with an electron microscope or a mass spectrometer that, truly, this is not the same food."*
> ~Michael Pollan, The Omnivore's Dilemma

The UN secretary general has called it a 'crisis in slow motion.' This is only the second time in its 65-year history that the UN has held such a high-level meeting to address a health topic.

It is believed that the incidence of cancer will continue to increase in the next decade, with the majority of cases appearing in the low- and middle-income countries. Furthermore, if you add cancer to other noncommunicable diseases, such as heart disease and diabetes, that death toll rises to a combined 36 million deaths per year, according to the latest World Health Organization report.

Cancer Epidemic - Present Assessment

One in three Americans will be diagnosed with cancer, often before the age of 65. Since 1940, we have seen in Western societies a marked and rapid increase in common types of cancer. In fact, cancer in children and adolescents has been rising by 1 to 1.5 percent a year since the 1960's.

For most common cancers - prostate, breast, colon, lung - rates are much higher in the West than in Asian countries. Yet Asians who emigrate to the United States catch up with the rates of Americans within one or two generations.

Dr. Sam Epstein, professor of Occupational & Environmental Medicine at the University of Illinois Medical Center, Chicago, is an internationally recognized authority in this field.

His work shows that since the 1950s, in North America, there has been a 55% increase in cancer, when the statistics are standardized for the fact that people are living longer. Childhood cancer of the brain and nervous system - 40% increase since 1975; male colon cancer - 60% increase; breast cancer - 60% increase; brain cancer

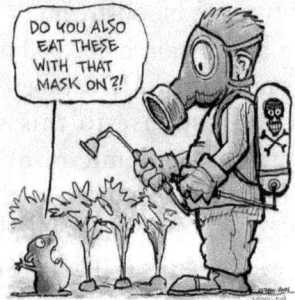

"There are scores of studies demonstrating that a diet rich in vegetables and fruits reduces the risk of dying from all the Western diseases; in countries where people eat a pound or more of vegetables and fruits a day, the rate of cancer is half what is in the United States."
~Michael Pollan

in adults - 80% increase; prostate cancer - 100% increase; testicular cancer - 100% increase; estrogen-receptor positive breast cancer -135% increase; testicular cancer among men aged 28-35 - 300% increase. In 1950, 1 in 20 women had breast cancer. Now it's 1 in 8.

What is driving the modern cancer epidemic? Study after study points to the role of runaway industrial technologies... producing a dizzying array of synthetic chemicals that have never been screened for human health effects. Worldwatch Institute founder Lester Brown concurs, noting, "Every human being harbors in his or her body about 500 synthetic chemicals that were nonexistent before 1920."

Cancer Epidemic - A Grim Future

Global cancer rates could increase by 50% to 15 million deaths per year by 2020, according to the World Cancer Report, the most comprehensive global examination of the disease to date. However, the report also provides clear evidence that healthy lifestyles and public health action by governments and health practitioners could stem this trend, and prevent as many as one third of cancers worldwide.

In many countries, more than a quarter of deaths are attributable to cancer. In 2000, 5.3 million men and 4.7 million women developed a malignant tumour and altogether 6.2 million died from the disease. The report also reveals that cancer has emerged as a major public health problem in developing countries, matching its effect in industrialized nations.

The World Cancer Report tells us that cancer rates are set to increase at an alarming rate globally. It calls on Governments, health practitioners and the general public to take urgent action.

The 351-page report is presented by the International Agency for Research on Cancer (IARC) which is part of the World Health Organization (WHO).

"It will not be long before the entire population will have to decide whether we will all die of cancer or whether we will have enough wisdom, courage, and will power to change fundamentally all our living and nutritional conditions." - Dr. Max Gerson

19.

Decreasing Life Expectancy

After much hype of increased life expectancy, we now have several documented episodes of declines in life expectancy. And some of them may be a terrifying warning for the developing world.

In Africa the decline occurred in after AIDS. By 2002, 22 million people had died of the disease. Life expectancy in southern Africa fell by as much as 10 years: in Botswana it dropped from 59 in 1995 to 49 in 2005.

For today's Chinese, Indians and urban Africans, the decline in life expectancy is alarming. Chronic diseases are afflicting these populations. Life expectancy in these regions is falling as the poor in these countries take to industrial lifestyle and Western diet.

Eastern Europe was hit after the Soviet Union's collapse. Health services and established social structures fell apart, and stress and depression increased. One result was that alcoholism soared. The average Russian man's life expectancy had been 64 years. By 2005, it was just 59.

In US, life expectancy of Americans fell for the first time in 15 years, as the nation's oldest adults died from heart disease, cancer and respiratory ailments, according to a report by the National Center for Health Statistics. The research found that the lifespan of men has decreased 4% since the 1980s and by 19% in women. Their children may be the first generation to not outlive their parents in many decades.

For Australians, they could be eating themselves to an early death, with new research suggesting life expectancy will decline for the first time in 100 years due to the obesity epidemic.

A paper published in the New England Journal of Medicine predicts a decrease in life expectancy, which rose slowly but steadily in last century. Obesity has been shown to reduce the length of life by about five to 20 years. About 68 per cent of Australian men and 52 per cent of Australian women are overweight or obese, which puts them at an elevated risk of diabetes, heart disease and cancer. Australia is tracking just behind the US in obesity trends.

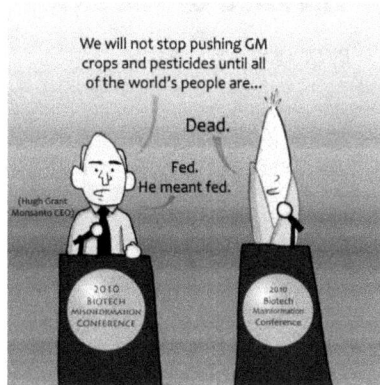

Its the same story with South Africa. International comparisons show that the average South African will not live longer than 50 years, according to the South African Institute of Race Relations (SAIRR).

According to its latest South Africa Survey, the country was part of a group of 37 developed and developing countries that had a decreasing life expectancy between 1990 and 2007. South Africa's life expectancy decreased from 62 years in 1990 to 50 years in 2007.

> "...every new genetically engineered plant is a unique event in nature, bringing its own set of genetic contingencies. This means that the reliability or safety of one genetically modified plant doesn't necessarily guarantee the reliability or safety of the next."
> ~Michael Pollan

20.

The Land Of The Sick

By Dr. Lynn Hardy, N.D.

Americans are sicker than ever! This is not my personal opinion but an undisputable fact. After examining the latest statistics and health forecasts, I am horrified about the future that lies before us. Even though most are preoccupied, and rightfully so, with the threat of terrorist attacks and other potential dangers, the phenomenon I'll be discussing also demands our immediate attention. Ending the atrocities of the world will not be enough to ensure a positive future for mankind. We must work just as hard to put a stop to the total deterioration of our food, water, and environment.

Based on scientific literature and the latest research, I will try to shine a light on the rapidly deteriorating state of health in America.

The Land Of The Sick

The United States, and on a smaller scale Europe, is being propelled towards total disaster through the deliberate poisoning of our most essential basic need - our food. Within the last hundred years food manufacturers, through their clever and aggressive marketing, have completely changed the way we look at food.

In fact, they've been so successful in their campaign that people actually believe they're getting a healthy nutritious meal

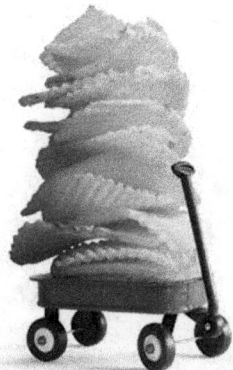

when they devour a McDonald's or Burger King hamburger. They don't realize that what they're actually eating is almost completely deficient of any nutrients and full of harmful ingredients.

These junk foods don't nourish the body in any way - as food should - they just barely keep the person from starving. (I mean this in a nutritional sense because the obese humans these foods produce look far from starved!) The situation has become so critical that the majority of people simply dismiss those of us fighting for clean food, water, and air as blind fanatics.

Paradoxically, supermarkets are actually starting to devote a tiny little section to so called "Health Food". But then what exactly are they selling in the remaining 99% of the store, "Sick Food"? My answer is "yes" and I will go on to prove my point and risk being called a fanatic or an idealist.

But am I, in fact, being fanatic when the latest statistics show that every second American is chronically ill? How could we have let things get so out of hand?

Partnership for Solutions, a new initiative of Johns Hopkins University and The Robert Wood Johnson Foundation, collects health statistics and calculates future projections. (See http://www.chronicnet.org.) They define "chronic illness" the following way:

"A chronic condition lasts a year or longer, limits what one can do and may require ongoing care. More than 125 million Americans have at least one chronic condition and 60 million have more than one condition. Examples of chronic conditions are diabetes, cancer, glaucoma and heart disease."

"The number of people with chronic conditions is growing at an alarming rate. In 2000, 20 million more people had one or more chronic conditions than the number originally estimated in 1996. By the year 2020, 25% of the American population will be living with multiple chronic conditions, and costs for managing these conditions will reach $1.07 trillion... The number of people with chronic conditions is projected to increase from 125 million in 2000 to 171 million in the year 2030."

These statistics are not only frightening but rather shocking as well! And even though data about the prevalence of chronic illness is available in many health publications, most people are simply not aware of it.

What's even more disturbing is that the average age of the "chronically ill" is on a constant decline. Nearly half are under the age of 45 and a staggering 15 percent of those are children. Millions of little ones are suffering from diabetes, asthma, developmental disabilities, cancer and other disorders. Unfortunately, this is just the beginning.

Asthma is the most common chronic disease of childhood, affecting an estimated 5 million children. Among the population, children now have the highest rate of asthma, and the numbers have increased 92% over the past decade. A growing number of children are also developing Type II (adult-onset) diabetes, which was primarily found only in adults.

Millions of young ones are being medicated for Attention Deficit Disorder (ADD) for their inability to concentrate. Cancer is still the leading cause of disease-related deaths in children under 15.

Along with countless others, all of the above-mentioned chronic conditions can be blamed on our polluted air and water, and the nutritionally deprived, chemically poisoned food we eat. Simply stated, if we were to eliminate these toxins from our lives we would not develop asthma, diabetes, ADD, cancer, etc.

Thus, does this mother who works so hard to fight for clean air, water and food for her child still seem like a fanatic? Or to phrase it in a different way: What can we say about the ignorance of the

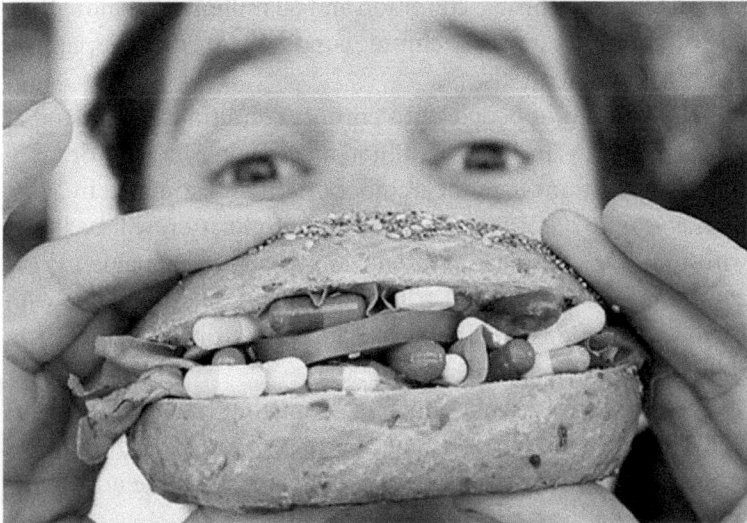

person who disregards the above statistics and continues to poison herself and her children on a daily basis?

Unfortunately, our modern health care system (or "sick care system" as my husband calls it) does not really believe in the health-preserving power nutrition plays in our lives. Instead, conventional medicine often blames heredity for diseases, which actually serves two purposes: It frees the industry from any liability and deems the patient helpless and not responsible for his own health (or lack thereof).

After all, anyone can change the way they eat, but we can't do anything about our genes! This is a very convenient and profitable standpoint.

(But as luck would have it, we have concrete evidence of what happens to a nation if it doesn't eat, drink and breathe garbage. We will present this "other side of the coin" to the reader in the next section of the book, so that the truth can be seen once and for all!)

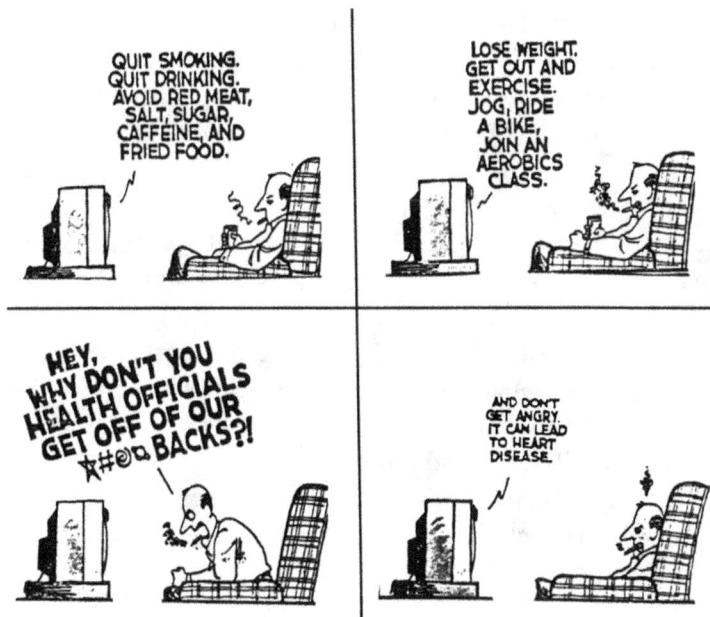

21.

Health Care

Misplaced Priorities

While governments are funding cash and devising plans to prevent a possible flu pandemic, critics say little is being done to tackle the World's biggest killers such as cancer, diabetes and respiratory and heart disease.

Professor Paul Zimmet, director of the International Diabetes Institute in Australia says, "There has been a preoccupation with AIDS and more recently bird flu, but diabetes has been escalating. It's a timebomb."

"In Australia, 170 million dollars (US$123 million) has been committed to tackle a (bird flu) epidemic which may or may not happen, but we have a huge diabetes problem and there may be five million dollars spent annually. It's completely disproportionate," he adds.

As the UN marks World Health Day, countries such as India are bracing for a worsening health crisis from chronic diseases that already claim more lives than infectious diseases such as malaria, AIDS and tuberculosis.

According to the World Health Organization (WHO), 270 million people in Asia will die from chronic disease between 2005 and 2015, mostly poor people in developing countries such as China, India, Pakistan and Indonesia.

Asia has an estimated 8.3 million HIV/AIDS cases, while bird flu has killed 108 people out of 191 cases worldwide since the outbreak began in Asia in late 2003.

Heart diseases, chronic respiratory conditions, cancer and diabetes are the world's top four killer diseases – more fatal than the much feared ailments like AIDS and influenza A (H1N1), according to UN.

The economic cost of chronic diseases will run into trillions of dollars, experts say. Many Asian governments, however, spend relatively little on public healthcare and a small percentage of that goes towards prevention of lifestyle diseases.

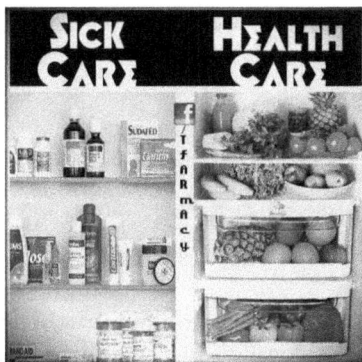

India at present spends 0.65 percent of GDP on health (defense spending almost touches 3 percent) and all other Asian governments devoted far less than 5 per cent of GDP to health,

The World Health Organization (WHO) in March 2010 called on governments across the Asia Pacific region to spend at least 4%-5% of gross domestic product (GDP) on health and put extensive safety-net provisions in place for vulnerable sections of the population.

But no one seems to be listening. India squandered $20 billion on Commonwealth games in 2011 while millions died from under-nutrition and chronic diseases during the same period. Most of the organizers are serving token jail sentences for corruption charges running into billions. So the problem is not exactly lack of resources but it's their gross mismanagement.

> "Though the industrial logic that made feeding cattle to cattle seem like a good idea has been thrown into doubt by mad cow disease, I was surprised to learn it hadn't been discarded. The FDA ban on feeding ruminant protein to ruminants makes an exception for blood products and fat; my steer will probably dine on beef tallow recycled from the very slaughterhouse he's heading to in June."
> ~Michael Pollan, The Omnivore's Dilemma: A Natural History of Four Meals

22.

Genetic Factors

Largely A Myth

Another common myth is that bad health is caused by bad genes. Therefore–other than having picked different parents–there's nothing you can do about your health as you grow older.

You've probably all heard a person say something like, "My Dad died of a heart attack at 54, and Grandpa died of one when he was only 49." Generally such explanations are offered with a look of deep resignation and regret.

The man speaking is doomed to an early death, and there's nothing he can do but accept the inevitable. And perhaps console himself with generous servings of barbecued ribs and French fries.

Obviously, there is a connection between genetics and aging. It's well known, for example, that the length of life of non-identical twins varies much more than that of identical twins who are genetically identical.

When there are similarities in a family, is it the results of genes or the environment or a combination of the two? To answer this perennial question, the MacArthur Research Network considered the role of genes in several aspects of aging:

Some genetic diseases do clearly shorten life. A few are caused by a single gene. For example, if a person has Huntington's disease, his or her children have a 50% chance of inheriting the gene from that parent. A child who inherits the gene will get the disease, unless, of course, he dies of some other cause before the disease manifests itself.

For all but a small number of conditions like Huntington's disease, however, the MacArthur studies show that a person's environment and lifestyle have a powerful effect on the likelihood that he will actually develop a disease.

It's true that a family history of heart disease, some cancers, high blood pressure, familial high cholesterol, rheumatoid arthritis, and certain other diseases may put a person at risk, but that doesn't mean that he or she will necessarily develop the disease.

We now know that diet, exercise, and even medications may delay or completely eliminate the emergence of the disease. Genes play a key role in promoting disease, but they are certainly less than half the story.

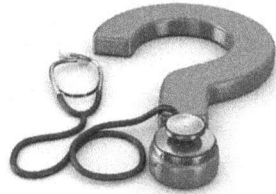

Effect Of Genes On Mental And Physical Function

To separate the effects of genetics from those of environment, the MacArthur researchers studied some twins who are reared apart.

Such studies clearly indicated that with rare exceptions, only about 30% of physical aging can be blamed on the genes and as we grow older, genetics becomes less important, and environment becomes more important.

Authors Rowe and Kahn, in their research conclude that the likelihood of conditions, such as obesity and hypertension, are largely not inherited and thus these risks are due to environmental and life style factors. How we live and where we live has the most profound impact on age-related changes in the function of many organs throughout the body, including the heart, immune system. lungs, bones, brain, and kidneys.

Diseases run into a family mainly because the diet pattern and life pattern of family members are often similar.

Also modern studies show that at most 15 percent of cancers are due - and only in part - to inherited genetic defects. Eighty-five percent are not.

However, cancer does run in families: A landmark New England Journal of Medicine study showed that children adopted at birth by parents who died of cancer before the age of 50 had the cancer risk of their adoptive parents, not of their biological ones. What gets passed on from one generation to the next are cancer-causing habits and environmental exposures, not just cancer-causing genes.

Racial Vulnerability To Diseases

Some races are prone to some particular diseases than the others. For example, Indians are more susceptible to develop type 2 diabetes than other nationalities. But this differentiation is only partly due to genes. Diet and lifestyle factors play a major role. *Every race has its own dietary and cultural patterns which define its susceptibility to a particular disease.*

The basis for this hypothesis is strengthened by results of studies showing that people who migrate from one country to another generally acquire the chronic disease rates of the new host country, suggesting that environmental [or lifestyle factors] rather than genetic factors are the key determinants of the international variation in chronic disease rates.

It was noted in the 1970s that people in many western countries had diets high in animal products, fat, and sugar, and high rates of cancers of the colorectum, breast, prostate, and lung; by contrast, individuals in developing countries usually had diets that were based on one or two starchy staple foods, with low intakes of animal products, fat, and sugar, and low rates of these cancers. So it was diet, rather than genes that led to variation in these cancer rates.

---

trimsad vimsati varsani
paramayuh kalau nrnam
The maximum duration of life for human beings in Kali-yuga will become fifty years.
(*Srimad Bhagavatam 12.2.11*)

23.

Precocious Puberty

Burden of Ageing on Tender Childhood

Puberty, usually occurring during adolescence, is when kids develop physically and emotionally into young men and women.

Just few decades ago, it occurred for girls at the age of 13 or 14 and in some traditional societies even later. For boys it was slightly later than girls. But it is no longer so. Puberty is striking much earlier now. Girls as young as 6 years are attaining puberty with serious social and health implications. Sudden changes in the body at such a tender age leave them traumatised.

Precocious puberty, defined as the onset of signs of puberty before age 7 or 8 in girls and age 9 in boys, can be physically and emotionally difficult for kids and can sometimes be the sign of an underlying health problem.

Heard of the shot that delays puberty? Well, many worried parents are now opting for these growth hormone injections for their child to either delay the early onset of menstrual cycle or stop monthly periods for a couple of years.

Doctors have seen a rise in this condition in the last several years. Doctors say this condition not only has implications on the child's height and overall growth but increases the exposure to oestrogen hormone which can lead to breast cancer at a later stage.

Early puberty also puts girls at a higher risk for teasing or bullying, mental health disorders and short stature as adults.

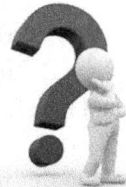

Early sexual maturation in boys can be accompanied by increased aggressiveness due to the surge of hormones that affect them.

Under these circumstances, health experts are urging people to watch what they eat.

Historical records show that puberty in girls in the United States and Europe changed dramatically from the mid-19th to mid-20th centuries. In the first part of the 20th century, the average age of menarche declined by two to three months each decade, falling from about 17 to 13, in both the United States and Europe.

Profit-seeking Leeches - Swallowing An Entire Generation

Our children are being destroyed in the name of profit by big industry and factory farms who feed their animals steroids, growth hormones and antibiotics to make them fatter, faster. More and more yield of meat from an animal means more and more profit, and if we need to sacrifice a generation of children along the way, so be it.

And these are not just the rantings of some liberal, tree-hugging vegan. According to Cornell University, hormones "reduce the waiting time and the amount of feed eaten by an animal before slaughter in meat industries." And that means bigger profit... faster.

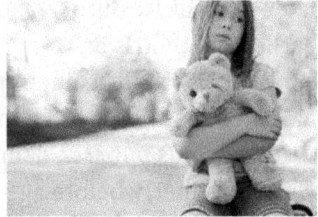

Meat, dairy and poultry lobbyists hide the real facts and peddle hormone, antibiotic and steroid-laced food to our children. And we wonder why little girls look like very big girls far before their time.

If hormones can make an animal fat, what do you think will happen to the children? We have always had access to junk food, but never in human history have we been the subjects of such an intense ingestion of chemicals and hormones.

Dr. Andrew Weil states that more than two-thirds of the cattle raised in the U.S. are given hormones, usually testosterone and estrogen to boost growth. According to Cornell, there are actually six hormones commonly used in meat and dairy production: estradiol, progesterone, testosterone, zeranol, trenbolone acetate and melengesterol. Another growth hormone to promote more milk production in dairy cows is rbGH.

Female Infants Growing Breasts

Female infants in China who have been fed infant formula have been growing breasts. According to the official *Chinese Daily* newspaper, medical tests performed on the babies found levels of estrogens circulating in their bloodstreams that are as high as those found in most adult women. These babies are between four and 15 months old. And the evidence is overwhelming that the milk formula they have been fed is responsible.

Chinese dairy association says the hormones could have entered the food chain when farmers reared the cows. Bovine growth hormones (invented by Monsanto) are used in China, as they are in the U.S., to promote greater milk production.

This isn't the first time something like this is happening. In the 1980s, doctors in Puerto Rico began encountering cases of precocious puberty. There were four-year-old girls with fully developed breasts. There were three-year old girls with pubic hair and bleeding. There were one-year-old girls who had not yet begun to walk but whose breasts were growing. And it wasn't just the females, young boys were also affected.

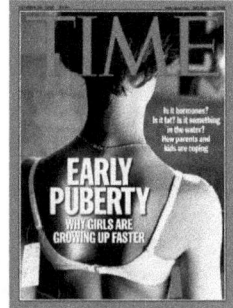

Writing a few years later in the Journal of the Puerto Rico Medical Association, Dr. Carmen A. Saenz explained the cause. "It was clearly observed in 97 percent of the cases that the appearance of abnormal breast tissue was...related to local milk in the infants."

> *"So this is what commodity corn can do to a cow: industrialize the miracle of nature that is a ruminant, taking this sunlight- and prairie grass-powered organism and turning it into the last thing we need: another fossil fuel machine. This one, however, is able to suffer. "*
> *~Michael Pollan, The Omnivore's Dilemma: A Natural History of Four Meals*

Along with China, the U.S. is today one of the few countries in the world that still allows bovine growth hormones to be injected into dairy cows. Though banned in Canada, Japan, Australia, New Zealand and most of Europe, the use of these hormones in U.S. dairy is not only legal, it's routine in all 50 states.

The problem is that dairy products made from cows injected with the hormone are not labeled. It's because Monsanto, the original manufacturer of BGH, has aggressively and successfully lobbied state governments in the past to make sure that no legislation is passed that would require such labeling.

As if that wasn't enough, Monsanto has also insistently sought to make it illegal for dairy products that are BGH-free to say so on their labels.

We also have to look at other options and invest in the health of our children before we lose an entire generation because we just want cheap, fast food. There are alternatives to these altered foods that can nourish our families and children healthfully and affordably.

In his book, Healing the Planet One Patient at a Time, Dr. Jozef Krops research indicates that breast milk in women in Western countries is so seriously contaminated that it would not pass American Food and Drug Administration standards if it were a packaged product. He adds, In the Eastern seaboard and southwestern United States (the most highly industrialized parts), mothers are not recommended to breastfeed past six months, as the baby by then already has the maximum lifetime amounts of carcinogens in its cells.

~ Michelle Schoffro Cook

24.

Druggernaut Rules

Big Pharma Boom - Even As The World Slows Down

Pharmaceuticals rank as the most profitable industry, again. In a year that saw a drop in employment rates, a plunge in the stock market and symbols of Global economy literally come crashing down, the pharmaceutical industry continued its reign as the most profitable industry in the annual Fortune 500 list.

While the overall profits of Fortune 500 companies declined by 53 percent - the second deepest dive in profits the Fortune 500 has taken in its 47 years - the top 10 U.S. drug makers increased profits by 33 percent.

Collectively, the 10 drug companies in the Fortune 500 topped all three of the magazine's measures of profitability in 2010, according to Fortune magazine's annual analysis of World's largest companies.

These companies had the greatest return on revenues, reporting a profit of 18.5 cents for every $1 of sales, which was eight times higher than the median for all Fortune 500 industries and easily more than the next most profitable industry, commercial banking (13.5 percent return on revenue).

The drug industry also dominated others by realizing a return on assets of 16.5 percent - almost six times the median (2.5 percent) posted by all industries. Pharmaceutical companies completed the sweep with a return on shareholders' equity (33.2 percent) that was more than three times the median of all Fortune 500 industries (9.8 percent).

Fortune 500 drug companies attained this triple crown, in part, by hiking pill prices, advertising some medicines more than Nike shoes and spending much less than the industry has suggested on R&D.

In addition, through its huge lobbying presence in Washington, D.C. the drug industry staved off congressional efforts to moderate rising drug prices. In fact, the industry went on the offensive last year in Congress, fighting for lucrative extensions of monopoly patents on drugs like Cipro, the antibiotic used to treat anthrax.

Congress was all too willing to help, as it approved a patent extension program for pediatric drugs that will give drug companies $592 million a year in added profits, according to the U.S. Food and Drug Administration (FDA). (The FDA acknowledges that this is a conservative estimate based on a limited sample of drugs.)

No wonder Fortune says that the pharmaceutical industry "showed some impressive gains."

These gains are nothing new. The latest figures reflect a trend that has been continuing for three decades. In the 1970s and 1980s, profitability of Fortune 500 medicine merchants (measured by return on revenues) was two times greater than the median for all industries in the Fortune 500. In the 1990s, when the intellectual property protections of the landmark Hatch-Waxman Act kicked in, the drug industry's profitability grew to almost four times greater than the median for all industries in the Fortune 500.

> "People are fed by the Food Industry, which pays no attention to health,
>
> and are treated by the Health Industry, which pays no attention to food."
>
> Wendell Berry

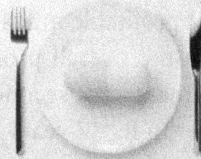

The industry begins the 21st century with even better prospects - a chronically sick population and annual increases in national spending on pharmaceuticals makes the future for top drug companies look healthier than ever.

Drug companies are recession proof and the best investment bet ever.

India - A Case Study

Notwithstanding the current global economic crisis, India's pharmaceutical industry and its health care market are expected to grow rapidly in the next few years, according to McKinsey, a global management consulting firm.

Driven by strong local demand, Indian health care market is expected to continue growing close to previously projected rates of 10 to 12 per cent, McKinsey said in its report 'New Opportunities for US-India Biopharma and Healthcare Collaboration'.

Released recently at the US India Biopharma and Healthcare Summit, the high growth of the Indian health care sector is primarily driven because of domestic reasons.

With average household consumption expected to increase by more than 7 per cent per annum, the annual healthcare expenditure is projected to grow at 10 per cent and also the number of insured is likely to jump from 100 million to 220 million.

Further hospital beds are expected to double from 1.5 per thousand to 2.9 per thousand and the diagnostic laboratories to grow by 20 to 25 per cent. There will be an addition of 3,00,000 to 4,00,000 doctors and another 2,50,000 to 3,00,000 nurses.

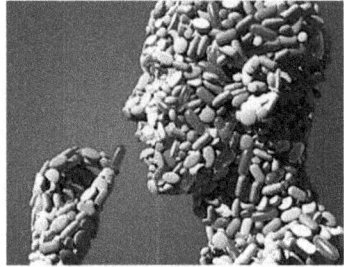

Uk Health Secretary Welcomes Greater Collaboration With India
On 24th October 2005, Ms Patricia Hewitt MP, Secretary of State for Health, met with captains of industry from India's health sector to discuss greater collaboration between India and Britain in the healthcare sector. Sonjoy Chatterjee, MD & CEO of ICICI Bank UK Ltd and Chairman of The India Group convened the meeting.

Mrs Hewitt in her formal comments welcomed the emergence of Indian companies and their attention on building partnerships in Britain. She said "We believe that long term relationships are important and recognise that our relations with India have shifted to one where both are seeking to be leaders in the global knowledge economy. There has been an explosion in healthcare services; it is the fastest growing and fastest changing sector in the world and we need to examine ways in which our medical model can be enhanced in this dynamic environment. With this in mind, I am sure our relationship with India can be enormously advantageous."

So pharmaceutical companies are liking what they see in India. Big pharma is poised for a big role in India.

Abbott Laboratories is leading the charge into the country, which now boasts the 10th largest economy in the world. In one fell swoop, Abbott recently became India's biggest drugmaker when it bought local generic manufacturer Piramal for $3.7 billion.

With that purchase, three of the largest pharmaceutical companies in India are now foreign multinationals. Outsiders already have 25% of the market, which grew by 16.5% in 2010 to an estimated $8 billion.

The market is expected to double by 2015, when the share of multinationals is expected to approach 50%. Look for at least two acquisitions of local companies in the near future, says one analyst.

Abbott is among those members of Big Pharma that are remodeling operations to suit emerging markets like India. In 2010 the company set up a stand-alone Established Products Division specifically for expanding the market for its well-known pharmaceutical portfolio outside the U.S.

> Medicine is not healthcare-- Food is healthcare. Medicine is sickcare. Let's all get this straight, for a change.

GlaxoSmithKline also wants a bigger piece of the Indian pie. It took an important step when it purchased the pipeline of India's biggest domestic pharmaceutical company, Dr. Reddy's Laboratories.

Glaxo also has shifted its strategy from a traditional blockbuster model toward driving growth from new products and its consumer business.

Then there are others like Merck, Pfizer and Novartis to name a few, who are competing for their share of the kill in a country already wracked by poverty, corruption and illiteracy.

Americans Drowning in Prescription Drugs

Nearly half of all Americans now use prescription drugs on a regular basis, says Mike Adams, quoting a CDC report of September 2010.

> "We are at once the problem and the only possible solution to the problem."
>
> ~Michael Pollan, Second Nature: A Gardener's Education

Nearly a third of Americans use two or more drugs, and more than one in ten use five or more prescription drugs regularly.

The report also revealed that one in five children are being regularly given prescription drugs, and nine out of ten seniors are on drugs.

All these drugs came at a cost of over $234 billion in 2008. The most commonly-used drugs were:

-Statin drugs for older people

-Asthma drugs for children

-Antidepressants for middle-aged people

-Amphetamine stimulants for children

America has become a nation of druggies. The seniors are being drugged for nearly every symptom a doctor can find, children are being doped up with (legalized) speed, and middle-aged soccer moms are popping suicide pills (antidepressants).

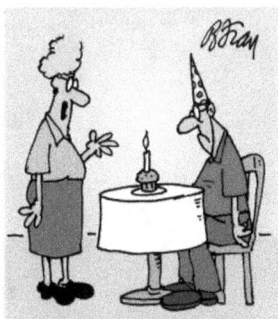

"IT'S WHEAT-FREE, DAIRY-FREE, FAT-FREE, NUT-FREE, SUGAR-FREE AND SALT-FREE...ENJOY!"

Prescription drug addictions are on the rise, too. Prescription drugs are so dangerous that now even the DEA (Drug Enforcement Agency) is hosting "take back your pills" day allowing citizens to anonymously surrender their unused prescription painkillers to DEA agents.

And It's Only Going To Get Worse

The percentage of Americans taking prescription drugs is expected to rise even further as the health reform insurance regulations kick in. Much of the bill was specifically designed to favor pharmaceutical industry interests by putting even more people on medication.

> "But human deciding what to eat without professional guidance - something they have been doing with notable success since coming down out of the trees - is seriously unprofitable if you're a food company, a definite career loser if you're nutritionist, and just plain boring if you're a newspaper editor or reporter."
> ~Michael Pollan, In Defense of Food: An Eater's Manifesto

The mass medication of American citizens has reached a disturbing tipping point where the future of the nation itself is at risk. That's because pharmaceuticals cause cognitive decline, and once you get to the point where over 50 percent of the voters can't think straight, you're trapped in a crumbling Democracy.

Primitive Races

Healthy, Happy And Peaceful

Evolution of Denatured Foods

And Impact

A History

25.

Primitive Man - His Food and His Health

Observations Of Early Explorers

By Dr. Stanley S. Bass

Columbus, in his 'discovery' of the Western World, was the beginning spark which ignited the interest of all the leading powers. This resulted in a series of expeditions sent forth for the purpose of acquiring these valuable lands, their rich natural resources and wealth. These countries included France, England, Spain, Portugal etc., who in competition with each other, explored North America, the Northlands, Central America, then South America, eventually spreading into Africa, Asia, Australia, the Pacific Islands and the entire world.

These expeditions were fully outfitted ships with supplies and crew, containing doctors to see after the health of all. Supplies for trading with the primitive Indians were in the form of white flour, white sugar, canned foods, salt, pepper, spices and other commodities which were exchanged for native furs, foods and other goods.

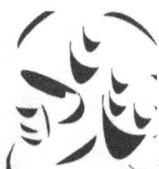

The accounts of early voyagers, explorers and missionaries are considered together with anthropological studies and knowledge gleaned from various nutritional surveys and medical inspections made in the primitive world. It is drawn from a literary survey of the people of many lands, including all continents and many islands. It covers centuries of time involving observations of racial groups living in the early 16th century to those of the modern day.

Shortlived And Diseased - A Myth?

The common view, that primitive man is generally short-lived and subject to many diseases is often held by physicians as well as layman, and the general lack of of sanitation, modern treatment, surgery and drugs in the primitive world is thought to prevent maintenance of health at a high physical level. The average nutritionist feels that any race lacking access to the wide variety of foods available, which modern agriculture and transportation now permit, could not be in good health.

Beauty, White Teeth, Long Life

But the facts are known, and they indicate that, when living under near-isolated conditions, apart from civilization and without access to the foods of civilization, primitive man lives in much better physical condition and health than does the usual member of civilized society. When his own nutrition is adequate and complete, as it most often is, his teeth are white without brushing, they are formed in perfect alignment and the dental arch is broad.

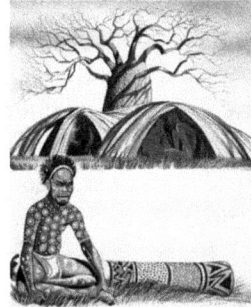

The face is finely formed, well-set and broad; the body development is also good, free from deformity, and desirably proportioned in beauty and symmetry. The respective members of the racial group reproduce in homogeneity from one generation to the next, with few deviations from the standard anthropological prototype.

Reproductive efficiency permits birth with no difficulty and little or no pain. There are no prenatal deformities. Resistance to infectious disease is high, few individuals are sick, and these usually rapidly recovering. The degenerative diseases are rare, even in advanced life, some of them being completely unknown and unheard of by the primitive.

Mental complaints are equally rare, and the usual state of happiness and contentment is one scarcely known by civilized man. The duration of life is long, the people being yet strong and vigorous as they pass the three score and ten mark, and living in many cases beyond a century.

These are the characteristics of the finest and healthiest primitive races living under the most ideal climatic and nutritional conditions. Even primitive races less favored by environment have better teeth and skeletal development than civilized man. We note that people living today, under the culture and environment of the "Stone Age", have far surpassed civilized man in strength, physical development and immunity to disease. This fact poses an important question to modern medicine and should arouse serious thought and consideration.

Contact With 'Civilization' - New Diet

The good health of the primitive has been possible only under conditions of relative isolation. As soon as his contact with civilization brings about changes in his dieting habits - with the introduction of refined white flour and white sugar, canned food, jams, marmalades, polished rice, etc. - within one generation he succumbs to disease very readily and loses all of the unique immunity of the past.

The teeth decay; facial forms cease to be uniform; deformities become common; reproductive efficiency is lowered; mental deficiency develops, and the duration of life is sharply lowered.

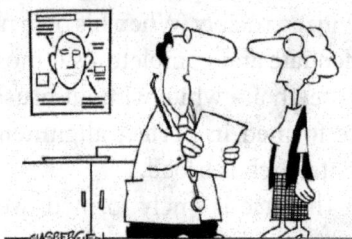

"You've got a rare condition called 'good health'. Frankly, we're not sure how to treat it."

It is the nutritional habits of primitive man that are responsible for the state of his health, and as long as his native foods remain in use, as important physical changes occur, and the bacterial scourges are absent - even though a complete lack of sanitation would indicate that pathogenic bacteria might be present.

When the native foods are displaced for those of modern commerce, the situation changes completely. And the finest sanitation, that the white man can provide, together with the best in medical services, is of no avail in preventing the epidemics that take thousands of lives.

Lessons To Learn

What is needed is the proper education of children in healthy nutrition, beginning in grade schools. And for those aspiring to become mothers, education in pre-parental, parental nutrition and proper feeding of children.

The direction should be in education and prevention, rather than in the treatment of disease symptoms with drugs and surgery, if we are to reverse the increasing of degenerative disease and the progressive deterioration of the human race.

There is need to learn from the dietary practices of the most magnificently healthful and successful primitive races from all parts of the world - as recorded by both ancient and modern explorers of these primitive cultures, who have accumulated their knowledge over a period of many thousands of years of experience.

"You are what what you eat eats."

"You are what you eat is a truism hard to argue with, and yet it is, as a visit to a feedlot suggests, incomplete, for you are what what you eat eats, too. And what we are, or have become, is not just meat but number 2 corn and oil."

~Michael Pollan, The Omnivore's Dilemma

26.

The Civilized Savage

And The Uncivilized Civilization

Wisdom From The Primitive People

In December 2004, a disastrous tidal wave struck several countries in Indian ocean. Thousands died and many thousands went missing in the massive tidal wave, called Tsunami. But the indigenous people on the Andaman and Nicobar islands are thought to have escaped the calamity, thanks to traditional warning systems that interpret bird and marine animal behaviour.

According to the director of the Anthropological Survey of India, V. R. Rao, no casualties were reported among five tribes - the Jarwas, Onges, Shompens, Sentenelese and Great Andamanese. He believes this is because the tribal people fled for safety at the first indications such as changes in bird calls that something was wrong.

According to a related BBC Online news story, wildlife officials in Sri Lanka reported that despite the large loss of human life, there were no reported animal deaths. It is thought that animals moved to safer ground having sensed vibrations or changes in air pressure in advance of the waves' arrival. In contrast to all this, modern civilized man suffered most in the hands of furious waves. So in a survival test, we are scoring rather low.

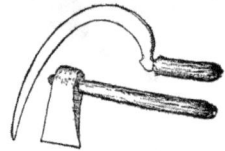

Another Island Survives The Tsunami

It is another remarkable story of how an entire population survives the 2004 tsunami.

Simeulue Island lies off the western coast of Sumatra in Indonesia. It is considered a backward place compared to the surrounding islands.

Most of the the people of Simeulue Island, just 40 miles from the epicenter of the earthquake, survived the 2004 tsunami.

Banda Aceh, the nearest city on another island lost over 100,000 people but most people on this island survived. These people have been taught a simple lesson by their grandmothers, "If an earthquake comes, we must always go and look at the beach. If we see a low tide, we must run for the hills."

In 2004, the locals new a "smong" was coming. On Simeulue island in the Defayan language the word for tsunami is smong. And when they felt the earthquake and saw the low tide, they ran. And their lives were saved. Most of the 83,000 people survived.

Even the buffalos knew something was wrong when the earthquake happened. They too ran for the hills.

Human tradition, coming down since time immemorial, has a lot to offer us and has answers to many a predicaments we face today.

Primitive races have avoided certain life problems and their life wisdom can be of great help to us.

As we study the primitives we find that they had an entirely different conception of the nature and origin of the controlling forces which have molded individuals and races.

After one has lived among the primitive racial stocks in different parts of the world and studied them in their isolation, few impressions can be more vivid than that of the absence of prisons and asylums. Few, if any, of the problems which confront modern civilization are more serious and disturbing than the progressive

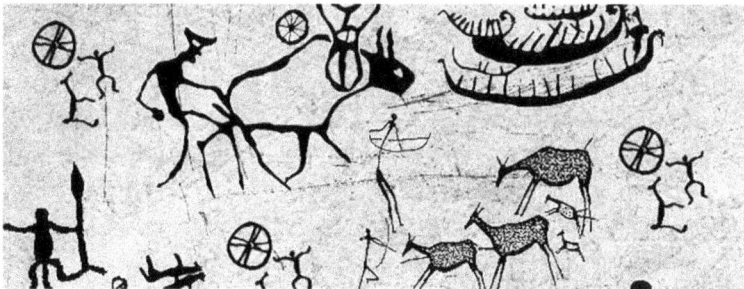

increase in the percentage of individuals with unsocial traits and irresponsible behaviour.

Criminal tendencies in isolated primitives are so slight that no prisons are required. There were hundreds of isolated tribes in different parts of the world and for the thousands of their inhabitants, there was no necessity of prisons. In Uganda, the Ruanda tribes estimated to number two and a half millions, had no prisons.

Much ancient wisdom, however, has been rejected and lost because of prejudice against the wisdom of so-called savages.

Nature must be obeyed, it is not an option. Apparently many primitive races have understood her language better than has our modern civilization.

While many of the primitive races have continued to thrive on the same soil through thousands of years, our modern human stock has declined rapidly within a few decades, as we saw in preceding chapters.

No era in the long journey of mankind reveals such a terrible degeneration of health as this brief modern period records. The

---

The members of the various primitive races that I have studied, are rapidly declining in health and numbers at their point of contact with our modern civilization. Since they have so much accumulated wisdom that is passing with them, it has seemed important that the elements in the modern contacts that are so destructive to them should be discovered and removed.

A critical examination of these groups revealed a high immunity to many of our serious affections so long as they were sufficiently isolated from our modern civilization and living in accordance with the nutritional programs which were directed by the accumulated wisdom of the group.

In every instance where individuals of the same racial stocks who had lost this isolation and who had adopted the foods and food habits of our modern civilization were examined, there was an early loss of the high immunity characteristics of the isolated group. These studies have included a chemical analysis of foods of the isolated groups and also of the displacing foods of our modern civilization.

~Dr. Weston A. Price

alternative seems to be a complete readjustment in accordance with the controlling forces of nature.

Modern science boasts the discovery of vitamin C. Thousands of white mariners died from scurvy due to lack of vitamin C. For centuries, its scourge continued.

But the native Indians in remote parts of Canada always knew how to avoid scurvy and many other dreaded diseases. When the British soldiers were dying in large numbers, the Indians taught them to use a tea made from the steeped tips of the spruce shoots. Over the centuries, not a single case of scurvy was ever detected in these natives.

Dr. Weston A. Price records his experience in the following words:

"As I have sojourned among members of primitive racial stocks in several parts of the world, I have been deeply impressed with their fine personalities, and strong characters. I have never felt the slightest fear in being among them; I have never found that my trust in them was misplaced. As soon as they had learned that I was visiting them in their interest, their kindness and devotion was very remarkable. Fundamentally they are spiritual and have a devout reverence for an all-powerful, all-pervading power which not only protects and provides for them, but accepts them as a part of that great encompassing soul if they obey Nature's laws."

Ernest Thompson Seton has beautifully expressed the spirit of the Red Indians in the opening paragraph of his book 'The Gospel of the Red Man':

The culture and civilization of the White man are essentially material; his measure of success is, "How much property have I acquired for myself?" The culture of the Red man is fundamentally spiritual; his measure of success is, "How much service have I rendered to my people?"

The civilization of the White man is a failure; it is visibly crumbling around us. It has failed at every crucial test. No one who measures things by results can question this fundamental statement.

The faith of the primitive in the all-pervading power of which he is a part includes a belief in immortality. He lives in communion with the great unseen Spirit, of which he is a part, always in humility and reverence.

27.

Hunza Valley

A Shangri-La Where Death Rides A Slow Bus

How would you like to live in a land where cancer has not yet been invented? A land where an optometrist discovers to his amazement that everyone has perfect 20-20 vision? A land where cardiologists cannot find a single trace of coronary heart disease? How would you like to live in a land where no one ever gets ulcers, appendicitis or gout? A land where men of 80 and 90 father children, and there's nothing unusual about men and women living a vigorous life at the age of 100 or 120?

In India during the 1920s, British researcher Sir Robert McCarrison conducted one of the most eye-opening experiments relative to the correlation between diet and health. Dr. McCarrison spent many years in the Himalayan Mountains including the picturesque Hunza Valley. This magical fairytale-like place is found between the borders of China, India, Pakistan and Russia at nearly 8000 ft. The natives of this valley, the Hunzakuts, captured Dr. McCarrison's attention because of the their excellent health and extremely long lifespan.

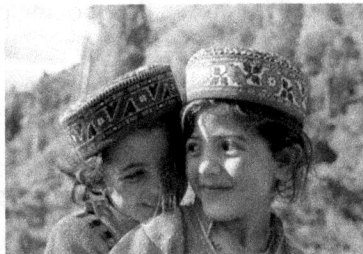

"In these Himalayan Mountains is Hunza; a country slightly more than a hundred miles long and perhaps just as wide, containing approximately thirty thousand inhabitants," writes Dr. Jay F. Hoffman, the author of the book Hunza - Secrets Of The

World's Healthiest And Oldest Living People, published in 1960. Dr. Hoffman was sent to Hunza under the auspices of the National Geriatrics Society.

He further writes, "Here the people lived to be 100, 110, 120, and occasionally as much as 140 years of age. Here lies the real Fountain of Youth... Hunza land is truly a Utopia if ever there was one. Just think of this! Here is a land where people do not have our common diseases, such as heart ailments, cancer, arthritis, high blood pressure, diabetes, tuberculosis, hay fever, asthma, liver trouble, gall bladder trouble, constipation or many other ailments that plague the rest of the world. Moreover, there are no hospitals, no insane asylums, no drug stores, no saloons, no tobacco stores, no police, no jails, no crimes, no murders, and no beggars."

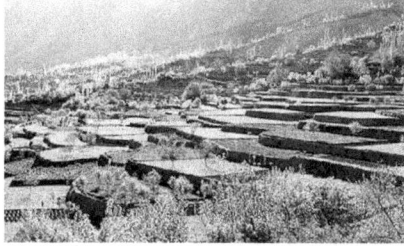

Any westerner who stepped foot on the tiny land of this friendly nation couldn't stop raving about their good nature, outstanding hospitality, not to mention the physical strength and stamina of

Hunzas are estimated to have lived in complete isolation for at least two thousand years. A British General and a garrison of solders on horseback investigated the Hunza River Valley in the 1870s. The pass to reach Hunza from Gilgit was 13,700 feet (4176 m) high, a difficult and treacherous trail. Upon entering the valley, the British found the steep, rocky sides of the valley lined with terraced garden plots, fruit trees, and animals being raised for milk and wool.

The gardens were watered with mineral-rich glacier water carried by an aqueduct system running a distance of 50 miles (80 km) from the Ultar Glacier on the 25,550 foot (7788 m) high Mount Rakaposhi. The wooden aqueduct trough was hung from the sheer cliffs by steel nails hammered into the rock walls. Silt from the river below was carried up the side of the valley to form and replenish the terraced gardens.

The difficult trail into Hunza kept the people isolated. As late as 1950, most of the children of Hunza had never seen a wheel or a Jeep even though airplanes were landing at the airport in Gilgit only 70 miles (112 km) away.

their men. "My own experience provides an example of a race unsurpassed in perfection of physique and in freedom from disease in general." Wrote Dr. McCarrison about the Hunzkuts. "Amongst these people the span of life is extraordinarily long... During the period of my association with these people I never saw a case of asthenic dyspepsia, of gastric or duodenal ulcer, of appendicitis, of mucous colitis, of cancer." (J.I. Rodale: The Healthy Hunza. Rodale Press)

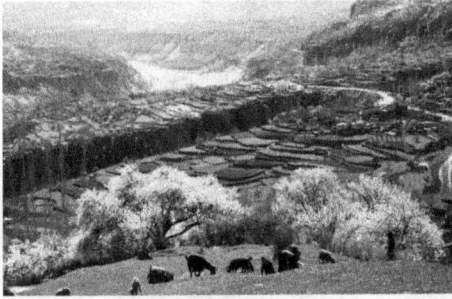

Not only are the Hunza people immune to serious diseases, they are also spared the discomfort of commonplace conditions such as the cold or the flu.

Dr. McCarrison, who specialized in nutritional diseases, was determined to learn their secret. The opportunity arose in 1927 when he was appointed the Director of Nutrition Research in India. Along with his designation he also received a well-equipped laboratory and qualified assistants.

Hunza food is completely natural, containing no chemical additives whatsoever. Unfortunately, that is not the case as far as most of our food is concerned. Everything is as fresh as it can possibly be, and in its original unsalted state. The only "processing" consists of drying some fresh fruits in the the sun, and making butter and cheese out of milk. No chemicals or artificial fertilizers are used in their gardens. In fact, it is against the law of Hunza to spray gardens with pesticides.

Renee Taylor, in her book Hunza health secrets (Prentice-Hall 1964) says that the Mir, or ruler of Hunza, was recently instructed by Pakistani authorities to spray the orchards of Hunza with pesticide, to protect them from an expected invasion of insects. But the Hunzas would have none of it. They refused to use the toxic pesticide, and instead sprayed their trees with a mixture of water and ashes, which adequately protected the trees without poisoning the fruit and the entire environment. In a word, the Hunzas eat as they live - organically.

The doctor designed a whole series of experiments to determine how big of a role the Hunzakuts' diet played in their supreme health and longevity.

Hunza meals don't consist of pre-cooked, over-processed, and nutritionally devoid industrial chemicals - like the average modern diet. Instead, they enjoy locally grown organic fruit, vegetables, unprocessed fresh milk products, and green or whole grains.

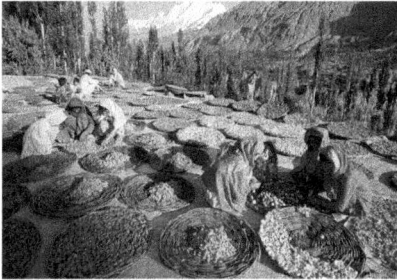

In the first experiment 1189 albino rats were fed the Hunza diet right from birth. This consisted of whole meal flatbread with a pat of fresh butter, sprouted legumes, fresh raw carrots and cabbage, whole milk, and once a week a tiny portion of meat and bones. Plenty of water was provided for drinking and bathing. The only thing the rats did not receive was fruit, which the Hunza people ate a great deal of.

No diseases, No Premature Death

The rats were fed this diet for 27 months, which would be the equivalent of approximately 45 human years. The rats were killed, and thoroughly examined at all stages leading up to 27 months. Remarkably, no trace of any disease could be found in their bodies! This astonishing consequence could best be explained through Dr.

An ordinary Hunza day starts early - around five a.m. Actually, the Hunzas rise with the sun, and go to bed at nightfall. The reason for this is simple: they possess no artificial means of illumination - no electricity, no gas, no oil. On the other hand, they are completely in tune with nature.

Of course it would be impossible for us to live that way. But you should be aware of one important point: your deepest hours of regenerating sleep occur before midnight.

The Hunzas do not seem to worry about the future, nor are they burdened with concerns about the past. Self doubt and the fear of failure, which tend to undermine the well-being of so many people, are unknown to the Hunzas.

McCarrison's words as he described his findings during a lecture at the College of Surgeons in 1931:

"During the past two and a quarter years there has been no case of illness in this 'universe' of albino rats, no death from natural causes in the adult stock, and, but for a few accidental deaths, no infantile mortality. Both clinically and at post-mortem examination this stock has been shown to be remarkably free from disease. It may be that some of them have cryptic disease of one kind or another, but, if so, I have failed to find either clinical or macroscopical evidence of it."

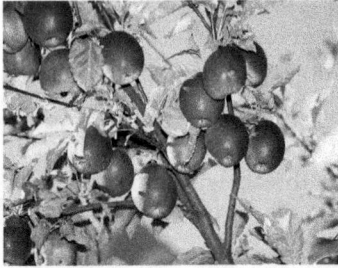

These results were truly staggering. But sadly, they did not have any real impact on the physicians present, who, much like the doctors of today, have a greater understanding of disease than the lack thereof.

There wasn't a sudden surge of articles and books propagating the Hunza diet and the avoidance of white rice, white flour, sugar and for the most part, meat.

As a follow up to his earlier experiment, Dr. McCarrison duplicated in his laboratory the low quality diet of a poor rural

---

The people there live long, happy, productive lives partly because they don't concern themselves much with time and age. This frees them from the hurry and worry that comes with alternately trying to rush time and hold it back -- both most fruitless and frustrating exercises. The people of Hunza have a grace that comes from flowing with time rather than trying to control it.

Renee Taylor writes, "Time is not measured by clocks or calendars (in Hunza). Time is judged by the changing of the seasons, and each season brings the feeling of newness, not a fear that time is slipping irrevocably away.

"In the West, on the other hand, where lives are dominated by clocks and calendars, we tend to view each passing moment as a little piece of life which has cruelly slipped away from us, never to return. Each such slipping bit of time brings us closer to old age and ultimately to death.

region of India. During this larger-scale experiment, 2243 rats were fed a diet deficient of vitamins, minerals and other important nutrients. The animal results matched the physical condition of the millions of people living in this region: Both groups developed diseases in every organ they possessed.

Diet and behavior

The most disturbing discovery of Dr. McCarrison was to come. In a later experiment, he set out to learn how the rats would react to the diet of the poorer class of England.

This consisted of white bread, margarine, sweetened tea, boiled vegetables, and cheap canned meats and jams. On this diet, not only did the rats not thrive physically, but they actually developed nervous disorders before things went from bad to worse: "They were nervous," writes the doctor, "and opt to bite their attendants; they lived unhappily together, and by the 16th day of the experiment they began to kill and eat the weaker ones amongst them."

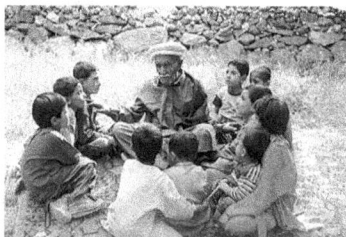

Shockingly, this diet of the lower-class English in the 1930s actually had a much greater nutrient value than the "food" the majority of well-to-do Americans stuff themselves with today.

First rule: frugality. In the west people eat too much - sometimes two or three times more than our organism actually needs. And we're not talking about people who have a weight problem either. Try to fashion your diet according to Hunza standards: remember that these mountain people eat only two light meals a day, even though they perform extremely laborious physical work for hours at a stretch, take part in demanding forms of physical exercise, and spend hours hiking along steep mountain paths each and every day. At the same time they do not feel in the least fatigued or anemic – on the contrary, their endurance and longevity is so great it has become almost legendary.

In fact, an excellent way to regenerate your organism and give your digestive system a rest is to fast, or drink only juice, for one day a week. Every spring the Hunzas fast for a number of days.

Following in the footsteps of Dr. McCarrison, cardiologists Dr. Paul D. White and Dr. Edward G. Toomey, made a difficult trip up the mountain paths to Hunza, toting along with them a portable, battery-operated electrocardiograph.

In the American Heart Journal for December, 1964, the doctors say they used the equipment to study 25 Hunza men, who were, "on fairly good evidence, between 90 and 110 years old." Blood pressure and cholesterol levels were also tested. They reported that not one of these men showed a single sign of coronary heart disease, high blood pressure or high cholesterol.

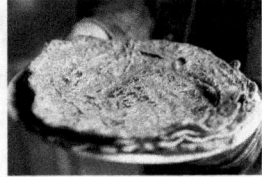

The Hunza people did not become a household name, even though they unintentionally came to possess the mental and practical skills needed to live long, joyous and disease-free lives. Of course, most of us are not able to move to the mountains and grow our own food but we can still learn a lot from this noble, peaceful and healthy nation. We can definitely start restoring our health by modifying our food selections.

Staying away from dead processed foods and turning towards natural, fresh, organically grown fruit and vegetables as much as

---

Milk and cheese are important sources of animal protein. Like grains, fruits and vegetables, yogurt is also a staple of the Hunza diet. Yogurt, which replenishes intestinal flora, is extremely beneficial for the human organism. Bulgarians, who also eat a lot of yogurt, are another people who live to a ripe old age. Bulgaria boasts 1,666 centenarians per million inhabitants, while in the West the number is only 9 per million inhabitants.

No discussion of the Hunza diet would be complete without mentioning their special bread, called 'chapatti,' which is eaten along with every meal. Since it is used so often, it would be logical to conclude that it is a determining factor - or at least a very important one - in causing their amazing longevity. In fact, chapatti bread contains all essential elements. It can be made from wheat, millet, buckwheat or barley flour, but what is most important is that the flour is whole, i.e. it is not refined, and has not had its germ removed, a common practice everywhere. It is this part of a grain which gives it its reproductive power, as well as its brown color.

possible is a good rule of thumb for everyone, regardless of his state of health. If enough people started demanding quality foods the food industry would have no choice but to alter its manufacturing processes and start supplying us with truly nutritious options instead of the falsely labeled junk we're subjected to. But since we can't foresee that day anytime in the near future, we all need to take responsibility for our own health and educate ourselves the best we can about the importance of nutrition.

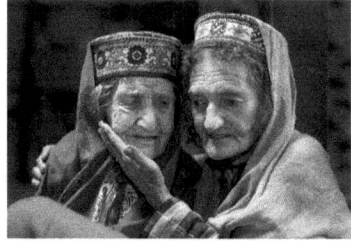

(Excerpts from a paper by Dr. Lynn Hardy, N.D., Director for the Global Institute For Alternative Medicine included here.)

Another important point to understand is that the health of the Hunzas is not characterized by the simple absence of disease, although that in itself is quite an accomplishment. More than just not being affected by diseases that strike down so many of our peers in the prime of life, the Hunzas seem to possess boundless energy and enthusiasm, and at the same time are surprisingly serene. Compared to the average Hunza, a westerner of the same age - even one who is considered extremely fit - would seem sickly. And not only seem sickly, but actually be sick!

All Hunzakuts are endurance athletes who practice all day. They have to work the fields and move long distances on foot. Every other day, a runner travels over the high mountain pass from Hunza to Gilgit. He picks up the mail and runs back. The round trip is about 120 miles. Other Hunzakuts frequently walk the distance, preferring walking to riding a horse.

28.

Abkhasia

The Land of Vitality

Abkhasia is a disputed territory on the eastern coast of the Black Sea and the south-western flank of the Caucasus. Abkhasia considers itself an independent state. This status is recognised by Russia and some other countries. However the Georgian government and the majority of the world's governments consider Abkhasia a part of Georgia's territory.

The status of Abkhasia is a central issue of the Georgian–Abkhasian conflict. This region formed part of the Soviet Union until 1991. As the Soviet Union began to disintegrate towards the end of the 1980s, ethnic tensions grew between Abkhaz and Georgians over Georgia's moves towards independence. This led to the 1992–1993 War in Abkhasia that resulted in a Georgian military defeat and de facto independence of Abkhasia.

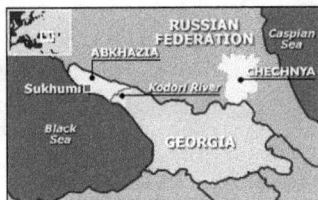

> *Shirali Mislimov was the world's oldest man when he died at 168. This Soviet citizen had this piece of advice for us, "There are two sources of long life. One is a gift of nature, and it is the pure air and clean water of the mountains, the fruit of the earth, peace, rest, the soft and warm climate of the highlands."*
>
> *"The second source is people. He lives long who enjoys life and who bears no jealousy of others, whose heart harbors no malice or anger, who sings a lot and cries a little, who rises and retires with the sun, who likes to work and knows how to rest."*

Abkhasia covers three thousand square miles between the eastern shores of the Black Sea and the crestline of the main Caucasus range. It is bordered on the north by Russia, and on the south by Georgia.

It is not unusual for the people of this region to live well into their 90s and 100s. Estimates suggest that almost 3 percent of the population of the Caucasus is over 90 years of age. In contrast, people over 90 in the United States represent only 0.4 percent of the population.

Not only do Caucasians live to a very old age, their physical and mental faculties remain remarkably intact. These people show the signs of aging—their hair is gray or white, and their skin in wrinkled—but they have good eyesight, excellent hearing, and unusually erect posture.

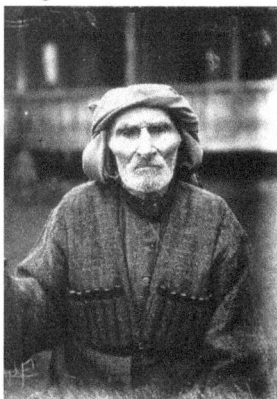

When high-quality machines break down, rarely is the breakdown the result of defective design or defective components. A motor car, carefully maintained and driven, will last for hundreds of thousands of miles. Yet many cars break down because of dirty ignition wires or distributor points and suffer early wear because of clogged filters and dirty oil. The car body may even look shiny and new but its vital mechanical components have been ruined by bad driving and poor maintenance.

Just as a reason can be found to explain the long life of one machine or the short life of another, so must there be reasons, perhaps just as simple, for different human life spans. Many researchers have spent their lives studying the subject.

Intrigued by the question of why the Caucasians live such long and healthy lives, American anthropologist Sula Benet undertook a study of the elderly people of Abkhasia. Benet's findings led her to suggest that the stability and continuity of the Abkhasians' culture is the major factor responsible for the Caucasians' long life expectancies. Below is a summary of her findings.

Benet found that the Abkhasians regard work as an activity vital to life and that the concept of retirement is completely foreign to them. From their early years to their old age, they work as hard as their ability and physical conditions allow. Obviously, as they grow older the amount of work they can do decreases. Even so, people in their 100s continue to work, often as much as four hours a day.

The Abkhasians also find time for exercise. An Abkhasian saying states that "it is better to move without purpose than to sit still." Consequently, Abkhasians usually begin each day by taking a long walk. They believe that these work and exercise habits greatly contribute to their long lives. Their doctors tend to agree with the Abkhasians, suggesting that the Abkhasians' slow, steady approach to work and their dedication to exercise help their bodies to operate more efficiently.

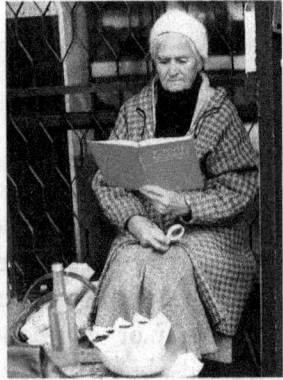

The Abkhasians believe that their diet also is a factor in their long lives. They never overeat, and they consider overweight people to be ill. When eating, they cut their food into small bites, which they chew very slowly. This habit greatly helps their digestion. Also, the type of food the Abkhasians eat varies little throughout their lives. They consume very little meat and practically no fish. Most of their protein comes from goat cheese and buttermilk. They never use sugar, although they do use honey as a sweetener. The bulk of their diet comes in the form of fresh fruits and vegetables and a bread substitute called abista.

Few Abkhasians smoke, and they do not drink tea or coffee. The only stimulant the Abkhasians use is a locally-produced red wine, which is low in alcoholic content. Doctors interviewed by Benet believe strongly that the Abkhasians' sensible diet and lack of "bad habits" add years to their lives.

Benet acknowledges that work, exercise, and diet all contribute to the Abkhasians' long life span. She argues, however that the Abkhasians' attitude toward aging is of equal importance.

Abkhasians over the age of 100 are called long-living people, not old people.

Further, Benet suggests, the structure of Abkhasian society and the role of the elderly in it also contribute to long lives. Abkhasian society is based on a complex kinship system. This system is so extensive that everyone with the same surname is considered kin.

Such interdependence is the basis of the strong sense of security and belonging that most Abkhasians—both young and old—possess. This sense of security and belonging is strengthened for older Abkhasian by the respect they receive. They are asked to lead major ceremonies and celebrations, are called on to settle disputes, and are consulted on all matters of importance.

In short, Benet found that the elderly of Abkhasia are life-loving, balanced people who believe that they are an important part of society. This, she notes, is in stark contrast to many older Americans who believe that they are burdens to themselves and to their families. Could such people—and all Americans—learn something from the Abkhasians? According to Benet, the answer is yes.

Sula Benet is the author of her famous book, Abkhasians: The Long Living People of the Caucasus (1974, New York).

What Do Abkhasians Eat?

According to John Robbins, the traditional Abkhasian diet is essentially lacto-vegetarian, with a rare serving of meat.

Abkhasians usually begin breakfast with vegetables [watercress, radishes in spring; tomatoes, cucumbers in summer and fall; pickled cucumber, tomatoes, radishes, cabbage in winter]. No dressings are used.

> In general, even at the end of their prolonged lives, these ancients, have their own teeth, fairly luxuriant hair, good eyesight, erect postures, and have never known illness or sickness. They look younger than their years, and Professor Benet, for instance, was once embarrassed in Abkhasia after making a toast to a man who looked about 70 years old. "May you live as long as Moses," she said. The man, it turned out, was already 119 and Moses had lived only to 120.
> ~David Wallechinsky

They drink one or two glasses a day of a fermented beverage called 'matzoni', made from the milk of goats, cows, or sheep.

At all three meals, the people eat their "beloved abista", a cornmeal porridge, always freshly cooked and served warm.

If they get hungry between meals, Abkhasians typically eat fruit in season from their own orchard or garden. Cherries and apricots are the choice fruits in the spring. Throughout the summer there are pears, plums, peaches, figs, and many kinds of berries. In the fall there are grapes and persimmons, as well as apples and pears. Fruit that is not eaten fresh is stored or dried for winter use.

With rare exception, vegetables are eaten raw.

Freshness of food is considered paramount.

Nuts [almonds, pecans, beechnuts, hazelnuts, chestnuts] play a major role in Abkhasian cuisine and are the primary source of fat in the Abkhasian diet. Virtually every meal contains nuts.

Abkhasians eat relatively little meat. ... Even then, the fat of the meat or poultry is never used. Abkhasians also consume no white sugar and very little salt.

Most Abkhasians consume less than 2000 calories a day. ... Overeating is considered both socially inappropriate and dangerous.

Abkhasians are universally very strong and slender people, with no excess fat on their bodies. They eat slowly and chew thoroughly.

John Robbins, a bestselling author, has discussed this region in his famous book - Healthy at 100: The Scientifically Proven Secrets of the World's Healthiest and Longest-Lived Peoples.

Dr. Alexander Leaf, a world-renowned physician is another person to shed light on this region. In the early 1970s, National Geographic magazine commissioned him to visit, study, and write an article about the world's healthiest and most long-living people.

Dr. Leaf, a professor of clinical medicine at Harvard University and Chief of Medical Services at Massachusetts General Hospital, had long been a student of the subject and had already visited and studied some of the

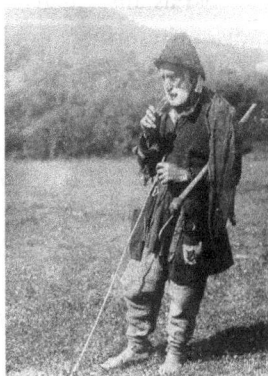

cultures known for the healthy lives of their elderly people. It was a time, unlike today, when these regions and their cultures were still somewhat pristine.

Dr. Leaf undertook a series of journeys that he subsequently described in an influential series of articles that appeared in National Geographic magazine beginning in 1973.

Dr. Leaf traveled to these remote areas to meet, photograph, examine, and appraise for himself the longevity and health of those who were reputed to be the world's oldest and healthiest people. Dr. Leaf listened to their hearts, took their blood pressure, and studied their diets and lifestyles.

"Certainly no area in the world," Leaf wrote, "has the reputation for long-lived people to match that of the Caucasus in southern Russia." And in all the Caucasus, the area most renowned for its extraordinary number of healthy centenarians (people above the age of 100) was Abkhasia. A 1970 census had established Abkhasia, then an autonomous region within Soviet Georgia, as the longevity capital of the world. "We were eager to see the centenarians," Leaf said, "and Abkhasia seemed to be the place to do so."

Prior to Dr. Leaf's visit, claims had been widely circulated for life spans reaching 150 years among the Abkhasians. Just a few years earlier, Life magazine had run an article with photos of Shirali Muslimov, said to be 161 years old. In one of the photos, Muslimov was shown with his third wife. He told the reporter that he had married her when he was 110, that his parents had both lived to be over 100, and that his brother had died at the age of 134.

> The legend of extraordinarily healthy and long-lived people in the Caucasus was being heavily promoted by U.S. corporations that manufactured and sold yogurt, attempting to connect the phenomenal longevity of people in the region to their consumption of yogurt. The Dannon yogurt company marketed a widely seen commercial showing a 110-year-old mother pinching the cheek of her 89-year-old son and telling him to eat his yogurt.
>
> This clever ad and others featuring Soviet centenarians were fabulously successful in the American market. They produced a generation of Americans who associated yogurt with extreme longevity.
>
> ~ John Robbins

Muslimov had passed away by the time of Leaf's studies. But a woman named Khfaf Lasuria had also been featured in the Life article. Leaf wanted to meet her, and he found her in the Abkhasian village of Kutol, where she sang in a choir made up entirely, he was told, of Abkhasian centenarians.

Though he was greatly impressed by this elderly lady's charm and spirit, Leaf did not simply take her word for her age. To the contrary, he went to significant efforts to assess it objectively. After laborious investigations, Leaf concluded that Mrs. Lasuria was close to 130 years old. He wasn't fully certain about that, saying only that he had arrived at a degree of confidence and this was his best estimate. But he was sure of one thing. She was one of the oldest persons he had ever met.

Everywhere he went in Abkhasia, Leaf met elders in remarkable health. The area seemed to warrant its reputation as the mecca of superlongevity.

Like others who have studied the elders of Abkhasia, Leaf had colorful stories to tell. All most all the elders examined by him had a youthful blood pressure of almost 120/85 and a pulse rate of 70. Also he learnt from local doctors that osteoporosis was nonexistent and fractures were rare.

There have been numerous controversies regarding the exact age of these elders but everyone accepts the unusual longevity in the region to be a genuine reality, and that the area is indeed home to an inordinate number of extremely healthy elders.

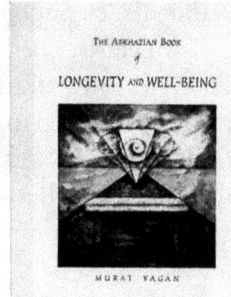

29.

Blue Zones

The Longest Living People On Earth Call These Places Home

The so-called "Fountain of Youth" is one of history's long sought-after mysteries: a legendary bubbling spring that restores a person's youth if he drinks its water. Spanish conqueror Juan Ponce de Leon, who sailed with Columbus on his second voyage to the New World in 1493, is most famous for his search for the fountain.

In his expedition, he would search the coasts of Florida and be the first European to discover the Gulf Coast. Unfortunately, he would die in Havana, Cuba before ever finding the mythical source of everlasting youth.

While most of us don't believe there's an actual fountain that spouts magic, life-giving water, the idea of the Fountain of Youth says a lot about our desire to cheat death and live as long as possible on Earth. Despite all of the hardships and minor annoyances, humans seem to enjoy life, and living a long, productive and healthy one is important and meaningful to many.

> *Your body is a living biological machine. Is it surprising our bodies suffer when we stuff them with inflammatory, chemically destructive diets high in saturated fat and sugar? The literature shows that heart disease and diabetes can often be almost 100% attributed to a lifetime of obesity and poor diet. It has been documented in thousands of trials and scientific studies that the incidence and severity of several major diseases, including cancer and Alzheimer's, can be severely restricted by a healthy diet.*

Some medicines, aptly nicknamed Fountain of Youth drugs, are making big waves in the pharmaceutical industry, as the company GlaxoSmithKline purchased anti-aging drug developer Sirtris for $720 million in June 2008. The multi-million dollar acquisition of Sirtris shows just how much GlaxoSmithKline, a giant in the pharmaceutical industry, believes in the potential of Fountain of Youth drugs.

Although these drugs may not provide immortality, scientists hope to offer longer life spans for people in the near future.

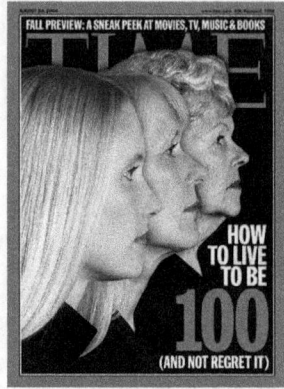

But some are worried about possible side effects that might come with taking a pill that slows the aging process, and others wonder if the drugs will even work at all. One way to combat old age, they argue, is to study blue zones -- places on Earth where people live longer and healthier lives on an average.

Where are these blue zones, and what are their inhabitants doing to gain a better chance of reaching 90, or even well past the age of 100? Is it medicine, genetics or lifestyle that determines blue zone life expectancy? And is it possible to create your own blue zone, a self-made Fountain of Youth?

Blue Zone is a concept used to identify a demographic and/or geographic area of the world where people live measurably longer lives, as described in Dan Buettner's book, "The Blue Zones: Lessons for Living Longer from people who lived the longest." The concept grew out of demographic work done by Gianni Pes and Michel

---

Especially in America, when we see those rare individuals that actually make it to 90 years old, they are often frail and weak, hunched over in wheelchairs and propped up with countless medications. Not so with the individuals in blue zones. Buettner shows us a man in his 90's who actually bests him in an arm wrestling match, and this is not just a special case. The individuals who are reaching 90 or even 100 years old in the blue zones are often able to live active, normal, medication free, mostly healthy lives all the way to the very end.

Poulain, who identified Sardinia's Nuoro province as the region with the highest concentration of male centenarians. As the two men zeroed in on the cluster of villages with the highest longevity, they drew concentric blue circles on the map and began referring to the area inside the circle as the Blue Zone.

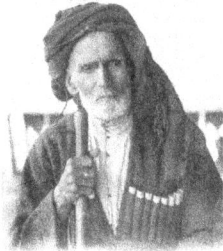

Dan Buettner identifies longevity hotspots in Okinawa, Japan; Sardinia, Italy; Nicoya, Costa Rica; Icaria, Greece; and among the Seventh Day Adventists in Loma Linda, California. He offers an explanation, based on empirical data and first hand observations, as to why these populations live healthier and longer lives.

The five regions identified and discussed by Buettner in the book Blue Zones:

Sardinia, Italy (specifically Nuoro province): One team of demographers found a hot spot of longevity in mountain villages where men reach the age of 100 years at an amazing rate.

The islands of Okinawa, Japan: Another team examined a group that is among the longest lived on Earth.

Buettner has found that those who live long and healthy in the blue zones unanimously live low stress, happy lives enriched with strong family ties, a sense of purpose, and a healthy dose of spirituality, and plenty of sleep. If we are generally happy with our place in life then we behave in ways that promote longevity and health. We are more likely to take good care of our bodies and our bodies are more often flooded with hormones and chemicals associated with happiness and health.

Stress is especially proven through mountains of data and studies to have serious harmful effects on the body. Cortisol, the hormone in our bodies produced in response to stress, is especially harmful to the body.

Those that are living a life constantly full of stress, anger, and resentment have high levels of cortisol constantly flowing in their bodies. The long term effects of this are dramatic, increasing blood pressure, and generally increasing the onset and severity of heart disease and several other major diseases.

Loma Linda, California: Researchers studied a group of Seventh-day Adventists who rank among America's longevity all-stars.

Nicoya Peninsula, Costa Rica: The Nicoya Peninsula was the subject of research on a Quest Network expedition which began on January 29, 2007.

Icaria, Greece: The April '09 expedition to the island of Ikaria uncovered the location with the highest percentage of 90 year-olds on the planet - nearly 1 out of 3 people make it to their 90s. Furthermore, Ikarians have about 80 percent lower rates of cancer, 50 percent lower rates of heart disease and almost no dementia.

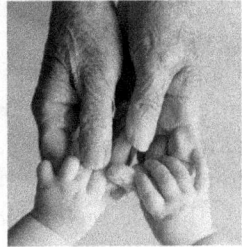

Residents of the first three places produce a high rate of centenarians, suffer a fraction of the diseases that commonly kill people in other parts of the developed world, and enjoy more healthy years of life.

Venn Diagram of Longevity

Venn Diagram of longevity clues from Okinawa, Sardinia, and Loma Linda. The Venn diagram at the right highlights the following shared characteristics among the Okinawa, Sardinia, and Loma Linda Blue Zones. These are some of the common lifestyle characteristics that contribute to their longevity.

Plant-based diet – The majority of food consumed is derived from plants. Fresh organic fruits and vegetables are consumed in large quantities in all these places.

Stress free life - People in these zones lead a slow paced and relaxed life style.

Run with the right crowd. "To make yourself healthier, the best thing you can do is to think about the kinds of people you spend time with. If you're involved with the right kind of people with the right kind of mindset, you get more dependable yourself—you have a reason to get up in the morning, so you're not out drinking late at night. One of the secrets of longevity is to join social groups and choose hobbies or jobs that lead you naturally to healthier patterns and activities. That's a gradual but effective way to change yourself."

Religion - People in these places attend faith based services on a regular basis. They seem to have a spiritual outlook on life.

Dairy - Except in Okinawa, milk, butter and cheese are always present in their diets. Unhealthy fats are conspicuous by their absence.

Family – Family is put ahead of other concerns.

No smoking – Smoking is not found in large quantities.

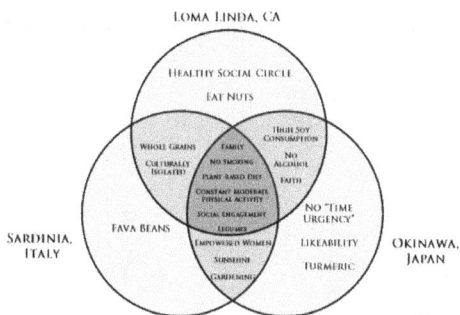

Constant moderate physical activity – Moderate physical activity is an inseparable part of life.

Social engagement – People of all ages are socially active and integrated into their communities.

Legumes – Legumes and nuts are commonly consumed.

Gardening - Except in Loma Linda, they all have some connection with gardening and cultivation.

> *"The secret of good health is to move," says 88-year-old Hoei Tabaru, who keeps in shape picking vegetables in his garden and by biking through his village on the island of Okinawa. Tabaru, who has never driven a car, hopes modern technology will not transform island life. "The world is too easy today," he says, "at least for an old man like me."*

30.

Ikaria, Greece

The Enchanted Island Of Centenarians.

Ikaria, an island of 99 square miles and home to almost 10,000 Greek nationals, lies about 30 miles off the western coast of Turkey. Its jagged ridge of scrub-covered mountains rises steeply out of the Aegean Sea. People here are three times more likely to reach age of 90 than anywhere else in the World.

Amid the lush green forests and beautiful waters, you find people who practically live longer than anywhere else on Earth.

Ikaria was the subject of repeated invasions by the Persians, Romans and Turks, causing the population to move away from the sea to the central area of the island. This created an isolated population, rich in tradition, family values, health and long life. Ikaria is also famous for its mineral thermal hot springs, which reportedly have numerous therapeutic benefits.

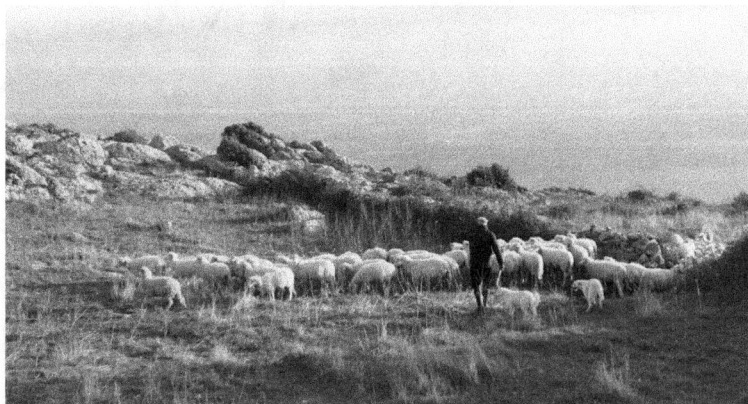

This island is mostly insulated from the mechanized conveniences and the fast-food culture of modern society. This has helped them to preserve age-old customs and lifestyle habits that scientists believe explain their exceptional lifespan.

Chronic diseases are a rarity in Ikaria. The biggest drain on our health care system are diseases like cardiovascular disease, cancer, and diabetes. The people here in Ikaria are eluding those diseases at incredibly high numbers.

Hidden somewhere on this remote, mountainous Greek island, may be the answer to one of life's most enduring questions: How can we live longer, healthier lives?

Ikaria seems to laugh in the face of modern life- the greedy rush through time, the loss of identity through globalization and homogenous life styles, consumerism, materialism and an official, or unofficial police state that observes and dictates the rules of living where there is meant to be freedom.

In the village of Raches, the police station that had been built has remained unused for the last seven years after the villagers got together and agreed that they didn't want or need cops to run their lives - they could do it perfectly well themselves. Yet the island remains one of the safest places to live, and local as well as foreign female residents emphasize that not only do they feel safe but that they feel free to live as they like.

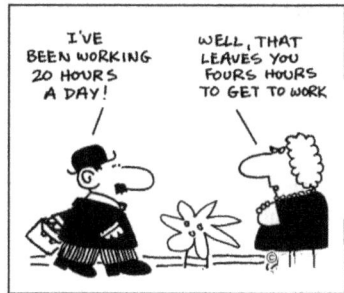

I'VE BEEN WORKING 20 HOURS A DAY!

WELL, THAT LEAVES YOU FOURS HOURS TO GET TO WORK

Ikarians are an impressively self-sufficient people, mainly shepards who own goats in the thousands. They farm their own land - with most households tending their own supply of organic

In the United States, when it comes to improving health, people tend to focus on exercise and what we put into our mouths — organic foods, omega-3's, micronutrients. They spend nearly $30 billion a year on vitamins and supplements alone. Yet in Ikaria and the other places like it, diet only partly explained higher life expectancy. Exercise — at least the way we think of it, as willful, dutiful, physical activity — played a small role at best. ~Dan Buettner

fruit, vegetables and herbs. Some others are shop or taverna owners. Youths start learning to tend the land and herd goats, as well as other traditional labour, as early as their adolescent years.

Towns here exist beyond the normal confines of time. In all Ikaria, the people live exclusively at their own pace; if a shop owner feels like opening his store at 18:00, so be it. After all, the mentality goes, it's their life, and their store, and there is no need to live life throttled by some artificial social compulsion.

These inhabitants live on average 10 years longer than the rest of Western Europe. Six out of 10 of people aged over 90 are still physically active. Experts says only about 20 percent of how long we live is dictated by genes; the rest is lifestyle.

Diet

Most food is cooked in extra-virgin olive oil. Large quantities of wild greens and herbs are gathered from the hillsides for both food and medicinal purposes.

Many older people make a daily brew of mountain tea from dried herbs such as sage, thyme, mint, and chamomile, and sweeten it with honey from local bees. It's supposed to cure everything. These

---

Seeking to learn more about the island's reputation for long-lived residents, I called on Dr. Ilias Leriadis, one of Ikaria's few physicians, in 2009. On an outdoor patio at his weekend house, he set a table with Kalamata olives, hummus and heavy Ikarian bread. "People stay up late here," Leriadis said. "And always take naps. I don't even open my office until 11 a.m. because no one comes before then." He took a sip of his wine. "Have you noticed that no one wears a watch here? No clock is working correctly. When you invite someone to lunch, they might come at 10 a.m. or 6 p.m. We simply don't care about the clock here."

Pointing across the Aegean toward the neighboring island of Samos, he said: "Just 15 kilometers over there is a completely different world. There they are much more developed. There are high-rises and resorts and homes worth a million euros. In Samos, they care about money. Here, we don't. For the many religious and cultural holidays, people pool their money and buy food. If there is money left over, they give it to the poor. It's not a 'me' place. It's an 'us' place."

~Dan Buettner

are rich in antioxidants and also contain diuretics which can lower blood pressure.

Probably it's this regular, ritualistic consumption of these herbal teas that explains low rates of heart disease and also low rates of dementia. Many of the teas are traditional Greek remedies.

Rates of smoking are relatively low. Goat's milk is available in plenty and its drunk warm from the goat's udder. It's rich in tryptophan, which lowers stress hormones and is a natural anti-depressant.

The Mediterranean Diet at its core is whole grains, vegetables, fruits, and olive oil. People who most strongly adhere to the Mediterranean Diet have 6 extra years of life expectancy than people who don't.

On a trip the year before, I visited a slate-roofed house built into the slope at the top of a hill. I had come here after hearing of a couple who had been married for more than 75 years. Thanasis and Eirini Karimalis both came to the door, clapped their hands at the thrill of having a visitor and waved me in. They each stood maybe five feet tall. He wore a shapeless cotton shirt and a battered baseball cap, and she wore a housedress with her hair in a bun. Inside, there was a table, a medieval-looking fireplace heating a blackened pot, a nook of a closet that held one woolen suit coat, and fading black-and-white photographs of forebears on a soot-stained wall. The place was warm and cozy. "Sit down," Eirini commanded. She hadn't even asked my name or business but was already setting out teacups and a plate of cookies.

The couple were born in a nearby village, they told me. They married in their early 20s and raised five children on Thanasis's pay as a lumberjack. Like that of almost all of Ikaria's traditional folk, their daily routine unfolded much the way Leriadis had described it: Wake naturally, work in the garden, have a late lunch, take a nap.

At sunset, they either visited neighbors or neighbors visited them. Their diet was also typical: a breakfast of goat's milk, sage tea or coffee, honey and bread. Lunch was almost always beans (lentils, garbanzos), potatoes, greens (fennel, dandelion or a spinachlike green called horta) and whatever seasonal vegetables their garden produced; dinner was bread and goat's milk. ~Dan Buettner

Included in that diet are lots of healthy greens. Over 150 varieties of wild greens grow on this island. Most Ikarians can walk out their front door to harvest a healthy feast.

There is very little consumption of white sugar, white flour, or meat. They consumed about six times as many beans a day as Americans. Food is mostly unprocessed and free from chemical fertilizers and pesticides.

Honey is treated as a panacea. They have types of honey here that you won't see anyplace else in the world. They use it for everything from treating wounds to curing hangovers, or for treating influenza.

During our time on Ikaria, my colleagues and I stayed at Thea Parikos's guesthouse, the social hub of western Ikaria. Local women gathered in the dining room at midmorning to gossip over tea. Late at night, after the dinner rush, tables were pushed aside and the dining room became a dance floor, with people locking arms and kick-dancing to Greek music.

Parikos cooked the way her ancestors had for centuries, giving us a chance to consume the diet we were studying. For breakfast, she served local yogurt and honey from the 90-year-old beekeeper next door. For dinner, she walked out into the fields and returned with handfuls of weedlike greens, combined them with pumpkin and baked them into savory pies. My favorite was a dish made with black-eyed peas, tomatoes, fennel tops and garlic and finished with olive oil that we dubbed Ikarian stew.

Despite her consummately Ikarian air, Parikos was actually born in Detroit to an American father and an Ikarian mother. She had attended high school, worked as a real estate agent and married in the United States. After she and her husband had their first child, she felt a "genetic craving" for Ikaria. "I was not unhappy in America," she said. "We had good friends, we went out to dinner on the weekends, I drove a Chevrolet. But I was always in a hurry."

When she and her family moved to Ikaria and opened the guesthouse, everything changed. She stopped shopping for most groceries, instead planting a huge garden that provided most of their fruits and vegetables. She lost weight without trying to. I asked her if she thought her simple diet was going to make her family live longer. "Yes," she said. "But we don't think about it that way. It's bigger than that." ~Dan Buettner

Old people here will start their day with a spoonful of honey. They take it like medicine.

In an interview, a 93 years old woman attributed her longevity to avoiding red meat and surrounding herself with friends.

Plenty of Rest

Wake up naturally, work in the garden, have a late lunch, take a nap. One cherished custom of Ikarians is the mid-day siesta or afternoon nap. You walk in one of these villages in mid-afternoon and it's like a ghost town. People are taking their naps and it's said that taking a 30-minute nap at least five times per week decreases the chance of heart attack by one-third. It also reduces stress and makes you look and feel younger.

People here have a low sense of time urgency. Take your time - is a popular slogan here.

When you ask people what time it is they say "late thirty." When you invite somebody to come to lunch you don't say come at noon you say come on Thursday and they may come any time between ten in the morning and six in the evening.

There is very little stress of any kind. People don't wear watches in Ikaria. Showing up late is socially accepted. This attitude reduces stress and wrinkles. They seem to prefer owning rather than being owned by time.

Although unemployment is high — perhaps as high as 40 percent — most everyone has access to a family garden and livestock, Parikos told me. People who work might have several jobs. Someone involved in tourism, for example, might also be a painter or an electrician or have a store. "People are fine here because we are very self-sufficient," she said. "We may not have money for luxuries, but we will have food on the table and still have fun with family and friends.

~Dan Buettner

Strong Sense Of Community

Ikaríans have preserved a traditional lifestyle that maintains the importance of family and strong social connections. Strong social connections have been shown to lower depression, body weight and chances of death.

Elders here stay busy and involved. Social structure and a cultural attitude that celebrates the elderly keeps them engaged in the community and in extended-family homes. Extended families give older people an important role in society. Levels of depression and dementia are low.

Children might see a grandparent every day, an arrangement that improves the health and well-being of both the younger and older generations.

Their relaxed sense of time, festive spirit (dance and song) and physical work in the great outdoors seem to make a huge difference to lifespan as well as their quality of life.

Studies have linked isolation and loneliness among some workers in industrialized economies to reduced life expectancy.

Natural Exercise

Due to the natural rugged terrain, Ikarians get their daily exercise without thinking about it. These islanders herd their own goats every day. It's a five-hour process that includes bringing the animals down from the mountain, feeding them and milking them. The milk is then filtered and prepared into local cheeses.

(Some edited excerpts from NBC News on Dan Buettner's research with National Geographic Society have been included here.)

"Do you know there's no word in Greek for privacy?" she declared. "When everyone knows everyone else's business, you get a feeling of connection and security. The lack of privacy is actually good, because it puts a check on people who don't want to be caught or who do something to embarrass their family. If your kids misbehave, your neighbor has no problem disciplining them. There is less crime, not because of good policing, but because of the risk of shaming the family. You asked me about food, and yes, we do eat better here than in America. But it's more about how we eat. Food here is always enjoyed in combination with conversation." ~Dan Buettner

31.

The Island Where People 'Forget to Die'

The New York Times, Dan Buettner

In 1943, a Greek war veteran named Stamatis Moraitis came to the United States for treatment of a combat-mangled arm. He'd survived a gunshot wound, escaped to Turkey and eventually talked his way onto the Queen Elizabeth, then serving as a troopship, to cross the Atlantic. Moraitis settled in Port Jefferson, N.Y., an enclave of countrymen from his native island, Ikaria. He quickly landed a job doing manual labor. Later, he moved to Boynton Beach, Fla.

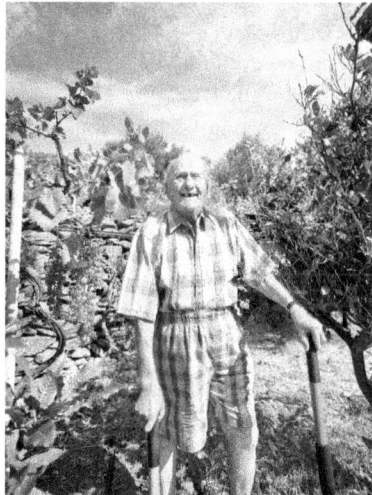

Along the way, Moraitis married a Greek-American woman, had three children and bought a three-bedroom house and a 1951 Chevrolet.

One day in 1976, Moraitis felt short of breath. Climbing stairs was a chore; he had to quit working midday. After X-rays, his doctor concluded that Moraitis had lung cancer. As he recalls, nine other doctors confirmed the diagnosis. They gave him nine months to live. He was in his mid-60s.

Moraitis considered staying in America and seeking aggressive cancer treatment at a local hospital. That way, he could also be close to his adult children. But he decided instead to return to Ikaria, where he could be buried with his ancestors in a cemetery shaded by oak trees that overlooked the Aegean Sea. He figured a funeral in the United States would cost thousands, a traditional Ikarian one only $200, leaving more of his retirement savings for his wife, Elpiniki.

Moraitis and Elpiniki moved in with his elderly parents, into a tiny, whitewashed house on two acres of stepped vineyards near Evdilos, on the north side of Ikaria.

At first, he spent his days in bed, as his mother and wife tended to him. He reconnected with his faith. On Sunday mornings, he

---

That's what the $70 billion diet industry and $20 billion health-club industry do in their efforts to persuade us that if we eat the right food or do the right workout, we'll be healthier, lose weight and live longer. But these strategies rarely work.

Not because they're wrong-minded: it's a good idea for people to do any of these healthful activities. The problem is, it's difficult to change individual behaviors when community behaviors stay the same. In the United States, you can't go to a movie, walk through the airport or buy cough medicine without being routed through a gantlet of candy bars, salty snacks and sugar-sweetened beverages. The processed-food industry spends more than $4 billion a year tempting us to eat. How do you combat that? Discipline is a good thing, but discipline is a muscle that fatigues. Sooner or later, most people cave in to relentless temptation.

As our access to calories has increased, we've decreased the amount of physical activity in our lives. In 1970, about 40 percent of all children in the U.S. walked to school; now fewer than 12 percent do. Our grandparents, without exercising, burned up about five times as many calories a day in physical activity as we do. At the same time, access to the processed food has exploded.

Despite the island's relative isolation, its tortuous roads and the fierce independence of its inhabitants, the American food culture, among other forces, is beginning to take root in Ikaria. Village markets are now selling potato chips and soda, which in my experience is replacing tea as the drink of choice among younger Ikarians.

As the island's ancient traditions give way before globalization, the gap between Ikarian life spans and those of the rest of the world seems to be gradually disappearing, as the next generations of old people become less likely to live quite so long. ~Dan Buettner

hobbled up the hill to a tiny Greek Orthodox chapel where his grandfather once served as a priest.

When his childhood friends discovered that he had moved back, they started showing up every afternoon. They'd talk for hours, an activity that invariably involved a bottle or two of locally produced wine. I might as well die happy, he thought.

In the ensuing months, something strange happened. He says he started to feel stronger. One day, feeling ambitious, he planted some vegetables in the garden. He didn't expect to live to harvest them, but he enjoyed being in the sunshine, breathing the ocean air. Elpiniki, his wife could enjoy the fresh vegetables after he was gone.

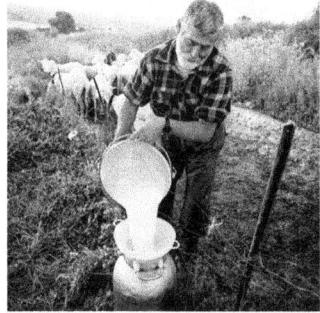

Six months came and went. Moraitis didn't die. Instead, he reaped his garden and, feeling emboldened, cleaned up the family vineyard as well. Easing himself into the island routine, he woke up when he felt like it, worked in the vineyards until midafternoon, made himself lunch and then took a long nap.

In the evenings, he often walked to the local tavern, where he played dominoes past midnight. The years passed. His health continued to improve. He added a couple of rooms to his parents' home so his children could visit. Today, three and a half decades later, he's 97 years old — according to an official document he disputes; he says he's 102 — and cancer-free. He never went through

The big aha for me, having studied populations of the long-lived for nearly a decade, is how the factors that encourage longevity reinforce one another over the long term. For people to adopt a healthful lifestyle, I have become convinced, they need to live in an ecosystem, so to speak, that makes it possible. As soon as you take culture, belonging, purpose or religion out of the picture, the foundation for long healthy lives collapses. The power of such an environment lies in the mutually reinforcing relationships among lots of small nudges and default choices.

~Dan Buettner

chemotherapy, took drugs or sought therapy of any sort. All he did was move home to Ikaria.

I met Moraitis on Ikaria this past July during one of my visits to explore the extraordinary longevity of the island's residents. For a decade, with support from the National Geographic Society, I've been organizing a study of the places where people live longest.

I called Moraitis a few weeks ago from my home in Minneapolis. Elpiniki died in the spring at age 85, and now he lives alone. He picked up the phone in the same whitewashed house that he'd moved into 35 years ago.

It was late afternoon in Ikaria. He had worked in his vineyard that morning and just awakened from a nap. We chatted for a few minutes, but then he warned me that some of his neighbors were coming over in a few minutes and he'd have to go. I had one last question for him. How does he think he recovered from lung cancer?

"It just went away," he said. "I actually went back to America about 25 years after moving here to see if the doctors could explain it to me."

I had heard this part of the story before. It had become a piece of the folklore of Ikaria, proof of its exceptional way of life. Still, I asked him, "What happened?"

"My doctors were all dead."

32.

Okinawa

The Land of 'Immortals'

Okinawa is the southernmost prefecture in all of Japan. It is the main island of a tropical chain of 160 coral islets called Ryukyu, has a volcanic soil, whipped by typhoons and torrential rains.

This island has a rich history. It is located in the center of the East China Sea relatively close to Japan, China and South-East Asia. Okinawa witnessed the largest amphibious assault in the Pacific War of World War II. A quarter of the civilian population died during the famous Battle of Okinawa.

After the end of World War II in 1945, Okinawa came under United States administration for 27 years. During the trusteeship

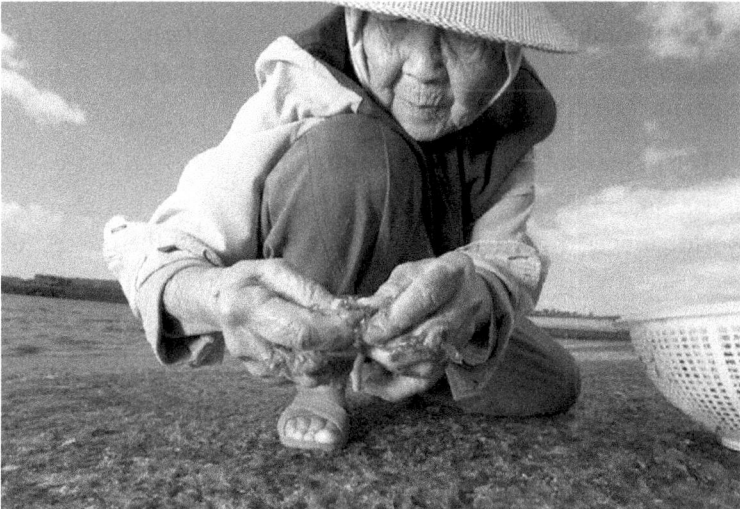

rule the United States Air Force established numerous military bases on the Ryukyu islands.

In 1972, the U.S. government returned the islands to Japanese administration. But under the Treaty of Mutual Cooperation and Security, the United States Forces Japan (USFJ) have maintained a large military presence.

Apart from the battle, Okinawa is known for the long life expectancy of its residents.

When the Japan Ministry of Health, Labor and Welfare conducted the Okinawa Centenarian Study in 1976, it was to investigate anecdotal reports of the long life expectancy of Okinawans.

What it found were low rates of cardiovascular disease and hormone-dependent cancers, low rates of dementia, strong bones and many other signs of vitality amongst the elderly in Okinawa.

The people of Okinawa live longer and are healthier than anyone else in the world. There are more than 900 centenarians living here and diseases like cancer, diabetes and hypertension are rare. Healthy seniors work actively in farming and community projects, seemingly immune to the effects of old age. The report mentioned an absence of stress and avoiding cigarettes and alcohol as being critical factors. This is besides their centuries old healthy dietary pattern.

"The calendar may say they're 70 but their body says they're 50," says Bradley Willcox, a scientist researching the extraordinary phenomenon. "The most impressive part of it is that a good lot of them are healthy until the very end."

The Okinawa Centenarian Study (OCS)

It's not only the world's longest life expectancy but also the world's longest health expectancy that has piqued the interest of the researchers.

Abstinence is the key for longevity: no liqueur, no smoking, no heavy fatty food. Plus to feel less stress;in this regard, the spiritual connection with God tremendously helps. I am already 77 but still going very well with original teeth.

~Sam Khan, Stratford, USA

The Okinawa Centenarian Study (OCS) is an ongoing population-based study of centenarians and other selected elderly that began in 1975.

The goal of the Okinawa Centenarian Study is to uncover the genetic and lifestyle factors responsible for this remarkable successful aging phenomenon for the betterment of the health and lives of all people.

Ages are validated through the koseki, the Japanese family registration system. At the baseline exam a full geriatric assessment is performed, including physical exam and activities of daily living.

Since the onset of the OCS, limited information on the demographics of the entire centenarian population of Okinawa has been collected and full assessments of a sub-sample of 900-plus centenarians have been performed.

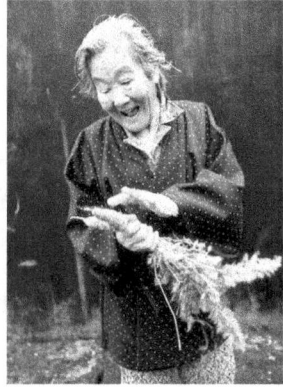

When Dr. Suzuki, the Principal Investigator of the OCS, first began his studies, he found an unusual number of centenarians to be in extraordinarily healthy shape. They were lean, youthful-looking, and energetic.

Diet

Explanations for this mostly centre around the dinner table. The Okinawans not only eat more tofu and soya products than any

Thousands of people saw it: 7 years ago Seikichi Uehara, 96, defeated an ex box champ in his 30's. Or the case of Nabi Kinjo, 105, that killed with a flyswatter a poisonous snake. Here you see 100 years old persons that do not even think about retirement.

Why are we cranking up people out of medical school to go and do cosmetic surgery for God's sake? This whole obsession with staying and looking young is not accepting basically, that we are biological creatures, we're ageing as a part of our lives.

If we took a leaf out of the Okinawans' book, we could grow old gracefully, without ever needing to go under the knife.

~Dr Suzuki

other population in the world, their diet also includes a vast range of different vegetables and fruit all rich in anti-oxidants. Scientists refer to it as a rainbow diet.

But it's what they don't eat that may be at the heart of their exceptionally long lives.

The Okinawan's most significant cultural tradition is known as hara hachi bu, which translated means eat until you're only 80% full.

In a typical day they only consume around 1,200 calories, about 20% less than most people in the US or UK. Culturally it is a million miles from attitudes in a lot of Western societies, where all-you-can-eat meal deals are offered in restaurants on most high streets. Scientists call it caloric restriction, but don't entirely understand how it works.

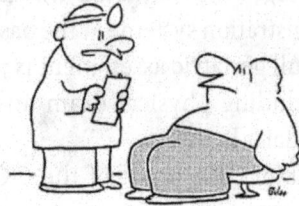

"LET'S EASE INTO THIS--I WANT YOU TO TRY FASTING BETWEEN MEALS."

Meat consumption is very rare and carbs are unprocessed and as natural as possible, like brown rice and whole wheat. Basically, it can be called a 'quasi-vegan' diet. While centenarian Okinawans do eat some pork, it is traditionally reserved only for infrequent ceremonial occasions and taken only in small amounts.

A weight-loss diet (which bears the name of Okinawa) has also been made based on this standard diet of the Islanders.

Generally, the traditional diet of the islanders contains 30% of the green/yellow vegetables. Although the traditional Japanese diet includes large quantities of rice, in Okinawa, rice is consumed in smaller amounts and the staple is instead the sweet potato.

Wilcox compared age-adjusted mortality of Okinawans versus Americans and found that, during 1995, an average Okinawan was

In the last century, 100,000 Okinawans migrated to Brazil, where they adopted the Brazilian diet, rich in meat. The result was that their average lifespan lowered by 17 years. When the Okinawan youth started to go to American Fast-Foods and Pizza Bars, which surround the American bases, the obesity levels, cardiovascular diseases and premature deaths in the young reached record levels.

8 times less likely to die from coronary heart disease, 7 times less likely to die from prostate cancer, 6.5 times less likely to die from breast cancer, and 2.5 times less likely to die from colon cancer than an average American of the same age.

The traditional Okinawa diet as described above has been practiced on the islands until about the 1960s. Since then, dietary practices have been shifting towards Western and Japanese patterns, with fat intake rising from about 10% to 27% of total caloric intake and the sweet potato being supplanted with rice and bread.

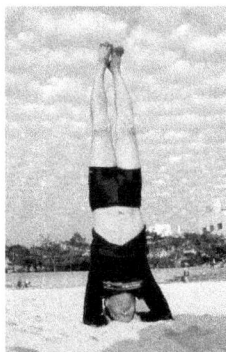

Genetics

Studies show that the genetics of the Okinawans help them in preventing inflammatory and autoimmune diseases. Siblings of long-lived Okinawans also tend to live long, healthy lives. However, when Okinawans move to new environments (causing changes in lifestyle habits), they lose their longevity. This indicates that other important factors are at play besides genetics.

Okinawa did not escape the trading trends: in the center of the island, there is now a big store with a big hanging poster "Okinawa, the world capital of the longevity" which offers the ingredients of the longevity: brown sugar "made of Okinawa cane", kombu, tofu and other products, supposed to prolong your life

Most of the over-85-years-old elderly I've ever met seem to be waiting to die, sick of dealing with their physical pains and of struggling to survive on small pensions, but not the Okinawans. They have a child-like zeal towards life, wanting to live more. Even a 100-year-old woman says she would like to live a few more years to spend with her grandchildren. As the old Okinawan saying goes, "At 70 you are still a child, at 80 a young man or woman.

Simply put, if Americans lived more like the Okinawans, we would have to close down 80 percent of the coronary care units and one-third of the cancer wards in the United States, and a lot of nursing homes would be out of business.

~From The Okinawa Program

Heart Health

The study participants have clean, healthy arteries, low cholesterol and low homocysteine levels. Researchers believe these low, healthy levels may decrease the risk of heart disease in Okinawans by as much as 80 percent. The reasons for these low levels are thought to be a good diet, high levels of physical activity, low alcohol use, not smoking, and positive attitude that reduces stress.

Low Cancer Risk

The Okinawans also have less risk for hormone-dependent cancers (breast, prostate, ovarian and colon cancers). Specifically, they have 80 percent less risk of breast and prostate cancer and 50 percent less risk of ovarian and colon cancers. Researchers attribute this risk reduction to eating fewer calories, consuming lots of fruits and vegetables, having good fats in the diet, eating plenty of fiber and staying physically active.

Bone Health

No surprise that Okinawans also have less risk of hip fractures than Americans. The bone density for the centenarians decreases at a slower rate than other Japanese people. This may be due to

---

Older Okinawans possess a strong sense of purpose, a concept contained in the word ikigai, which translates roughly to "that which makes one's life worth living." Here, 84-year-old Fumiyasu Yamakawa practices his ikigai—daily exercises, including yoga, to train for an annual decathlon. Some centenarians find that a moai—a group of lifelong friends—provides a sense of purpose. These secure social networks serve as financial safety nets and provide emotional support in times of need.

The ritual of daily offerings to ancestors is a cornerstone of religious life on Okinawa. Families worship their ancestors at the family tomb on the Okinawan island of Taketomi. Once a year, families on Taketomi gather to worship their ancestors with a feast for the living as well as the dead.

An 88-year-old farmer who still works 11-hour days at the field, says, "I hardly ever get angry. I'm happy at work and I think that's the medicine for a long life."

---

a higher calcium intake in the Okinawan diet, more exposure to vitamin D in sunlight and higher levels of physical activity.

Positive Outlook

When the personalities of Okinawans was tested, it was found that they were generally unstressed and maintained a positive outlook on life. They had strong coping skills and a deep sense of spirituality, meaning and purpose. Positive outlook in the Okinawans is thought to explain their reduced risk for dementia.

Unfortunately, the secrets accumulated by the elderly aren't being imbibed with much enthusiasm by the present generation Okinawans. As in many other countries, Western fast food joints have invaded the island, which the youth prefer over traditional foods.

One youngster chomping down on a burger says: "I like thick, greasy food." "Goya is bitter," says another, "so I don't like it much." The degradation of the healthy eating habits has taken its toll on the island, considerably reducing life expectancy. The rates of obesity and lung cancer in the new generation are higher in Okinawa than compared to anywhere else in Japan.

It appears that when the western world is awakening to the benefits of living life like the Okinawans, their very own youth are leaving it behind. It's sad really, but the truth is the healthy people of Okinawa are nothing but living relics whose secrets of a truly healthy life will be lost in just a few years time.

> *Okinawa is one of the world's best kept secrets. The culture is complex, yet simple, comfortable and classy. Healthy food there is plentiful, readily available and delicious. Okinawan's are humble, shy, and interesting. I never found a single dark street or alley that I could not walk safely at night. No guns, overall. Low violent crime. Okinawans socialize well. The extensive variety of fresh fruits, seafood and vegetables dishes lack boredom. Politeness and service are no better anywhere in the world. Whether you are low, middle or high income hardly matters when it comes to customer service. Okinawans are awesome. I found living there to be extremely enjoyable. Okinawa is a true paradise. The scenery is gorgeous, overall. Okinawa is the land of peace, uniqueness, creativity and vibrance. ~ Tom, New York.*

33.

Vilcabamba

The Valley of Longevity.

Vilcabamba is a village in the southern region of Ecuador, in the Loja province, about 45 km from the city of Loja. The area has been referred to as the "Playground of the Inca" which refers to its historic use as a retreat for Incan royalty. The valley is overlooked by a mountain called Mandango whose presence is said to protect the area from earthquakes and other natural disasters.

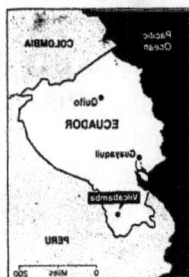

Located in a historical and scenic valley, it is a common destination for tourists, in part because it is widely believed that its inhabitants grow to a very old age. Locals assert that it is not uncommon to see a person reach 100 years of age and it is claimed that many have gotten to 120, even up to 135. It is often called the Valley of Longevity. As proof, there is one person over 100 years old for every 2.7 million Americans; In Vilcabamba, it is one in 68.

> *Jose Maria Roa was 132 years old when we met, married for the third time to a woman who was then 66, and who had given birth to Roa's youngest son 24 years earlier. The Ecuadorian government verified these facts and the Spanish interpreters supplied to us by the Ministry of Health, presented Roa's birth certificate that indicated he was born in 1850. Also, his name is carved into the foundation stone of the church sitting in the center of Vilcabamba; Roa helped erect that church in 1866.*
> ~ Dr. Morton Walker

In 1973, Dr. Alexander Leaf of Harvard Medical School introduced these remarkable people to the world for the first time in his cover story for National Geographic Magazine. In 1981, the Ecuadorian government hired medical journalist Dr. Morton Walker to study these people in depth. Medical researchers have confirmed that the retinas of 100 year-old residents are often comparable with those of 45 year-old city-dwellers.

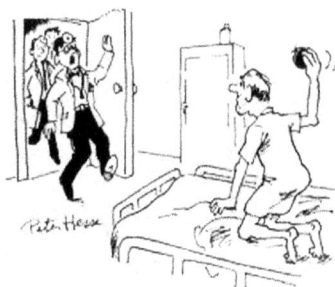

"HOLD ON GUYS, HE'S GOT AN APPLE!"

Several books published in the mid-1970s further enhanced the town's reputation. In 1975, Dr. David Davies, an English gerontologist, published The Centenarians of the Andes which contains his research in Vilcabamba. In 1976 the popular author Grace Halsell published Los Viejos: Secrets of Long Life from the Sacred Valley, about her experience living in Vilcabamba for a year.

Halsell's picturesque account of life in Vilcabamba emphasized the simple virtues of the villager's way of life. She wrote, "I lived in a dirt-floor mountain hut with Gabriel Erazo, who matter-of-factly says, 'I am 132.' Halsell described how Erazo stayed healthy by composing poetry in his head while hiking in the mountains. She also wrote of 113-year-old Gabriel Sanchez who "climbed the steep El Chaupi mountain to work all day with his crude hoe or lampa, cultivating a small plot of ground."

It was also in the 1960s that one of the first foreign residents— Johnny Lovewisdom— found his way to the Vilcabama Valley. An eccentric spiritual seeker, he was looking for his own version of Nirvana, a place with a near-perfect climate where food could be grown unsullied by chemicals or the threat of nuclear fallout that was then top-of-mind in the post-World-War-II world. He brought an eclectic mix of alternative lifestyle pursuits, including some out-of-the-ordinary (at least for back then) dietary and religious beliefs.

This tendency to attract the more interesting and offbeat among us continues to this day. ~Suzan Haskins

Halsell concluded that the secret to long life was to stay active: "The viejos apparently do not suffer from bad arteries or heart attacks. I saw no examples of fractured legs or arms. They stay flexible and hardy by a simple rule: Keep moving, don't stop, now or ever."

Members of this community also appeared in Ripley's Believe It or Not and were featured in National Geographic, Reader's Digest and other popular press outlets. These books and articles about Vilcabamba led to a sharp rise in tourism to the area.

Dietary pattern is similar to other Blue Zone areas. They eat only fresh fruits and vegetables. Although the sacred valley is almost exactly on the equator, it's not hot because Vilcabamba is so high up. There's plenty of rainfall and sun, and plant life grows in abundance. You need but reach out your hand to gather bananas, mango, papaya, grapes, lemons, oranges, apple, pineapple, crab-apples and berries of all kinds. A variety of vegetables grows everywhere without cultivation; there are avocados, zucchini, legumes, potatoes,

High up among the surrounding mountain peaks lies an area of primevial tundra, which is made up of great masses of vegetation .... layer upon layer of these grasses and vegetation of many types and colors. There are also some fourteen lakes, each containing the melt of this uncontaminated glacier ice. Come the rainy season, these lakes overflow and flood the tundra, which then acts as a filter for any undesirable heavy metals or minerals. After seeping through these countless layers of tundra, this purest of waters flows down into thousands of pools, then into hundreds of cascading waterfalls .... and remember this part for a little later, because the countless waterfalls contributes to the extremely high negative ion count in the valley.

Modern science has also demonstrated that the inhabitants of Vilcabamba have something else going for them, besides pristine water. Dr. Richard Laurence Millington Synge, a Nobel Peace Prize winner and the man who discovered amino acids, claims that there are medicinal remarkable qualities to be found in the plant-life in certain places near the Equator .... with the valley of Vilcabamba being one of these areas. Due to scientific chemical assay techniques, analysis has now shown that the fruit, roots and herbs of this particular Equatorial sub-area offer the strongest anti-oxidant protection in the world!

rice, all of the grains, tomatoes, cabbage, eggplant, squash, and much more. Canned foods are never used. Meat is hardly eaten except on feast days. There is no refrigeration. Food is eaten fresh.

This hardy race of indiginous Vilcabambans attribute their long-lived heritage to "being touched by the hand of God." There is no degenerative disease in Vilcabamba – no heart attacks, no cancer, never diabetes, no stroke - they didn't even know the word senility.

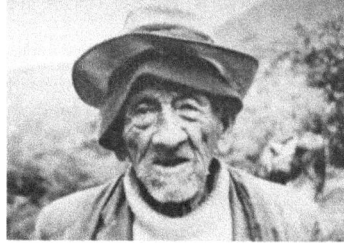

No doubt it's so, thanks to all these ingredients...and to the fact that it was only a short time ago (in the 1960s) that "civilization" came to this part of the world...in the form of a reliably drivable road that connected it with the outside world.

It was even only more recently that the telephone, television, and the Internet forced their versions of stress into this valley. Foreigners and other tourists are increasingly buying property in the region for spa and vacation homes. Tourists have created problems for the locals, including rising prices as well as increasing drug and alcohol use. Some locals say that the peace and simplicity of their lives, to which they attributed their longevity, has been lost.

If your energy is all engaged in manufacturing tires and wheels, then who will go to the... Actually I have seen in your country. Now the farmers' son, they do not like to remain in the farm. They go in the city. I have seen it. The farmers' son, they do not like to take up the profession of his father. So gradually farming will be reduced, and the city residents, they are satisfied if they can eat meat. And the farmer means keeping the, raising the cattle and killing them, send to the city, and they will think that "We are eating. What is the use of going to..." But these rascals have no brain that "If there is no food grain or grass, how these cattle will be...?" Actually it is happening. They are eating swiftly.

-Srila Prabhupada (Room Conversation with Dr. Theodore Kneupper, November 6, 1976, Vrindavana)

34.

Sardinia

An Epicenter Of Longevity

Sardinia is the second largest island in the Mediterranean Sea (after Sicily) and an autonomous region of Italy. It is situated 120 miles off the coast of Italy. The island has a typical Mediterranean climate.

Of 1.6 million Sardinians, there are at least 220 who have reached 100, twice the typical ratio. Five of the world's 40 oldest people live on the island. Sardinia shares with the Japanese island of Okinawa the highest rate of centenarians in the world. In a cluster of 17 white washed villages in island's highland Nuoro Province, you find nearly 10 times the number of centenarians per 1000 people than you do in America.

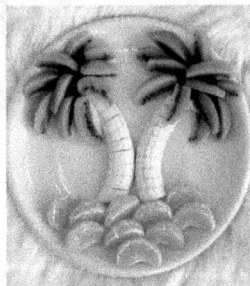

The epicenter of longevity in Sardinia is located around the mountainous region of Barbagia and the Province of Nuoro. This is where Sardinians fled to escape the invading Barbarians in Roman times, isolating themselves from outside influences and creating a pocket of especially resilient and proud people who are some of the healthiest in the world.

Here you will find octogenarians running after sheep up steep hillsides, nonagenarians climbing nut trees and chopping wood, and calendars depicting 'centenarian of the month'. These centenarians walk long distances their entire lives

This region has traditionally been home to shepherds, who pasture their sheep across the rugged, sun-beaten terrain. The steep, rocky terrain is not suited to wide-scale agriculture.

Sardinian women are known to complain that they are the ones who have to do the domestic drudgery and the worrying back at home whilst their men spend the day roaming around in nature and often sleep out under the stars with hardly a care in the world.

A Danish study concluded that longevity here was mainly due to lifestyle choices and environmental factors, with genetics accounting for only about a quarter of the picture.

Historically, Sardinians have made sure to maintain their way of life as a way of protecting themselves from the constant invaders coming in from the sea wanting a slice of this wild and beautiful island. This has meant that they have kept family close and honored family customs such as respecting their elders and looking out for each other.

Sardinian Longevity Foods

Sardinians consume milk and cheese from goats. The goats in this region have a unique quality. They eat dwarf curry, a plant currently used in the U.S. to make anti-inflammatory drugs. The most common variety of goat's cheese is pecorino. Sardinians also consume large quantities of fava beans and barley. This cheese made from grass-fed goats—a traditional part of the Sardinian diet—is high in omega-3 fatty acids. Goat's milk, another staple, contains

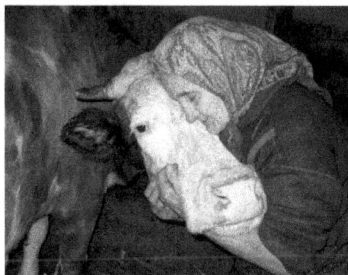

Sir Arbuthnot Lane, one of England's distinguished surgeons, and a student of public welfare, has made this comment: (2)

Long surgical experience has proved to me conclusively that there is something radically and fundamentally wrong with the civilized mode of life, and I believe that unless the present dietetic and health customs of the White Nations are reorganized, social decay and race deterioration are inevitable.

components that might help protect against inflammatory diseases of aging such as heart disease and Alzheimer's disease.

Needless to say, the food eaten by long-lived Sardinians is plant-based, organic, and free from junk food, preservatives, or anything else that comes from outside. The classic Sardinian diet consists of whole-grain bread, beans, garden vegetables, fruits, and, in some parts of the island, mastic oil. Meat is largely reserved for special occasions. Consumption of locally made Cannonau wine is moderate. Islanders traditionally eat sugary foods sparingly, with desserts and pastries reserved for saints' days and festivals. Herbs and infusions are part of the daily fare.

People regularly attend church. Family is revered and grandparents provide love, child care, financial help, wisdom, and motivation to perpetuate traditions and push children to succeed in their lives. In turn, elders feel a sense of belonging in their families and communities. They live at home, where they're likely to receive better care and remain more engaged than they would in a nursing home or assisted-living facility. These grandparents help raise a healthier and better adjusted generation. They are respected as the living memories of their communities. People with strong family ties have lower rates of depression and stress.

The World's Oldest Family

The Melis family on the island are officially the world's oldest with nine brothers and sisters clocking up a total of 818 years between them.

The oldest sibling, Consolata, who turned 105 recently, has nine children, 24 grand-children and 25 great-grandchildren.

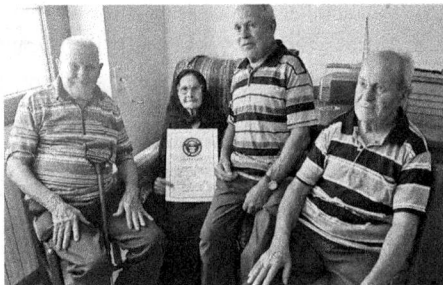

The next oldest are Claudia (99), Maria (97), Antonio (93), Concetta (91), Adolfo (89), Vitalio (86), Vitalia (81), and Mafalda (78).

The longevity of the Melis had been recognised as a Guinness World Record. The Guinness certification followed a seven-year review around the world.

Claudina attends morning Mass every day. Her doctor has tried to give her medicine, but she has always refused, telling "I only have one illness, old age, and nobody can cure that!"

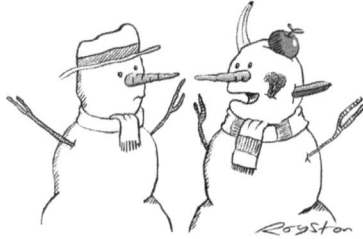

Consolata, who received little schooling and speaks in the Sardinian dialect, says, "In

"I'm making sure I get my five daily portions."

my time women had to wash clothes in the river. My granddaughters have washing machines and dishwashers, when I hear this new word 'stressed,' I just don't understand."

Luca Deiana, a professor of clinical biochemistry at the local university has studied some 2500 centenarians on the island since 1996 says the longevity of local inhabitants was due to various factors.

"On the one hand it is about genetics, about inherited longevity ... but there is also the bounty of the land and the local fruit, particularly pears and prunes. Minestrone soup is another suspect."

Alfonso, 89 says, "Every free moment I have I am down at my vineyard or at the allotment where I grow beans, aubergines, peppers and potatoes."

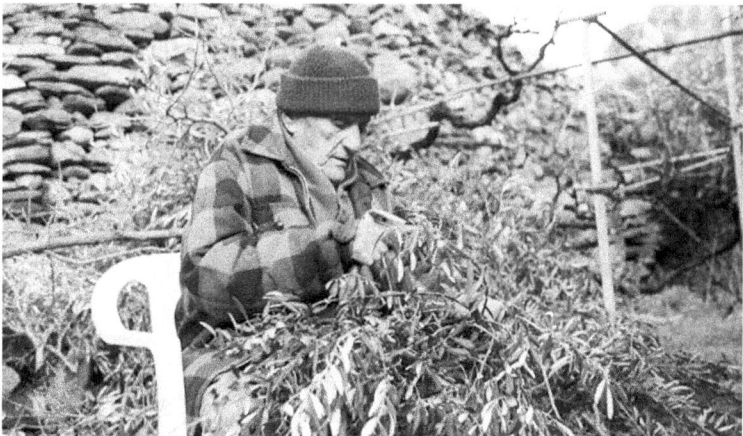

35.

Loma Linda, California

Highest Longevity In USA

Loma Linda (Spanish for Beautiful Hill) is a city in San Bernardino County, California, United States. The population was 23,000 at the 2010 census. The city is located about 60 miles east of Los Angeles.

Loma Linda was featured by National Geographic Magazine as one of the five places in the world with the highest longevity. Dan Buettner considers this community to be a Blue Zone. Residents of this small community routinely live to 100. Majority of the residents are Seventh Day Adventists.

The National Institute of Health funded a study of 34,000 California Adventists from 1976 to 1988 to learn if there is a link between their lifestyle and their life span. The study found that their diet, which includes tomatoes, fruits, soymilk and beans, lowered their likelihood of developing certain cancers. Eating whole wheat bread, drinking plenty of water and eating at least four servings of nuts per week lowered their risk of heart disease. The study also correlated lower cancer rates and the avoidance of red meat.

The Seventh Day Adventist faith prohibits caffeine, alcohol, smoking and unhealthy eating. Most practitioners are vegetarians, and the city requires all food establishments to offer vegetarian choices. Sylvie, a clinical nutritionist is currently leading a fight to

"Being able to define your life meaning adds to your life expectancy."
~ *Dr. Robert Butler, Director, National Institute on Aging*

keep McDonald's out of the community. One restaurant, Demiana Deli offers salads, pasta and other non-meat dishes. "They are prepared like my grandmother used to cook," the owner claims.

Normally, eating healthy is thought to be expensive, but the price of foods are relatively inexpensive in Loma Linda because most of their beans and nuts are locally grown and sold in big bins. That way the buyers don't have to pay a lot of money for marketing and packaging.

A new study shows American woman are not living as long these days as they did a generation ago, but Loma Linda is bucking the trend. A casual visit to a grocery store explains why the residents here live such long and healthy lives. It's full of bins of locally grown beans and nuts and aisles of fresh fruits and vegetables.

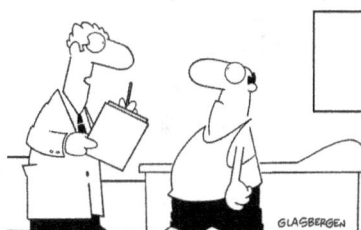

GLASBERGEN

"If you lose weight, you'll have more energy. Why do you think they call it FATigue?"

A light dinner early in the evening is another Adventist practice. It avoids flooding the body with calories during the inactive parts

---

"It does certainly raise the question if there's something about spiritual life that also has an impact on longer life," says Dr Gary Fraser, who is researching the community.

"At this moment we don't really know that but there's been one interesting fact that's been known now for 20 or 30 years and that is that people that go to church regularly - whatever faith they have - live longer and there's no question about that."

It seems that regular churchgoers have significantly lower levels of stress hormones and so may be better equipped to cope with the challenges in life, say scientists.

"Religion and connection to something higher than oneself, connection to the sacred, connection to a tight-knit religious community allows you to modulate your reactions and your emotions to believe there is a broader purpose," says Dr Kerry Morton, who is involved in a longer-term study on Adventist health.

"Therefore your body can stay in balance and not be destroyed by those stressors and traumas over time." -BBC News

of the day and seems to promote better sleep and a lower BMI (body mass index).

Seventh Day Adventist Church emphasizes a very strict observance of the sabbath. "For 24 hours every week no matter how stressed out, no matter where the kids need to be driven to, they stop everything," Dan says. "From Friday night until Saturday night, they focus on their God, their family, their community and nature."

Loma Linda is also home to Loma Linda University, a Seventh-day Adventist health sciences institution of higher learning with a world-renowned medical center. Notable firsts at this center include baboon-to-human heart transplant and the first split-brain surgery.

Maintaining a healthy body mass index (BMI) is equally important. Adventists with healthy BMIs who keep active and avoid meat, have lower blood pressure, lower blood cholesterol, and less cardiovascular disease than heavier Americans with higher BMIs.

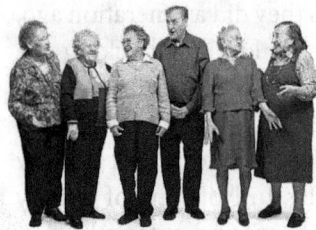

The healthful plant-based diet that Seventh-day Adventists eat has been associated with an extra decade of life expectancy. It has also been linked to reduced rates of diabetes and heart disease. Adventists' diet is inspired by the Bible — Genesis 1:29. ("And God said: 'Behold, I have given you every herb yielding seed . . . and every tree, in which is the fruit of a tree yielding seed; to you it shall be for food.' ")

But again, the key insight might be more about social structure than about the diet itself. While for most people, diets eventually fail, the Adventists eat the way they do for decades. How? Adventists hang out with other Adventists. When you go to an Adventist picnic, there's no steak grilling on the barbecue; it's a vegetarian potluck. No one is drinking alcohol or smoking. As Nicholas Christakis, a physician and social scientist at Harvard, found when examining data from a long-term study of the residents of Framingham, Mass., health habits can be as contagious as a cold virus. ~ Dan Buettner

Work Outs At 103

While investigating the longevity of the Loma Lindans, Dan Buettner met Marge Jetton who was 103 at the time. Marge's secret to staying healthy is daily exercise, prayers and volunteerism.

Marge's daily exercise routine consisted of weight lifting and riding a stationary bicycle for 7 or 8 miles at 25 mph! Marge demonstrated her dumbbell workout and how strong her arms looked

After 77 years of marriage, Marge's husband passed away. As most people would do, Marge mourned her loss, but then realized that there was more for her to do. She realized the world was not going to come to her, she needed to go to the world. At the time of the interview, she was still volunteering for seven organizations.

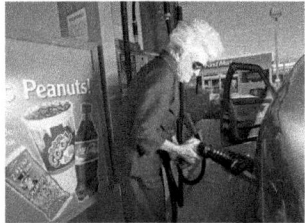

Dan Buettner believes that being a member of a community where everyone has the same values can add quality years to your life. Also showing gratitude is another reason why people in these communities have such long and healthy lives.

> *Heart surgeon Ellsworth Wareham is a 94-year-old Adventist who can still be found in the operating room. "I think it's important for an individual to have some security and peace in his life. And I get that from believing in a loving, caring God, you see. And so if he's in charge of my life, why sit around and worry? I mean, he takes care of the universe, he can certainly take care of me, so I don't worry."*
>
> *Dr. Wareham also follows a vegan diet, which means he doesn't eat any meat, fish or eggs. He also spends about 10 hours a week working in his garden. "I've been fortunate, first, but I do try to follow a good lifestyle," he says. Having performed more than 12,000 operations in his life, Dr. Wareham says it may not just be the work that's keeping him heathy. "It's more about a sense of purpose".*

36.

Nicoya Peninsula

An Idyllic Oasis Of Peace

Nicoya is a peninsula on the Pacific coast of Costa Rica. It is divided into two provinces: Guanacaste Province in the north, and the Puntarenas Province in the south. It is known for its beaches and is a popular tourist destination. The main commercial centre in the region is Nicoya, one of the oldest settlements in Costa Rica. Its located about a two-hour trip on bumpy roads from the national capital of San Jose.

In 2005, Dr. Rosero-Bixby, a Costa Rican demographer trained in the United States, presented a paper at an international conference claiming to have discovered that 60-year-old Costa Ricans have the longest life expectancy of anyone in the world. In other words, if you are middle aged and live in Costa Rica, you are more likely to reach, say, a healthy age 90 than your counterparts worldwide.

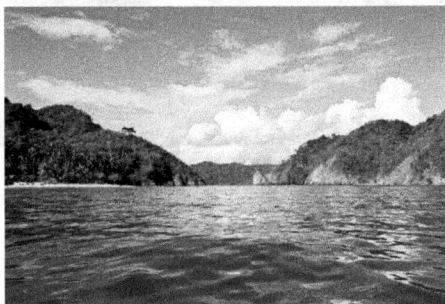

Many centenarians eat less and avoid meat.
You look in the blue zone in Okinawa, these people are consistently eating off of small plates. One of the cues for fullness is an empty plate, so stock your cupboard with smaller plates. ~Dan Buettner

The academics at the conference did not believe Dr. Rosero-Bixby. After all, Central America is still considered 'Third World,' a place of poverty, tropical disease, and, during the 1990s, terrible wars. How could the people here live longer than 'First World' countries.

Centenarians and Census Records

In August, thanks to a grant from National Geographic and Allianz Life, Dan Buettner traveled with a world-renowned longevity expert, Dr. Michel Poulain, to meet Dr. Rosero-Bixby and examine his data. They interviewed 90-to-100-year-olds to verify their ages, and then doubled-checked in the archives (Costa Rica has an excellent record-keeping system that has recorded everyone born since 1888) to make sure these subjects weren't lying or misguided about their dates of birth.

They found that not only was Rosero-Bixby's data accurate, but in looking at it more closely they noticed something extraordinary -- a Blue Zone: In northwestern Costa Rica, residents live even longer than people in the rest of the country.

This area -- the Nicoya Peninsula -- is about 70 miles long and 30 miles wide. Surfer beaches and upscale resorts hem the peninsula's western edge. But inland, forest-covered hills and cow pastures blanket most of the terrain.

For the 75,000 or so people who live here, life proceeds much the way as it has for hundreds of years. Nicoyans make their living as small farmers, laborers or sabaneros -- cowboys who work the area's huge cattle ranches. Judging by the dusty villages where neighbors hang out on porches, or the rural homes where women still cook on ancient wood-burning stoves, one can never guess that the Nicoya is the longest-life place in the Americas.

"We know that people who make it to a hundred tend to be nice. They ... drink from the fountain of life by being likeable and drawing people to them."

Set up your life, your home environment, your social environment, and your workplace so that you're constantly nudged into behaviors that favor longevity.

~Dan Buettner

Costa Rica indeed does celebrate its elderly citizens; every person who has a 100th birthday is featured on the national news. As of June 2012, this tiny country reported 417 citizens over the age of 100; the country's official population is more or less 4.5 million. Costa Rican Photographer Mónica Quesada is creating a book and video documenting natives who have lived a century.

So what's the secret? Buettner's team of researchers and specialists found interesting similarities among the Nicoyan centenarians that are common characteristics in all of the other Blue Zones: There are so many Centenarians in Nicoya that The Blue Zone team spent 9 months in research in 2007.

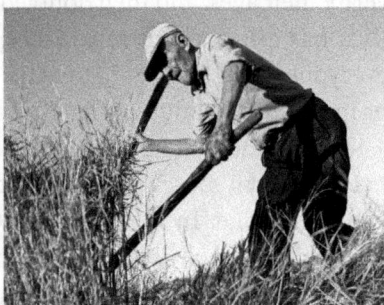

Have a "plan de vida," or reason to live; it also can be called "why I get up in the morning". Centenarians say they feel needed, with a sense of purpose that often centers on their family.

Have Faith. The Nicoyans' strong belief in God and their "faith routines" help relieve stress and anxiety. Almost all of the centenarians interviewed around the world for Buettner's book belonged to a faith-based community of some form.

Healthy diet. Most of the various Blue Zone residents in the world eat a primarily plant-based diet, especially legumes (all kinds

While visiting Patrone, 107, Dan and Dr. Oz enjoyed a meal prepared by his 65-year-old daughter. Families stay together in Nicoya, which is another important key to living a long life.

For lunch, she made corn tortillas from scratch. First, she soaks the corn in ash and lime to break it down. Then, she smashes it in a metate—a Central American stone mortar. Then, she cooks the corn patties without oil. "It's a lot of hard work, and there's no electricity, so she can't do it any other way," Dr. Oz says. "And it's a good workout."

This daily process of cooking tortillas is like an automatic workout. "You know, most Americans don't really exercise. A very small proportion," Dan says. "But in Nicoya, they'll be making lunch and it's like doing 25 reps with the free weights."

of beans, peas and lentils). They also eat rich, colorful fruits – in Nicoya, they eat marañon, the red-orange cashew tree fruit that has more vitamin C than oranges, and noni, a pear-like fruit rich in antioxidants. Another indigenous diet is Chorotega, consisting of high-fortified corn and beans—healthy and high in fiber.

Another important aspect of the Nicoyan diet is that they tend to eat their larger meals in the morning, with progressively smaller meals throughout the day. This not only leaves Nicoyans craving fewer calories during the day, it also lets them transition into sleep much more easily when darkness falls. "A hundred years ago, when the sun went down, the brain would start making more melatonin. And with more melatonin, you'd get tired, you'd get drowsy,"

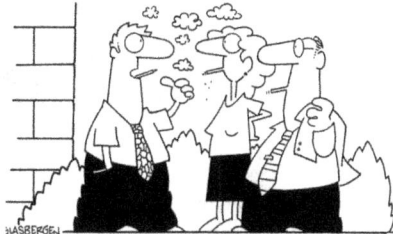

"Smoking may kill us. On the other hand, the non-smokers are inside working themselves to death!"

Dr. Oz says. "Today, the reason half of us don't sleep normally is because the last thing we see is a computer screen or the tube. That actually does the opposite to your brain—it stimulates it. So of course you can't fall asleep. You've got to glide to sleep."

Get some sun. Climate allows Nicoyans to get plenty of sunshine. Regular sun exposure helps their bodies produce vitamin D for strong bones and healthy body function. Vitamin D deficiency is associated with a host of problems, such as osteoporosis and heart disease, and regular, "smart" sun exposure (about 15 minutes on the legs and arms) can help supplement nutrients received through diet. Nicoya is the driest part of Costa Rica, and in dry climates people get fewer respiratory diseases.

> *"The natural food of man, judging from his structure, appears to consist principally of the fruits, roots, and other succulent parts of vegetables. His hands afford every facility for gathering them; his short but moderately strong jaws on the other hand, and his canines being equal only in length to the other teeth, together with his tuberculated molars on the other, would scarcely permit him either to masticate herbage, or to devour flesh, were these condiments not previously prepared by cooking."*

Get Sleep. Nicoyans sleep an average of at least 7 hours per day. They more or less go to sleep soon after nightfall and wake with the sun. They spend one-fifteenth the amount developed countries do on public health

No smoking. Smoking is not common in Blue Zone communities.

Having a good relationship with their family and maintaining a strong social network contributes greatly to centenarians' sense of purpose and well-being. People of all ages are socially active and integrated into their communities.

Nicoyan centenarians maintain a strong work ethic, which keeps them active and healthy while contributing to their sense of purpose. Moderate physical activity is a normal part of daily life – walking, bicycling, gardening, cooking, keeping up the house, taking care of animals, etc.

Researchers met 102-year-old Panchita, who still chops wood every day for cooking; 86-year-old Filippa, who sells her homemade tamales; and 95-year-old Serillo, who was cruising by on his bike as he visited his neighbors.

In a broader context, Costa Rica represents an idyllic oasis of peace and stability in a region otherwise battered by poverty and civil wars.

Dan says one of the secrets of Nicoyans' lifespan can be found in the water that flows through the hills. Their water is among the hardest in Costa Rica—which means it's chock-full of minerals. "Hard water means stronger bones. It also means your muscles are probably working better, especially when you get old," Dan says.

Hard water has proven benefits. "Calcium, magnesium and water—it relaxes your arteries, it builds bone strength and it has a huge benefit across the board in how your body functions.

Having strong bones is actually one of the most important ways to live a long life. One of the biggest killers of older people is simply falling down and breaking a bone. If you take calcium and couple it with vitamin D, your bones don't deteriorate as quickly.

To re-create the benefits of the Nicoyans' calcium-rich water, dairy and leafy green vegetables like kale and broccoli can be suggested.

Indeed, Costa Rica enjoys a well-developed social welfare system, possesses no standing army (having abolished it in 1948) and high living standards.

It is for these reasons that Costa Rica is often referred to as the Switzerland of Central America.

37.

Kalenjins And Tarahumara

Power of Natural, Chemical Free, Plant Based Diet

In this chapter we reproduce two articles about two different tribes whose dietary habits and lifestyle have endowed them with exceptional physical abilities. This shows in order to achieve optimum health, we don't need anything super-extraordinary. A simple, natural, chemical free, unprocessed plant based diet is all that we need.

Secrets From The Savannah: The Diets Of Elite Kenyan Runners
By Jonathan Bechtel

East african runners have a record of dominance in elite distance running. Since pushing themselves into the spotlight by steamrolling the competition in the 1968 olympics, Kenyans and Ethiopians have enjoyed a peculiar success at international events. Since that time they've grabbed 10 of the 20 top times for middle and long distance cross-country races. This success naturally led to curiousity about these runners' origins and practices.

Studies of their biology, conditioning, and nutritional habits have been both illuminating and confusing. A surprising fact discovered by western researchers was that running prowess is not evenly distributed in these countries. Within Kenya and Ethiopia are different geographies, cultures, and tribes that create very different lifestyles from one region to the next.

It was eventually discovered that the majority of Kenyan runners came from a small ethnic group called the Kalenjins, who live in the Great Rift Valley in northern Kenya. They make up less than

10% of the Kenyan population, but won a staggering 40% of middle and long distance races in international competition from 1987 to 1997. Such a story naturally stokes the imagination. What is it about this band of people that makes them world-class runners? Is it in their genes? Was it a culture that glorified running? Was it something special in their diet? Ensuing research provided some answers, but no silver bullet.

You could write a book (and some have) about all the unique wrinkles in Kalinjin life that led to their running prowess, but this article will slice one important variable: their diet. Any runner knows the importance of nutrition in a training regimen, and studies of Kalinjin eating habits both re-affirmed currently held beliefs while raising doubts about others.

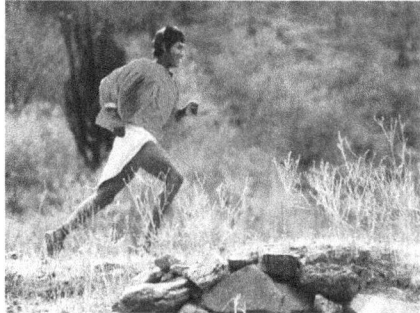

Ingredients

Whenever a mysterious tribe or part of the earth is discovered, rumors quickly spread about a new superfood or diet with extraordinary health properties. Acai berries, mangosteen fruit, and chia seeds are the products of such hype. Did the Kalinjin diet have a special ingredient? Would their eating habits shed new light into running and nutrition the same way the Okinawans did for longevity? The answer is a decisive no. The Kalinjin diet, it turns out, is pretty plain.

Surveys and observations done in person confirmed that a typical day's food consists of cabbage, potatoes, kidney beans, boiled rice, and ugali, a paste made from corn maize. Drinks usually consisted of water and tea. The nutritional quality of all these foods was high, but none were out of the ordinary. Overall macronutrient intake among Kalinjins conformed to traditional canons of athletic nutrition, and studies of their diet confirmed conventional beliefs about the macronutrients you should consume in your diet and did not turn over any new leaves.

(Jonathan Bechtel is a lifelong marathoner. He covers health, nutrition, and benefits of a whole foods diet in his writings).

Secrets of the Tarahumara Runners

Adapted from Born to Run by Christopher McDougall.

The man in the shot may look like an ancient Aztec goofy-footing his way down a rockslide. But he's actually a Tarahumara Indian, a member of a tribe living deep in Mexico's remote Copper Canyons. When it comes to going ultra-distances, nothing could beat the Tarahumara – not a racehorse, not a cheetah, not an Olympic marathoner. Very few outsiders had ever seen the Tarahumara in action, but amazing stories of their superhuman toughness and tranquillity have drifted out of the canyons for centuries. One explorer spent 10 hours crossing a mountain by mule; a Tarahumara runner made the same trip in 90 minutes.

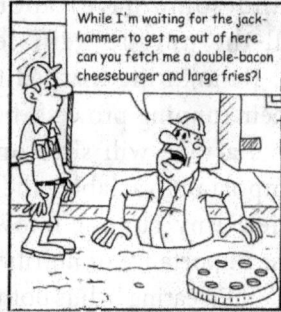

When it comes to the top 10 health risks facing American men, the Tarahumara are practically immortal: Their incidence rate is at or near zero in just about every category, including diabetes, vascular disease, and colorectal cancer. Age seems to have no effect on them, either: The Tarahumara runner who won the 1993 Leadville ultramarathon was 55 years old. Plus, their supernatural invulnerability isn't just limited to their bodies; the Tarahumara have mastered the secret of happiness as well, living as benignly as bodhisattvas in a world free of theft, murder, suicide, and cruelty.

So how do they do it? How is it that we, in one of the most technologically advanced nations on Earth, can devote armies of scientists and terabytes of data to improving our lives, yet keep getting fatter, sicker, and sadder, while the Tarahumara, who haven't changed a thing in 2,000 years, don't just survive, but thrive? What have they remembered that we've forgotten?

-Christopher McDougall

Tony Ramirez, a horticulturist in the US, who's been obsessed with Tarahumara foods for decades. "Anything the Tarahumara eat, you can obtain easily," says Ramirez. "It's mostly beans, squash, chilli peppers, wild greens, ground corn and chia." (Chia is a seed that can absorb more than 12 times its weight in water.)

The Tarahumara's favourite drink, apart from home-brewed corn beer, is a little concoction whipped up by dissolving chia seeds in water and adding a little sugar and a squirt of lime. As tiny as those seeds are, they're packed with omega-3s, protein, fibres and antioxidants. And there's no arguing with its pedigree: On a diet like that, a 55-year-old Tarahumara runner won a 160km race through the Colorado Rockies.

"Sooner or later your fingers close on that one moist-cold spud that the spade has accidentally sliced clean through, shining wetly white and giving off the most unearthly of earthly aromas. It's the smell of fresh soil in the spring, but fresh soil somehow distilled or improved upon, as if that wild, primordial scene has been refined and bottled: eau de pomme de terre. You can smell the cold inhuman earth in it, but there's the cozy kitchen to, for the smell of potatoes is, at least by now, to us, the smell of comfort itself, a smell as blankly welcoming as spud flesh, a whiteness that takes up memories and sentiments as easily as flavors. To smell a raw potato is to stand on the very threshold of the domestic and the wild."

~ Michael Pollan, The Botany of Desire: A Plant's-Eye View of the World

38.

Irulas

A Treasure House Of Traditional Knowledge

India is a repository of ancient traditions. It's a land seeped in history with a glorious past.

Science and technology in ancient India covered all major branches of knowledge like mathematics, astronomy, physics, chemistry, medical science, surgery, fine arts, mechanical and production technology, civil engineering, architecture, shipbuilding and navigation, sports and games etc.

Coming to medicine, India is rich in ethnic diversity and traditional knowledge has resulted in a considerable body of ethnobotanical research. There are over 537 different aboriginal groups in India with extensive knowledge of plants. Many qualitative surveys have recorded detailed utility of specific plants for many aboriginal groups such as the Malasars, Malamalasars, Malayalis, Irulas, Gonds, Koysd, Konda reddis, Valmikis, Koyas, Chenchus, Lambadis, Jatapus, Savaras, Bagatas, Kammaras, Khondas, Nukadoras, Porjas, Jatapus and host of others.

In India, it is reported that traditional healers use 2500 plant species as regular sources of medicine. Traditionally, this treasure of knowledge has been passed on orally from generation to generation without any written documentation. This is apart from the mainstream medicinal systems such as Ayurveda, Siddha and Unani.

In this chapter we take up the case of the Irulas, a tribe in South India. India is home to the world's largest tribal population.

The Irulas reside in the Kodiakkarai Reserve Forest (KRF) in the Coromandal coast of Thanjavur district, India. They are one among the six oldest tribes in the region. Their population in this region is estimated to be between 1000 to 2000.

Early 20th century anthropological literature classified the Irulas under the Negrito ethnic group. The term Irula means being capable of finding one's path in dark forests, according to an Irula lore. This is characteristic of the Irulas.

They are known to be exceptional healers and keepers of traditional knowledge of the flora in the coastal forest. Furthermore, the Irulas are an example of a culture that has preserved a highly diverse ecosystem that sustains their healthy life-styles.

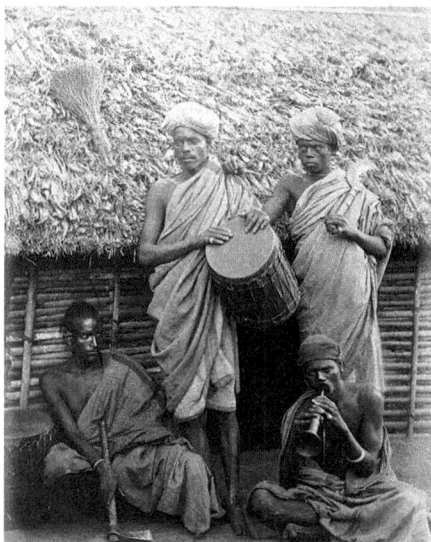

Born in nature's lap, Irulas share a symbiotic relationship with Mother Earth. Irula healers, mostly women, practice traditional healing systems, which use over 320 medicinal herbs.

They treat several new-age diseases with a high success rate. People around the world realize that traditional healing practices must have a place in modern medicine.

The Irula Tribal Women's Welfare Society (ITWWS), established in 1986, focuses on this traditional science.

It empowers Irula women by promoting their medicinal products. This revival of traditional healing systems addresses public health needs as well as conserves Irula culture and expertise.

The Irulas' Natural Products Corporation is a partnership firm located in the ITWWS campus, which produces, promotes and markets Irula health-care products. It provides employment to several hundred Irula women. This project is supported by the

Ministry of Tribal Affairs and Ministry of Rural Development. These products are made from medicinal plants grown naturally without any chemical additives or pesticides.

Ethnomedicine - Emerging Trends

A mounting body of critical research is raising the credibility of traditional knowledge in scientific studies and natural resource management. The lack of recognition of the place and value of traditional knowledge in science has prevented real engagement of this knowledge in scientific endeavours including nutrition, medicine, environmental assessment and resource management practices. These studies have gained credibility because their claims are supported by methods that are repeatable and provide data for quantitative analyses that can be used to assess confidence in the results.

Throughout history aboriginal people have been the custodians of bio-diversity and have sustained healthy life-styles in an environmentally sustainable manner. However this knowledge has not been transferred to modern society.

It was recently this aboriginal group, Irulas chose to share this knowledge with society-at-large in order to promote a global lifestyle of health and environmental sustainability. They believe that a healthy lifestyle is founded on a healthy environment.

They found themselves virtually bonded labourers in 1976 when the Forest Protection Bill was passed. It became very difficult for them to lead their traditional lifestyle.

The culture of the Irulas has changed little over the last one thousand years. Their staple food consists of minor millets, grain legumes, and wild yams supplemented with rice. They do not practice agriculture and therefore wholly depend on forest produce and wild animals. The Irulas settlements are located within or on the edge of the forests and consist of tiny scattered huts. The community is divided into several exogamous clans.

More recently, some Irulas go to local villages to trade or sell honey, honey wax, firewood, wild fruits, yams, berries and other native herbal products. This supports a productive and localized non-timber forest product industry, which supports many families.

The Irulas trade these products for local farm produce. Before this, their interaction with civilization was very limited.

A variety of plant morphological structures are utilized as medicine by the Irulas of which leaves are used most frequently, followed by roots, bark, seeds, whole plants, flowers, fruits and latex/sap. The preparation for utilization of these plant parts can be grouped into several categories based on the mode of preparation; decoction, extract, fresh or cooked plant, juice, latex, paste, and powder.

These herbs can be used as mosquito repellents, antibiotics, antidotes, appetizers or simply, as food compliments. Plant remedies are utilized for various illnesses such as asthma, blood flow, body pain, weak or feeble body, cold, cough, diabetes, diarrhoea, earache, eye pain, fever, general medicine, hydrocoele, hypothermia, intestinal worms, jaundice, leprosy, pregnancy pain, purgative, rheumatism, skin disease, skin-shine, spiritual, toothache and wounds.

With a rise in lifestyle diseases, many patients are flocking them in search of a cure. Native healing practitioners provide a source of income for many Irulas families.

The Irulas share the concept 'Neenda aauil', which translates to "living a long healthy life". The Irulas believe that the treatment of ailments can be preempted by a healthy lifestyle. The Irulas routinely consume these herbs for good health.

A great variety of plants are collected from the wild and distributed among the community or sent off to local markets for trading with other communities.

An ancient tradition of the Irulas is to eat certain plants on a regular basis according to the seasons in order to prevent certain diseases. It is a common practice for the Irulas to consume plants in the wild throughout their daily routine. While trekking or hunting, they routinely grab some leaves or chew on some twigs. They seem know exactly what and when to eat for good health.

The Forest Is A Natural Pharmacopeia/Grocery Store For Them

Not unlike our modern society they encourage good hygiene from a young age. This may include cleaning or brushing your teeth with various types of twigs. The Irulas believe that brushing your teeth with the roots of thumbai (Leucas aspera Willd.) for 40 consecutive days makes you immune to any snake venom. However this is a very complicated procedure and only few elders know how to do it right. Irulas are expert in catching snakes and they are being engaged in venom extraction for medicinal purposes. Young children playing with snakes is a common sight in their communities.

They treat diabetes with a preparation called 'Sirukurinjan', which appears to be made from Gymnema sylvestre leaves. They grow many medicinal plants in their backyard. They may consume some herbs first thing in the morning or routinely add others in their cooking. Rheumatoid arthritis is treated with Diplocyclos palmatus and Boerhavia diffusa. Some of their medicines make use of plants which are otherwise extremely poisonous. Begonia malabarica Roxb. is used to treat blood cancer.

Every household has a bunch of twigs tied on the doorway to ward off evil influences. They even know how to communicate with spirits.

The Irulas are an excellent example of a culture that has preserved a highly diverse area while harvesting their food and medicine from it for thousands of years. These communities are a treasure house of traditional knowledge that can greatly benefit our civilization. However this priceless knowledge is disappearing very fast and it is an urgent necessity to document and preserve it as soon as possible.

(Source: Valorizing the 'Irulas' traditional knowledge of medicinal plants in the Kodiakkarai Reserve Forest, India, Subramanyam Ragupathy and Steven G Newmaster)

39.

Diseases of Faulty Nutrition

By Major-General Robert McCarrison, M.D.

(Paper Read Before The Far Eastern Association of Tropical Medicine, England, 1927)

More than 2,000 years ago Hippocrates wrote as follows:
'... it appears to me necessary to every physician to be skilled in nature, and to strive to know, if he would wish to perform his duties, what man is in relation to the articles of food and drink, and to his other occupations, and what are the effects of each of them to every one.

'Whoever does not know what effect these things produce upon a man, cannot know the consequences which result from them.

'Whoever pays no attention to these things, or paying attention, does not comprehend them, how can he understand the diseases which befall a man? For, by every one of these things a man is affected and changed this way and that, and the whole of his life is subjected to them, whether in health, convalescence, or disease. Nothing else, then, can be more important or more necessary to know than these things.'

It is strange that, although these words were written so long ago, it is only within the last quarter of a century that we have begun to pay attention to 'what man is in relation to the articles of food and drink', to 'know what effect these things produce upon a man', and, 'to understand the diseases which befall a man' in consequence of them.

In the time at my disposal I can do no more than give a very brief outline of the present state of knowledge of the nutritional

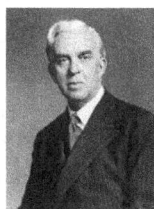

or, as I prefer to call them, the malnutritional diseases. I shall not, therefore, concern myself with morbid states which result from the ingestion of food in insufficient quantity, nor with those which may be associated with over-eating, but will confine myself to ailments whose genesis is directly or indirectly dependent upon the improper quality and or the improper balance of food ingested in sufficient quantity.

Since the functions of food are to rebuild the living tissues, to supply energy and to preserve a proper medium in which the biochemical processes of the body can take place, it follows that derangements of nutrition -- and, therefore, of health -- must result if the food ingested fails adequately to subserve these functions.

Then the architecture of the living tissues becomes imperfect; transformation of energy in the body becomes deranged; and, metabolic processes become disordered, with the consequent production of abnormal or, it may be, of toxic metabolites.

The failure of food to subserve these functions may be brought about in a number of ways; but the one which chiefly concerns us here is the insufficient provision in the diet of one or other or all of three of its essential constituents: suitable protein, inorganic salts and vitamins. Foods which are unsatisfactory in these regards give rise to sub-optimal, or to subnormal states of health, or even to actual disease, the character and the severity of which depend upon the nature and degree of the food faults and the length of time the organism has been subjected to their influence.

The first effect of such unsatisfactory foods to which reference must be made is the *low standard of physical efficiency* which they induce both in man and his domestic animals. In no country in the world is this more clearly manifested than in India where malnutrition is so widespread.

No one who has traveled far in India can have failed to notice the great differences in physique of different Indian races. The poor physique, the lack of vigour and of powers of endurance of certain southern and eastern races provide a remarkable contrast to the fine physique and hardiness of certain stalwart races of the north: these differences are in the main attributable to differences in biological value of their national diets.

The low standard of physical efficiency of man's domestic animals in certain parts of India is common knowledge: it has the same malnutritional basis, and the gravity of its influence on the well-being of the people can hardly be over-estimated.

In addition to lowering the standard of physical efficiency (a matter of vast economic importance to India) food which is faulty with respect either to suitable protein, to mineral elements, to vitamins or to all three gives rise to many minor manifestations of ill health.

It inevitably leads to some deviation from the normal histological structure, and to a corresponding reduction in functional efficiency, of one or other of the various organs and tissues of the body: the nervous, the osseous, the muscular, the endocrine, the gastro-

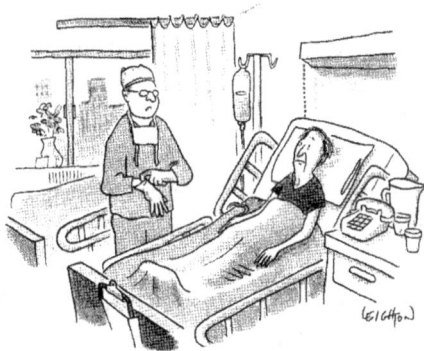

"I'll have someone come in and prep you for the bill."

intestinal, the respiratory and the circulatory systems. It leads also to some deviation of the body fluids from their normal constitution; the blood, the lymph, the digestive juices, the secretions, the excretions, even the tears, are all altered in one way or another, each alteration contributing to, or being indicative of, impaired wellbeing.

The lesser manifestations of malnutrition often escape our observation altogether, although they 'affect the health of individuals to a degree most important to themselves.'

If we closely observe animals subsisting on faulty food -- even though the fault be not so great as to cause such wreckages of health as scurvy, beri-beri, pellagra, rickets or keratomalacia -- we notice many signs of impaired well-being which have their counterpart in human subjects similarly situated with respect to the quality and balance of their food.

Thus, we may notice sub-normal or, as I prefer to say, sub-optimal states of growth or of unbalanced growth; or we may find that the animals' 'condition' is not so good as it might be, that their coats lack lustre, or that they are dull-eyed and devoid of the beauty of the well-nourished animal; we may notice, also, that their excreta are not wholly normal, that they age prematurely, that their fertility is impaired, that they have but poor success in rearing their young, that their offspring when reared are very prone to disease and that the mortality amongst them is high.

We may find, too, that they are apprehensive and timid, peevish, or it may be ill-natured, and that they resent handling which the well-nourished animal rarely does: all of which is unmistakable evidence of an unstable nervous system. Yet such animals may be suffering from no nameable disease though they are obviously not well.

Similar symptoms of sub-normal health are common enough in human beings; but since they may conform to no stereotyped disease, have no 'microbe' nor any 'toxin' associated with them, nor be accounted for by any laboratory tests which we apply to them, we are apt to find nothing wrong with sufferers from them and to mistake their malnutritional meaning.

Obsessed by the idea of the microbe, the protozoa, or the invisible virus as all important excitants of disease, subservient to laboratory methods of diagnosis, and hidebound by our system of nomenclature, we often forget the most fundamental of all rules for the physician, that *the right kind of food is the most important single factor in the promotion of health and the wrong kind of food the most important single factor in the promotion of disease.*

I emphasize these minor manifestations of malnutrition because they represent the beginnings of disease, and their recognition is, to my way of thinking, vastly more important than that of the wreckages of health.

The mention of lamziekte in cattle, introduces us to a novel sequence of events in disease production. This condition is due to a pathogenic agent -- the Parabotulinus bovis -- which has its habitat in decaying bones. The primary cause of the disease is, however,

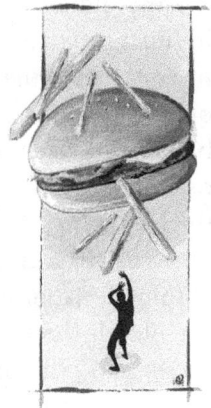

a deficiency of phosphorus in the food of cattle which induces in them so great a craving for this element that, to satisfy it, they eat the bones in which the pathogenic agent resides, thereby becoming infected. It may be that in this observation there lies a general principle which has an application to mankind.

This brings me to one of the most important means by which disease is brought about both in man and animals by faulty nutrition: namely, by increasing their susceptibility to infectious agents.

During the past two-and-a-half years (1925-7) 2,463 rats, living in my laboratories under conditions of perfect hygiene, have been fed on various faulty foods, while the daily average of control or well-fed stock rats was 865.

The mortality in the ill-fed animals (excluding those that were killed on the conclusion of experiments) was 31.4 per cent, while in the well-fed animals it was less than 1 per cent; the chief causes of death being lung diseases, pneumonia or broncho-pneumonia and acute gastrointestinal disease.

In the course of my own work I have seen dysentery arise in ill-fed monkeys while well-fed monkeys living in the same animal room escaped; and I have seen ill-fed pigeons become infected with Bacillus suipestifer and with the invisible virus of epithelioma contagiosum, while well-fed birds living in their immediate vicinity escaped these infections.

Other workers have had like experiences; the bacillus of mouse typhoid kills, on injection, over 90 per cent of ill-fed mice while it kills less than 10 per cent of well-fed mice; the ill-fed mice are likewise less resistant to B. pestis cavide and to botulinus toxins. Birds are rendered susceptible to infection by anthrax when fed on food deficient in vitamin B and rats to septic broncho-pneumonia when fed on food deficient in vitamin A; guinea-pigs, when fed on food deficient in vitamin C, die more readily from tuberculosis, new-born calves deprived of colostrum develop interstitial nephritis due to B. coli infection; swine suffer from tuberculosis, which can be eradicated from the herds by well-balanced vitamin-rich food; stock animals develop sarcosporidia from the same malnutritional cause.

Man himself provides many examples of a like kind: I need but mention two: In Northern Melanesia, the native's modern diet has been shown to be deficient in suitable protein, mineral elements and vitamins and the poor physique of the natives and their high death-rate from respiratory and intestinal diseases has been correlated with these deficiencies in the food; outbreaks of broncho-pneumonia in children have been definitely traced to the inadequate ingestion of fat-soluble A, and have been caused to disappear by the adequate provision of this vitamin.

This list of infectious diseases, to which animals and man are rendered highly susceptible by faulty food, is comprehensive enough including, as it does, infections by such diverse organisms as protozoa, bacilli and invisible viruses.

There is good reason, therefore, for the assumption that such death-dealing diseases as tuberculosis, leprosy, cholera, dysentery, plague and malaria have often in this country (India) a malnutritional element in their genesis and course.

Within recent years 'the spectacular results which have attended the experimental study of vitamins have overshadowed much else in nutrition both in the minds of the profession and the public' (Mendel, 1923).

It may not be inappropriate, therefore, to refer to a class of disease which results under experimental conditions in animals from the lack of balance of various components of the food, each component in itself good.

One example of the kind is afforded by the hyperplastic goitre which may result from an excess in the food of so homely a substance as butter. The excess of butter, or of unsaturated fatty acid, causes thyroid hyperplasia by reason of the relative deficiency of iodine brought about by this excess; similarly, enlargements of the thyroid gland of the colloid type may be induced by an excess of lime; they are preventable by increasing the iodine ingested proportionately to this excess.

Another example of much the same sort is that of stone-in-the-bladder which is brought about in rats by ill-balanced diets containing much oatmeal, or whole-wheat flour.

To avoid 'stone' the excess of these cereals must be compensated for by the consumption of appropriate amounts of milk. Those most excellent foods, oatmeal and whole-wheat flour -- the staple articles of diet of such vigorous races as the Scots and the Sikhs -- may likewise prove harmful, by causing disturbance in the normal processes of calcification, when, but only when, the diets containing them are poor in vitamin D.

These cereals are not in themselves complete foods; a fact of which the races using them as staple articles of diet are not wholly in ignorance: the Sikh does not attempt to subsist on atta (whole-wheat flour) alone, nor the Scot on oatmeal. Any ill effect which these two foods may exercise is due to the failure suitably to combine them with other food materials which compensate for their defects. They are not to be condemned nor to be displaced from their prominent place in the dietaries of mankind for this reason.

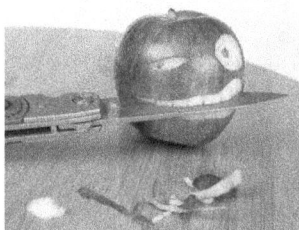

As well might we condemn the perfectly good fuel, petrol, for the over-heating of the engines of our cars when we fail to supply them with sufficient oil, as condemn the excellent wheat and oats when we fail to consume with them sufficient quantities of milk or other vitamin-rich foods, which are required by the human machine for its smooth and efficient running.

Next, then, in importance to the quality of the various ingredients of our food is their right combination.

Of all the constituents of food on which normal health is dependent, vitamins are the most remarkable. We know neither what they are nor yet how much of them we need, though knowing that normal metabolism is impossible without them.

We are accustomed to think of them in such infinitesimal terms that we have come to believe that the amounts we need of them are almost imponderable. I do not know whether they are ponderable or not, nor whether science will ultimately succeed in encompassing them all within chemical formulae; but I do know that for optimum well-being we need much more of them than is generally supposed.

At all events, races like the Sikhs, whose physical development and vigour are equal to those of any race of mankind, and superior to many, consume these substances in large quantities as compared with races whose physique is poor.

I find that for rats the wellbalanced, vitamin-rich diet of the Sikhs is superior to any synthetic diet I can devise and to which vitamins in the form of yeast and cod-liver oil are added. I do not believe that human beings can have too much vitamins when they are taken in the form in which Nature provides them in well-balanced combinations of unsophisticated food materials.

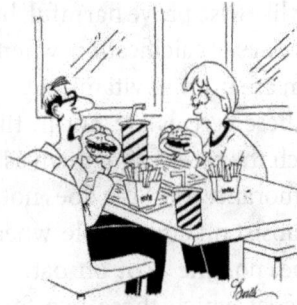

"Is it just me or is it a bad idea to eat at a place that prints CPR instructions on their placemats?"

Some individuals appear to require more vitamins than others, size being an important factor in determining their requirements; some species of animals require more of a particular kind of vitamin than do others; more are required by the lactating than by the non-lactating animal and more for longevity than for a shorter life.

The amount needed varies with the composition of the food, with its balance in other essentials and with its digestibility; more of one vitamin is required when the food is very rich in another as, for instance, more vitamin C when the food is rich in vitamin D; there is for optimum nutrition an ordered balance even amongst the vitamins themselves.

> *"Eating is an agricultural act," Wendell Berry famously wrote, by which he meant that we are not just passive consumers of food but cocreators of the systems that feed us. Depending on how we spend them, our food dollars can either go to support a food industry devoted to quantity and convenience and "value" or they can nourish a food chain organized around values--values like quality and health. Yes, shopping this way takes more money and effort, but as soon as you begin to treat that expenditure not just as shopping but also as a kind of vote--a vote for health in the largest sense--food no longer seems like the smartest place to economize." ~Michael Pollan*

In short, the amount of vitamins needed varies with the metabolic requirements of the individual; the attainment and maintenance of physical perfection, reproduction, lactation, heavy work, exposure to cold, infectious and debilitating diseases are all indications for their liberal supply.

Before bringing this brief survey to an end I may, perhaps, refer to another aspect of the matter: the effect of vitamin-deficiency in increasing the susceptibility to certain poisons, which the work of Smith, McClosky and Hendrick has recently brought into prominence.

It has been mentioned that deficiency of vitamin A increases the susceptibility of mice to botulinus toxin; it also increases their susceptibility to mercuric chloride. The same deficiency induces in rats an enormously increased susceptibility to morphine, to ergotoxine and, in lesser degree, to histamine. Deficiency of vitamin B likewise increases greatly the susceptibility of rats to ergotoxine and to pilocarpine. Stimulants of the central nervous system are all more toxic to rats receiving too little vitamin A than to well-fed animals.

WE NEED TO TEACH OUR CHILDREN **TO EAT REAL FOOD.** NO FAST FOODS. NO JUNK FOODS. NO PROCESSED FOODS. JUST HONEST, NUTRITIOUS, REAL FOOD.

Observations of this kind suggest forcibly that the ability of the tissues to detoxify certain poisons -- both bacterial and other -- is reduced by diets deficient in vitamins; while indicating that such diets increase the sensitivity of the nervous system and of its autonomic division to toxic agents.

Not only may this be so, but the disturbances of metabolism which result from vitamin-insufficiency may themselves give rise to toxic metabolites which exercise specific effects on certain organs and tissues of the body.

This I believe to be the case in beri-beri, about which malady we shall presently engage in argument. Most of us will probably agree

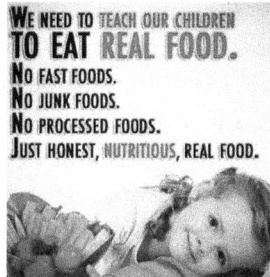

"The whole of nature is a conjugation of the verb to eat, in the active and passive." ~Michael Pollan

that there is such a thing as a specific beri-beri producing poison; though disagreeing as to whether it be produced in rice before this food is ingested, or in the intestine by some bacterial agent introduced with rice, or in the course of a disordered metabolism arising out of vitamin-insufficiency.

Our disagreements will not greatly matter so long as we recognize the prime importance of a sufficiency of the anti-neuritic fraction of vitamin B in preventing beri-beri.

In looking through the pages I have just written, I find mention of a host of diseases and departures from health which make up an imposing array. But amongst them there are none that I have not myself seen to arise as the direct or the indirect result of faulty nutrition or which are not vouched for by investigators of repute. I know of no disease producing agency which reaps so rich a harvest of ill health as this: though like others it has its limitations.

Perfectly constituted food is not a panacea for all diseases, but it is an agent as potent in preventing a host of them as is the mosquito-net in preventing one or inoculation in preventing another; while it is no mean coadjutor even to these.

The newer knowledge of nutrition is, I am convinced, the greatest advance in medical science since the days of Lister, and the sustained success of our profession in its conquest of disease depends, in no small measure, on the extended study of this vitally important subject and on the application in practice of the results reached by that study.

When physicians, medical officers of health and the lay public learn to apply the principles which the newer knowledge of nutrition has to impart, when they know what malnutrition means, when they look upon it as they now look upon sepsis and learn to avoid the one as much as they now avoid the other, then will this knowledge do for Medicine what asepsis has done for Surgery.

40.

Dr. Weston A. Price

Pioneering Research In Nutrition And Modern Foods

Dr. Weston A. Price was an American dentist who traveled around the world, camera and film in hand, in the late 1920s and early 1930s.

Dr. Price had the wisdom and persistence to study the dietary habits of healthy nonindustrialized people before they disappeared from the face of the earth. His research led to the radical conclusion that the diet that supports good health is in all respects the very opposite of the dietary recommendations given by all those smart people who work for the medical/ agricultural complex and the government.

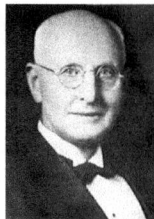

His travails took him to many isolated human groups which included sequestered villages in Switzerland, Gaelic communities in the Outer Hebrides, Eskimos and Indians of North America, Melanesian and Polynesian South Sea Islanders, African tribes, Australian Aborigines, New Zealand Maori and the Indians of South America.

Price specifically sought out native peoples who were still eating their native foods. He asked about their dietary habits, then examined and took photographs of their teeth. At the same time, he undertook similar studies and took similar photos of people from the same cultures who had become exposed to Western foods, and who had begun to substitute foods like white flour, white sugar, marmalade and canned goods for their native diets.

The differences, as shown in Price's 1939 book Nutrition and Physical Degeneration, were startling. Time and again, Price found that those people who were still eating their native diets had very few if any dental caries (decay or crumbling of teeth), and appeared to be in radiant health, while their counterparts who were now eating refined and processed foods from the West were exhibiting massive tooth decay and malformation of their dental arches, and were suffering from a growing cascade of illness and dysfunction.

Price came to believe that dental decay was caused primarily by nutritional deficiencies, and that the same conditions that promote tooth decay also promote disease elsewhere in the body.

Price photographed the teeth and dental arches of the people he encountered. He found that as long as these people consumed their native diet, their mouths and jaws developed so that they never experienced crowded teeth, overbites, underbites, or tooth decay. When their wisdom teeth came in, they always had plenty of room.

But as his photographs poignantly showed, once they left the wisdom of their native foods for "civilized" foods the results were ruinous. Now all kinds of dental problems that had been previously unknown became rampant.

And it wasn't just dental problems Price found that as people shifted to refined foods, birth defects increased, and people became more susceptible both to infection and to chronic disease. As people ate ever more refined and devitalized foods, he said, they and their offspring became increasingly weaker and more prone to all kinds of illnesses.

"Me and the folks who buy my food are like the Indians -- we just want to opt out. That's all the Indians ever wanted -- to keep their tepees, to give their kids herbs instead of patent medicines and leeches. They didn't care if there was a Washington, D.C., or a Custer or a USDA; just leave us alone. But the Western mind can't bear an opt-out option. We're going to have to refight the Battle of the Little Big Horn to preserve the right to opt out, or your grandchildren and mine will have no choice but to eat amalgamated, irradiated, genetically prostituted, barcoded, adulterated fecal spam from the centralized processing conglomerate."

~Michael Pollan, The Omnivore's Dilemma: A Natural History of Four Meals

---

Today, Price's work has attracted a loyal and devoted following among those who rebel against processed foods and who seek a way of life more in tune with nature's laws.

Some of the most zealous of his followers now run an organization called the Weston A. Price Foundation. They are heavily into meat eating. Dr. Price gave no such indications in his works. It is clearly a speculation on their part. No traditional culture uses meat as a staple but these followers seem to be promoting that. It appears they have found a convenient excuse to go on a meat eating spree.

Not a single culture examined by Price had a regular slaughterhouse operating in their community. Slaughterhouse culture is unique to our modern civilization. These tribals had to go to great lengths to obtain their meat supply.

Price discovered many native cultures that were extremely healthy while eating a lacto-vegetarian diet. Describing one lacto-vegetarian people, for example, he called them, "The most physically perfect people in northern India… the people are very tall and are free of tooth decay."

41.

Pristine Valleys And Prized Cows

A Comparison Of Isolated And Modernized Swiss

By Dr. Weston A. Price

(This is the third chapter of Dr. Price's travelogue, Nutrition And Physical Degeneration. It deals with his research, both in the isolated valleys as well as the modernized districts of Switzerland.)

In order to study the possibility of greater nutritive value in foods produced at a high elevation, as indicated by a lowered incidence of morbidity, including tooth decay, I went to Switzerland and made studies in two successive years, 1931 and 1932.

It was my desire to find, if possible, groups of Swiss living in a physical environment such that their isolation would compel them to live largely on locally produced foods.

Officials of the Swiss Government were consulted as to the possibility of finding people in Switzerland whose physical isolation provided an adequate protection. We were told that the physical conditions that would not permit people to obtain modern foods would also prevent us from reaching them easily.

However, owing to the completion of the Loetschberg Tunnel, eleven miles long, and the building of a railroad that crosses the Loetschental Valley, a group of about 2,000 people had been made easily accessible for study, shortly prior to 1931.

Practically all the human requirements of the people in that valley, except a few items like sea salt, have been produced in the valley for centuries.

The people of this valley have a history covering more than a dozen centuries. The architecture of their wooden buildings, some of them several centuries old, indicates a love for simple stability, adapted to expediency and efficiency. Artistically designed mottoes are expressive of devotion to cultural and spiritual values rather than to material values.

These people have never been conquered, although many efforts have been made to invade their valley. Except for the rugged cleft through which the river descends to the Rhone Valley, the Loetschental Valley is almost completely enclosed by three high mountain ranges which are usually snow-capped. This pass could be guarded by a small band against any attacking forces since artificial landslides could easily be released. The natural occurrence of these landslides has made passage through the gorge hazardous, if not impossible, for months of the year.

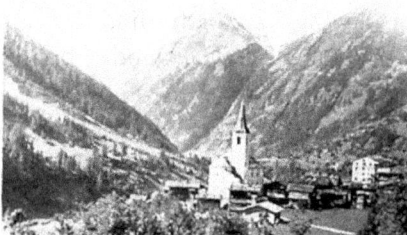

Beautiful Loetschental Valley about a mile above sea level. About two thousand Swiss live here. In 1932 no deaths had occurred from tuberculosis in the history of the valley.

At the altitude of the Loetschental Valley the winters are long, and the summers short but beautiful, and accompanied by extraordinarily rapid and luxuriant growth. The meadows are fragrant with Alpine flowers, with violets like pansies, which bloom all summer in deepest hues.

The people of the Loetschental Valley make up a community of two thousand who have been a world unto themselves. They have neither physician nor dentist because they have so little need for them; they have neither policeman nor jail, because they have no need for them.

The clothing has been the substantial homespuns made from the wool of their sheep. The valley has produced not only everything that is needed for clothing, but practically everything that is needed for food.

It has been the achievement of the valley to build some of the finest physiques in all Europe. This is attested to by the fact that many of the famous Swiss guards of the Vatican at Rome, who are the admiration of the world and are the pride of Switzerland, have been selected from this and other Alpine valleys. It is every Loetschental boy's ambition to be a Vatican guard.

Notwithstanding the fact that tuberculosis is the most serious disease of Switzerland, according to a statement given to me by a government official, a recent report of inspection of this valley did not reveal a single case.

The people live largely in a series of villages dotting the valley floor along the river bank. The land that is tilled, chiefly for producing hay for feeding the cattle in the winter and rye for feeding the people, extends from the river and often rises steeply toward the mountains which are wooded with timber so precious for protection that little of it has been disturbed.

Fortunately, there is much more on the vast area of the mountain sides than is needed for the relatively small population. The forests have been jealously guarded because they are so greatly needed to prevent slides of snow and rocks which might engulf and destroy the villages.

The valley has a fine educational system of alternate didactic and practical work. All children are required to attend school six months of the year and to spend the other six months helping with the farming and dairying industry in which young and old of both sexes must work.

The school system is under the direct supervision of the Catholic Church. The girls are also taught weaving, dyeing and garment making. The manufacture of wool and clothing is the chief homework for the women in the winter.

No trucks nor even horses and wagons, let alone tractors, are available to bear the burdens up and down the mountain sides. This is all done on human backs for which the hearts of the people have been made especially strong.

We are primarily concerned here with the quality of the teeth and the development of the faces that are associated with such splendid hearts and unusual physiques. I made studies of both adults and growing boys and girls, during the summer of 1931, and arranged to have samples of food, particularly dairy products, sent to me about twice a month, summer and winter.

These products have been tested for their mineral and vitamin contents, particularly the fat-soluble activators. The samples were found to be high in vitamins and much higher than the average samples of commercial dairy products in America and Europe, and in the lower areas of Switzerland.

Hay is cut for winter feeding of the cattle, and this hay grows rapidly. The hay proved, on chemical analysis made at my laboratory, to be far above the average in quality for pasturage and storage grasses.

Almost every household has goats or cows or both. In the summer the cattle seek the higher pasturage lands and follow the retreating snow which leaves the lower valley free for the harvesting of the hay and rye.

The turning of the soil is done by hand, since there are neither plows nor draft animals to drag the plows, in preparation for the next year's rye crop. A limited amount of garden stuff is grown, chiefly green foods for summer use. While the cows spend the warm summer on the verdant knolls and wooded slopes near the glaciers and fields of perpetual snow, they have a period of high and rich productivity of milk.

The milk constitutes an important part of the summer's harvesting. While the men and boys gather in the hay and rye, the women and children go in large numbers with the cattle to collect the milk and make and store cheese for the following winter's use. This cheese contains the natural butter fat and minerals of the splendid milk and is a virtual storehouse of life for the coming winter.

From Dr. Siegen, I learned much about the life and customs of these people. He told me that they recognize the presence of Divinity in the life-giving qualities of the butter made in June when the cows have arrived for pasturage near the glaciers. He gathers the people together to thank the kind Father for the evidence of his Being in the life-giving qualities of butter and cheese made when the cows eat the grass near the snow line.

This worshipful program includes the lighting of a wick in a bowl of the first butter made after the cows have reached the luscious summer pasturage. This wick is permitted to burn in a special sanctuary built for the purpose. The natives of the valley are able to recognize the superior quality of their June butter, and, without knowing exactly why, pay it due homage.

The nutrition of the people of the Loetschental Valley, particularly that of the growing boys and girls, consists largely of a slice of whole rye bread and a piece of the summer-made cheese (about as large as the slice of bread), which are eaten with fresh milk of goats or cows.

Meat is eaten about once a week. In the light of our newer knowledge of activating substances, including vitamins, and the relative values of food for supplying minerals for body building, it is clear why they have healthy bodies and sound teeth. The average total fat-soluble activator and mineral intake of calcium and phosphorus of these children would far exceed that of the daily intake of the average American child.

The sturdiness of the child life permits children to play and frolic bareheaded and barefooted even in water running down from the glacier in the late evening's chilly breezes, in weather that made us wear our overcoats and gloves and button our collars.

Of all the children in the valley still using the primitive diet of whole rye bread and dairy products the average number of cavities per person was 0.3. On an average it was necessary to examine three

---

It is clear from this verse that the residents of Vrndavana had become highly prosperous simply by protecting cows. Well-tended cows produce large quantities of milk, from which come cheese, butter, yogurt, ghee and so on. These foods are delicious by themselves and also enhance other foods, such as fruits, vegetables and grains. Bread and vegetables are delicious with butter, and fruit is especially appetizing when mixed with cream or yogurt. Dairy products are always desirable in civilized society, and the surplus can be traded for many valuable commodities. Thus, simply by a Vedic dairy enterprise, the residents of Vrndavana were wealthy, healthy and happy, even in the material sense, and most of all they were eternal associates of the Supreme Lord Krishna.

~ Srila Prabhupada (Srimad Bhagavatam 10.25.6)

---

persons to find one defective deciduous or permanent tooth. The children examined were between seven and sixteen years of age.

One understands why doors do not need to be bolted in the Loetschental Valley.

How different the level of life and horizon of such souls from those in many places in the so-called civilized world in which people have degraded themselves until life has no interest in values that cannot be expressed in gold or money, which they would obtain even though the life of the person being cheated or robbed would thereby be crippled or blotted out.

One immediately wonders if there is not something in the life-giving vitamins and minerals of the food that builds not only great physical structures within which their souls reside, but builds minds and hearts capable of a higher type of manhood in which the material values of life are made secondary to individual character. In succeeding chapters we will see evidence that this is the case.

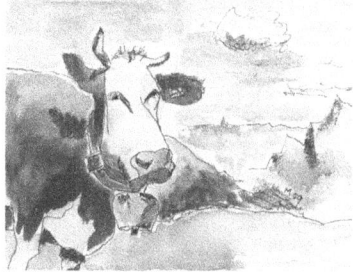

Our quest has been for information relative to the health of the body, the perfection of the teeth, and the normality of development of faces and dental arches, in order that we might through an analysis of the foods learn the secret of such splendid body building and learn from the people of the valley how the nutrition of all groups of people may be reinforced, so that they, too, may be free from mankind's most universal disease, tooth decay and its sequelae.

These studies included not only the making of a physical examination of the teeth, the photographing of subjects, the recording of voluminous data, the obtaining of samples of food for chemical analysis, the collecting of detailed information regarding daily menus; but also the collecting of samples of saliva for chemical analysis.

These children will, it is hoped, be reexamined in succeeding years in order to make comparative studies of the effect of the changes in the local nutritional programs. Some of these changes are already in progress. There is now a modern bakery dispensing white bread and many white-flour products which was in full operation in 1932.

I inquired of many persons regarding the most favorable districts in which to make further studies of groups of people living in protected isolation because of their physical environment, and decided to study some special high Alpine valleys between the Rhone Valley and Italy, which I included in 1932.

Our first expedition was into the valley of the Visp which is a great gorge extending southward from the Rhone River, dividing into two gorges.

We left the mountain railroad, which makes many of the grades with the cog system, at the town of St. Nicholas, and climbed the mountain trail to an isolated settlement on the east bank of the Mattervisp River, called Grachen, a five-hour journey.

The settlement is on a shelf high above the east side of the river where it is exposed to southern sunshine and enjoys a unique isolation because of its physical inaccessibility. An examination made of the children in this community showed that only 2.3 teeth out of every hundred had been attacked by tooth decay.

The hardihood of the people was splendidly illustrated by a woman of 62 years who carried an enormous load of rye on her back at an altitude of about 5,000 feet. We met her later and talked to her, and found that she was extraordinarily well developed and well preserved. She showed us her grandchildren who had fine physiques and facial developments.

The rye is so precious that while being carried the heads are protected by wrapping them in canvas so that not a kernel will be lost. The rye is thrashed by hand and ground in stone mills which were formerly hand-turned. Recently water turbines have been installed. Water power is abundant and the grinding is done for the people of the mountain side in these water-driven mills. Only whole rye flour is available. Each household takes turns in using the community bake-oven. A month's supply of whole-rye bread is baked at one time for a given family. Here again the cows were away in the midsummer, pasturing up near the glaciers. Grachen has an altitude of about 5,000 feet. The church at Grachen was built several hundred years ago.

The children have goat's milk in the summer when the cows are away in the higher pastures near the snow line. Certain members of the families go to the higher pastures with the cows to make cheese for the coming winter's use.

The problem of identifying goats or cattle for establishing individual ownership is a considerable one where the stock of all are pastured in common herds. It was interesting to us to observe how this problem was met.

The president of the village has what is called a "tessel" which is a string of manikins in imitation of goats or cattle made of wood and leather. Every stock owner must provide a manikin to be left in the safekeeping of the president of the village with whom it is registered. It carries on it the individual markings that this member of the colony agrees to put on every member of his animal stock. The marking may be a hole punched in the left ear or a slit in the right ear, or any combination of such markings as is desired. Thereafter all animals carrying that mark are the property of the person who registered it; similarly, any animals that have not this individual symbol of identification cannot be claimed by him.

As one stands in profound admiration before the stalwart physical development and high moral character of these sturdy mountaineers, he is impressed by the superior types of manhood, womanhood, and childhood that Nature has been able to produce from a suitable diet and a suitable environment.

Surely, the ultimate control will be found in Nature's laboratory where man has not yet been able to meddle sufficiently with Nature's nutritional program to blight humanity with abnormal and synthetic nutrition.

When one has watched for days the childlife in those high Alpine preserves of superior manhood; when one has contrasted these people with the pinched and sallow, and even deformed, faces and distorted bodies that are produced by our modern civilization and its diets; and when one has contrasted the unsurpassed beauty of the faces of these children developed on Nature's primitive foods with the varied assortment of modern civilization's children with their defective facial development, he finds himself filled with an earnest desire to see that this betterment is made available for modern civilization.

Again and again we had the experience of examining a young man or young woman and finding that at some period of his life tooth decay had been rampant and had suddenly ceased; but, during the stress, some teeth had been lost. When we asked such people whether they had gone out of the mountain and at what age, they generally replied that at eighteen or twenty years of age they had gone to this or that city and had stayed a year or two. They stated that they had never had a decayed tooth before they went or after they returned, but that they had lost some teeth in the short period away from home.

The village of Ayer lies in a beautiful valley well up toward the glaciers. It is still largely primitive, although a government road has recently been developed, which, like many of the new arteries, has made it possible to dispatch military protection when and if necessary to any community. In this beautiful hamlet, until recently isolated, we found a high immunity to dental caries. Only 2.3 teeth out of each hundred examined were found to have been attacked by tooth decay. Here again the people were living on rye and dairy products.

We wonder if history will repeat itself in the next few years and if there, too, this enviable immunity will be lost with the advent of the highway. Usually it is not long after tunnels and roads are built that automobiles and wagons enter with modern foods, which begin their destructive work.

This fact has been tragically demonstrated in this valley since a roadway was extended as far as Vissoie several years ago. In this village modern foods have been available for some time. One could probably walk the distance from Ayer to Vissoie in an hour. The number of teeth found to be attacked with caries for each one hundred children's teeth examined at Vissoie was 20.2 as compared with 2.3 at Ayer.

We had here a splendid opportunity to study the changes that had occurred in the nutritional programs. With the coming of transportation and new markets there had been shipped in modern white flour; equipment for a bakery to make white-flour goods; highly sweetened fruit, such as jams, marmalades, jellies, sugar and syrups—all to be traded for the locally produced high-vitamin dairy products and high-mineral cheese and rye; and with the exchange there was enough money as premium to permit buying machine-made clothing and various novelties that would soon be translated into necessities.

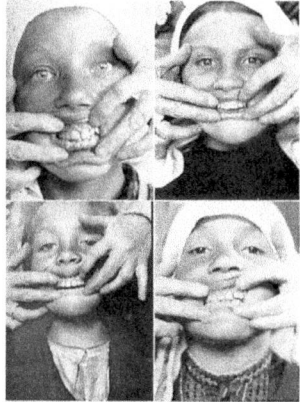

Each valley or village has its own special feast days of which athletic contests are the principal events. The feasting in the past has been largely on dairy products. The athletes were provided with large bowls of cream as constituting one of the most popular and healthful beverages, and special cheese was always available. Practically no wine was used because no grapes grew in that valley, and for centuries

Normal design of face and dental arches when adequate nutrition is provided for both the parents and the children. Note the well developed nostrils.

the isolation of the people prevented access to much material that would provide wine.

It is reported that practically all skulls that are exhumed in the Rhone valley, and, indeed, practically throughout all of Switzerland where graves have existed for more than a hundred years, show relatively perfect teeth; whereas the teeth of people recently buried have been riddled with caries or lost through this disease.

It is of interest that each church usually has associated with it a cemetery in which the graves are kept decorated, often with beautiful designs of fresh or artificial flowers. Members of succeeding generations of families are said to be buried one above the other to a depth of many feet. Then, after a sufficient number of generations have been so honored, their bodies are exhumed to make a place for present and coming generations. These skeletons are usually preserved with honor and deference. The bones are stacked in basements of certain buildings of the church edifice with the skulls facing outward. These often constitute a solid wall of considerable extent. In Naters there is such a group said to contain 20,000 skeletons and skulls.

These were studied with great interest as was also a smaller collection in connection with the cathedral at Visp. While many of the single straight-rooted teeth had been lost in the handling, many were present. It was a matter of importance to find that only a small percentage of teeth had had caries. Teeth that had been attacked with deep caries had developed apical abscesses with consequent destruction of the alveolar processes. Evidence of this bone change was readily visible. Sockets of missing teeth still had continuous walls, indicating that the teeth had been vital at death.

The reader will scarcely believe it possible that such marked differences in facial form, in the shape of the dental arches, and in the health condition of the teeth as are to be noted when passing from the highly modernized lower valleys and plains country in Switzerland to the isolated high valleys can exist.

Photo with the healthy teeth shows four girls with typically broad dental arches and regular arrangement of the teeth. They have been born and raised in the Loetschental Valley or other isolated valleys of Switzerland which provide the excellent nutrition that we have been reviewing.

They have been taught little regarding the use of tooth brushes. Their teeth have typical deposits of unscrubbed mouths; yet they are almost completely free from dental caries, as are the other individuals of the group they represent.

In a study of 4,280 teeth of the children of these high valleys, only 3.4 per cent were found to have been attacked by tooth decay. This is in striking contrast to conditions found in the modernized sections using the modern foods.

In Loetschental, Grachen, Visperterminen and Ayer, we have found communities of native Swiss living almost exclusively on locally produced foods consisting of the cereal, rye, and the animal product, milk, in its various forms.

When we move on to a place where modern nutrition is available, there is a complete change in the level of immunity to dental caries. St. Moritz is one of such places.

It is situated in the southeastern part of the Republic of Switzerland near the headwaters of the Danube. This world-famous watering place attracts people of all continents for both summer and winter health building and for the enjoyment of the mountain lakes, snow-capped peaks, forested mountain sides, and crystal clear atmosphere with abundance of sunshine.

It is of significance that a study of the child life here, as reported by Swiss officials shows that practically every child had tooth decay and the majority of the children had decay in an aggravated form. People of this place are provided with adequate railroad transportation for bringing them the luxuries of the world.

Here almost everyone wears one of English walking coats and the most elegant of feminine attire. Everyone shows the effect of contact with culture. The hotels in their appointments and design are reminiscent of Atlantic City.

Immediately one sees something is different here than in the primitive localities: the children do not have the splendidly developed features, and the people give no evidence of the great physical reserve that is present in the smaller communities.

Through the kindness of Dr. William Barry, a local dentist, and through that of the superintendent of the public schools, we were invited to use one of the school buildings for our studies of the children. The summer classes were dismissed with instructions that the children be retained so that we could have them for study.

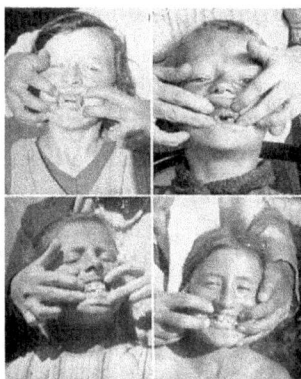

In the modernized districts of Switzerland tooth decay is rampant. The girl, upper left, is sixteen and the one to the right is younger. They use white bread and sweets liberally. The two children below have very badly formed dental arches with crowding of the teeth. This deformity is not due to heredity.

Several factors were immediately apparent. The teeth were shining and clean, giving eloquent testimony of the thoroughness of the instructions in the use of the modern dentifrices for efficient oral prophylaxis. The gums looked better and the teeth more beautiful for having the debris and deposits removed.

Surely this superb climate, this magnificent setting, combined with the best of the findings of modern prophylactic science, should provide a 100-per-cent immunity to tooth decay. But in a study of the children from eight to fifteen years of age, 29.8 per cent of the teeth had already been attacked by dental caries.

Our study of each case included careful examining of the mouth; photographing of the face and teeth; obtaining of samples of saliva for chemical analysis; and a study of the program of nutrition followed by the given case. In most cases, the diet was strikingly modern, and the only children found who did not have tooth decay proved to be children who were eating the natural foods, whole rye bread and plenty of milk.

I was told by a former resident of this place that in one of the isolated valleys only a few decades ago the children were still carrying their luncheons to school in the form of roasted rye carried dry in their pockets. Their ancestors had eaten cereal in this dry form for centuries.

St. Moritz is provided with modern nutrition consisting of an abundance of white-flour products, marmalades, jams, canned vegetables, confections, and fruits—all of which are transported to the district. Only a limited supply of vegetables is grown locally.

We studied some children here whose parents retained their primitive methods of food selection, and without exception those who were immune to dental caries were eating a distinctly different food from those with high susceptibility to dental caries.

In the section lying to the north and east, and near Lake Constance, there is a considerable district where it is reported that 100 per cent of the people are suffering from dental caries. In almost all the other parts of Switzerland, 95 to 98 per cent of the people suffer from dental caries.

Many individuals in the modernized districts bore on their faces scars which indicated that the abscess of an infected tooth had broken through to the external surface where it had developed a fistula with resultant scar tissue, thus producing permanent deformity.

We found an occasional child with much better teeth than the average. Usually the answer was not far to seek. For example, in one of the St. Moritz groups, in a class of sixteen boys, there were 158 cavities, or an average of 9.8 cavities per person (fillings are counted as cavities). In the cases of three other children in the same group, there were only three cavities, and one case was without dental caries. Two of these three had been eating dark bread or entire-grain bread, and one was eating dark bread and oatmeal porridge. All three drank milk liberally.

When looking here for the source of dairy products one is impressed by the absence of cows at pasture in the plains of Switzerland, areas in which a large percentage of the entire population resides. True, one frequently sees large creameries, but the cows are not in sight.

On asking the explanation for this, I found that a larger quantity of milk could be obtained from the cows if they were kept in the stables during the period of high production. Indeed, this was a necessity in most of these communities since there were so few fences, and during the time of the growth of the crops, including the stock feed for the winter's use, it was necessary that the cows be kept enclosed. About the only time that cows were allowed out on pasture was in the fall after the crops had been harvested and while the stubble was being plowed.

Since so many cattle were stall-fed in the thickly populated part of Switzerland, and since so low a proportion of the children used milk even sparingly, I was concerned to know what use was made of the milk. Numerous road signs announcing the brand of sweetened milk chocolate made in the several districts suggested one use. This chocolate is one of the important products for export and a popular beverage.

When I asked a government official what the principal diseases of the community were, he said that the most serious and most universal was dental caries, and the next most important, tuberculosis; and that both were largely modern diseases in that country.

When I visited the famous advocate of heliotherapy, Dr. Rollier, in his clinic in Leysin, Switzerland, I wondered at the remarkable results he was obtaining with heliotherapy in nonpulmonary tuberculosis. I asked him how many patients he had under his general supervision and he said about thirty-five hundred. I then asked him how many of them come from the isolated Alpine valleys and he said that there was not one; but that they were practically all from the Swiss plains, with some from other countries.

I inquired of several clinicians in Switzerland what their observations were with regard to the association of dental caries and tuberculosis among the people of Switzerland. I noted that the reports indicated that the two diseases were generally associated. We will find a corollary to this in many studies in other parts of the world.

These studies in Switzerland, as briefly presented here, seem to demonstrate that the isolated groups dependent on locally produced natural foods have nearly complete natural immunity to dental caries, and that the substitution of modern dietaries for these primitive natural foods destroys this immunity whether in ideally located elevated districts like St. Moritz or in the beautiful and fertile plains of lower Switzerland. The question seems to answer itself in a general way, without much laboratory data, from the results of a critical examination of the foods.

High immunity to dental caries, freedom from deformity of the dental arches and face, and sturdy physiques with high immunity to disease were all found associated with physical isolation, and with forced limitation in selection of foods. This resulted in a very liberal use of dairy products and whole-rye bread, in connection with plant foods, and with meat served about only once a week.

The individuals in the modernized districts were making liberal use of refined cereal flours, sweets, canned goods, sweetened fruits, chocolate; and a greatly reduced use of dairy products.

Anthropocentric as [the gardener] may be, he recognizes that he is dependent for his health and survival on many other forms of life, so he is careful to take their interests into account in whatever he does. He is in fact a wilderness advocate of a certain kind. It is when he respects and nurtures the wilderness of his soil and his plants that his garden seems to flourish most. Wildness, he has found, resides not only out there, but right here: in his soil, in his plants, even in himself...

But wildness is more a quality than a place, and though humans can't manufacture it, they can nourish and husband it...

The gardener cultivates wildness, but he does so carefully and respectfully, in full recognition of its mystery."

~Michael Pollan, Second Nature: A Gardener's Education

42.

Remnants of Swiss Milk Culture

In the Footsteps of Dr. Weston A. Price

By Linda Joyce

In his global travels during the 1930s, Weston A. Price sought out locations where people were not yet eating what he called the "displacing food of modern commerce." One of the places Price visited was Switzerland's Lötschental--an isolated valley then only accessible by a footpath. It was so isolated from the rest of Switzerland, let alone the world, that the residents existed on what they could grow in the valley, with no food brought in from outside, with the exception of salt.

Their diet primarily consisted of dairy products (raw milk, butter, cream and raw milk cheese) from cows grazing on lush alpine slopes, and rye bread, or roggenbrot, from rye grown in the valley. They ate little meat about once a week and some vegetables during the summer months. The raw milk, butter and cream from cows eating lush green grass were a rich source of vitamins A and D.

With the help of a Swiss dentist who was his travel companion and the community elders, Price was able to examine the mouths of many valley inhabitants. He reported that the majority of the residents had healthy, straight teeth. Price only found one cavity in every three mouths, which was about 1 percent tooth decay.

Both adults and children had broad, well-developed faces and palates, good dispositions and sturdy bodies. He noted that the children played barefoot in frigid streams during cold weather and that there were no cases of TB in the valley.

In other parts of Switzerland, Price studied the "modernized Swiss," who lived in towns accessible by roads and therefore got their food from stores selling sugar, white flour, pastries, jams and jellies, canned condensed milk, canned foods and vegetable oils.

They were experiencing dental caries in one tooth in three, or 33 percent tooth decay, and the younger generations had dental deformities, overlapping, crowded and crooked teeth and narrow faces. TB was a huge problem in these communities.

Revisiting The Valley

In June of 2003, about 70 years after Price's visit, I revisited the Lötschental. The valley consists of four small picturesque towns accessible by car and bus from the entrance of the valley near the train station. At the far end of valley is a glacier.

Price described the good health and sturdiness of the Lötschental men who often took jobs in the Pope's Swiss Guard. They also served the kingdoms of Versailles and Naples and were mercenaries in foreign countries.

The day after I arrived, the locals were constructing mini altars to honor the Virgin Mary, several in each of the valley towns. The backdrop for each altar was pine branches cut from the alpine forest. On the next day, the townspeople assembled and ceremonially marched to the church for a special mass.

Despite all this religious activity, there was no evidence of an ancient ceremony recalled by Price--lighting a wick in a bowl of the first spring butter--to honor the life-giving force contained therein.

According to Price, the wick was permitted to burn in a special sanctuary built for the purpose. At least back then, the natives recognized the superior quality of their June butter, perhaps without really understanding why. At first impression, it seems that this ceremony is now forgotten.

Vanishing Agriculture

The tourism authority for the valley, Lötschental Tourism, always ends their emails with the signature, "Friendly Greeting from the Valley of Valleys." It is a beautiful valley and one to be proud of for its majestic scenery and beautiful architecture.

However, what I saw in the valley was a culture in danger of losing its agricultural roots. To be blunt, junk foods abounded. While our half-board arrangement at the hotel gave us a good breakfast with cheese and bread in the morning and a hot meal for the evening meal, it was hard to find good food in the stores. And we were served pale, commercial butter with each meal instead of golden alpine butter, rich in nutrients.

Some restaurants still serve rye bread and raw milk cheese as an entrée or appetizer, but most of the small stores are filled with processed foods like chips, candy and soft drinks. Oftentimes, alpine butter sat next to ultra-high temperature pasteurized (UHT) milk on the grocery shelf. Switzerland is, after all, headquarters to Nestlé.

Dwindling Dairies

During our stay in the valley, we learned that the inhabitants are slowly abandoning farming due to the fact that they cannot make a living wage. Over the past few decades a large exodus from the valley to look for work has left the older inhabitants to take care of the dwindling dairies. Most of these workers are women.

When I finally sufficiently explained my desire to the valley tourism officials to see "cows and milk," I was taken to a spot off the main valley road called Chiemad--Kühmad, or "cow path."

With our guide in lead, we walked up a very long steep hill through a pasture towards a lean-to in the far distance. I was told this is where we would find some cows and hopefully some signs of activity and someone to interview. I was rapidly loosing steam and were out of breath, when we saw a dairywoman approaching at fast pace down the path we were struggling so hard to ascend.

I asked the tourism official to ask her to stop so I could take a picture, but he would not. So, I tried to get her attention, but she just kept moving--either ashamed or shy of getting her picture taken. Hence, I got pictures of her coming and going, with a 50-pound container of milk strapped to her back.

As she continued to descend, we kept going up the pasture towards the aforementioned lean-tos. When we arrived, we found a couple of cows in the shack resting after having been milked. I was told they would probably stay there the night and be let out the morning to forage on the alpine grass and flowers again. By the time we were finished looking around, the woman had disappeared.

The morning of my departure, I was determined to make a deeper connection to what appeared to be the vanishing dairy culture of the valley. Unable to persuade the tourism officials to take me to a high-alpine dairy above 3,000 meters, I decided to camp out at the valley's main cheese factory in Wiler to see who came to deposit their morning milk.

First, a local milk lady arrived with milk cans on a humble pull cart. After about a half hour, a muscular and tanned woman arrived with several milk cans piled in the back of her SUV. She had just milked her cows on the high-alpine pasture and had driven the milk down to the dairy. She only spoke German, so I interviewed her with my intermediate German skills. I found out that she only had six cows and spent the summer living with them at high altitude. I so wished I had been introduced to her on the day of my arrival.

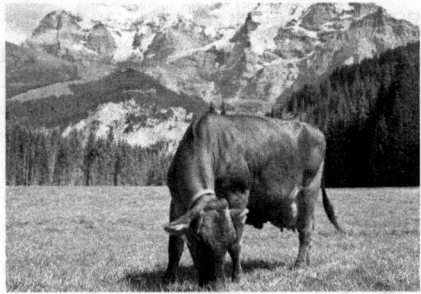

Through my research, I learned that the main Lötschental dairy makes three kinds of cheese. First, there is Lötschental Mutschli, which is made from both raw and pasteurized milk and is formed into small wheels weighing one-half to one kilogram, and then aged 6-12 weeks. It is championed as a cheeese that captures the taste of alpine flora.

The bulk of the valley's milk goes into cut cheese, a second kind of cheese in which the curdled milk is cut to produce curds and then pressed to express the whey and form 2-5 kg wheels or logs.

My favorite is the third kind of Lötschental cheese, Hobel käse, a hard cheese made exclusively from raw milk that is typically fashioned into large wheels and then aged 1-3 years. Unfortunately, the dairy store was never open for business when I passed by--and definitely not early in the morning when the dairywomen come to deposit their milk.

When I got home, I decided to contact the Swiss government to obtain agriculture data about the valley. Although it took a few months, I was finally presented with some astoundingly interesting data from the Census of Agricultural Establishment that dates back to the 1920s.

Since agriculture has historically been very important to Switzerland, the government has gathered agricultural data for decades. That data includes the number of agriculture establishments in the Lötschental, obtained by combining data from all four villages.

In 1929, the Lötschental was home to 205 farms and employed 690 farm workers aged 15 or older, but by the year 2000, the official number of farms had fallen to 75 and the full-time workers to 13. Also, the valley has made some steps to embrace ski tourism as a path to economic development and some of the pastures have been lost to ski chalets.

Year	No. of farms	Full-time Workers
1929	205	690
1939	228	742
1955	215	374
1965	185	86
1975	143	29
1985	128	26
1996	104	20
2000	75	13

Another source of data was the Federal Population Census, which counts not only people but livestock as well. Although the dates don't quite match, these figures show the number of "milking cows" in the Lötschental over almost seven decades--and tell a similar story.

Year	No. Of Cows Producing Milk
1936	357
1951	349
1966	347
1978	214
1985	143
1996	126
2000	89

I did not find one person who knew who Dr. Weston A. Price was or had heard of his travels to the valley. Although the valley and region has tourist offerings all year long, I believe summer is the best time to see the remnants of its milk culture.

"People have traditionally turned to ritual to help them frame and acknowledge and ultimately even find joy in just such a paradox of being human - in the fact that so much of what we desire for our happiness and need for our survival comes at a heavy cost. We kill to eat, we cut down trees to build our homes, we exploit other people and the earth. Sacrifice - of nature, of the interests of others, even of our earlier selves - appears to be an inescapable part of our condition, the unavoidable price of all our achievements.

A successful ritual is one that addresses both aspects of our predicament, recalling us to the shamefulness of our deeds at the same time it celebrates what the poet Frederick Turner calls "the beauty we have paid for with our shame." Without the double awareness pricked by such rituals, people are liable to find themselves either plundering the earth without restraint or descending into self-loathing and misanthropy. Perhaps it's not surprising that most of us today bring one of those attitudes or the other to our conduct in nature."

~Michael Pollan, A Place of My Own: The Education of an Amateur Builder

43.

Secrets Of Survival - Frozen In Time

Isolated And Modernized Eskimos

By Dr. Weston A. Price

During the rise and fall of historic and prehistoric cultures that have often left their monuments and arts following each other in succession in the same location, one culture, the Eskimo, living on until today, brings us a robust sample of an ancient race. The Maya race is gone, but has left its monuments.

The Indian race is rapidly changing or disappearing in North America. The Eskimo race has remained true to ancestral type to give us a living demonstration of what Nature can do in the building of a race competent to withstand for thousands of years the rigors of an Arctic climate.

Like the Indian, the Eskimo thrived as long as he was not blighted by the touch of modern civilization, but with it, like all primitives, he withers and dies.

In his primitive state he has provided an example of physical excellence and dental perfection such as has seldom been excelled by any race in the past or present. We are concerned to know the secret of this great achievement since his circumscribed life greatly reduces the factors that may enter as controlling units in molding this excellence.

While we are primarily concerned in this study with the characteristics of the Eskimo dentition and facial form and the effect upon it of his contact with modern civilization, we are also deeply concerned to know the formula of his nutrition in order that we may learn from it the secrets that will not only aid the unfortunate modern or so-called civilized races, but will also, if possible, provide means for assisting in their preservation.

It is a sad commentary that with the coming of the white man the Eskimos and Indians are rapidly reduced both in numbers and physical excellence by the white man's diseases. We have few problems more urgent or more challenging than that means shall soon be found for preventing the extermination of the primitive Americans.

Many reports have been made with regard to the condition of the teeth of the Eskimos. Doubtless, all have been relatively authentic for the groups studied, which have been chiefly along the routes of commerce. Clearly those people would not represent the most primitive groups, which could only be located beyond the reach of contact with modern civilization.

The problems involved strongly suggested the desirability of locating and studying Eskimos in isolated districts. While dog teams could furnish means of approach in the winter season, they would not be available for summer travel.

Through the kindness of Dr. Alexis Hrdlicka, who has made anthropological studies of the Eskimos in many of the districts of Alaska, I learned that the most primitive groups were located south of the Yukon in the country between it and Bristol Bay including the Delta and mouth of the Kuskokwim River.

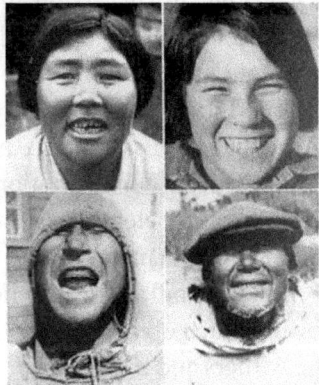

Typical native Alaskan Eskimos. Note the broad faces and broad arches and no dental caries (tooth decay). Upper left, woman has a broken lower tooth. She has had twenty-six children with no tooth decay.

A government station has been established on the Kuskokwim River for which a government boat enters the mouth of the Kuskokwim to deliver supplies. It carries officials, but not passengers.

This contact with civilization has made available modern foods for a limited district, chiefly at the point at which the boat lands, namely, Bethel. A portion of these supplies is transported by a stern-wheel river boat to settlements farther up the river.

A great number, however, of Eskimos live between the mouth of the Kuskokwim and the mouth of the Yukon River, on the mainland and islands, a distance of several hundred miles, and have little or no contact with this food.

Accordingly, our program for making these field studies among the Eskimos in 1933 required transportation over long distances and into districts where travelling facilities were practically non-existent by other means than by modern aeroplane. Mrs. Price accompanies and assisted me with my records.

Our itinerary included steamship service to Seward in western Alaska and railway to Anchorage, where an aeroplane was chartered which carried us to various districts in western and central Alaska. This plane carried our field equipment, and travelled to the points selected.

The great Alaska mountain range, culminating in the magnificent Mt. McKinley, stretches across Alaska from

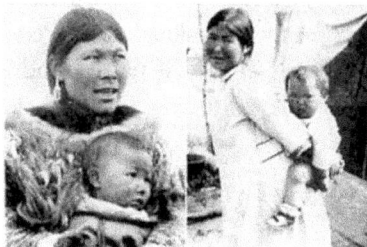

These primitive Alaskan mothers rear strong, rugged babies. The mothers do not suffer from dental caries.

the Aleutian Peninsula at the southwest far into the heart of this vast territory.

The highest mountain in the United States proper is Mt. Whitney, 14,502 feet. The highest mountain in Canada is Mt. Logan, 19,539 feet. Alaska, however, boasts many mountains that are higher than any of these, many of which are in this range. Mt. McKinley is 20,300 feet.

It was necessary for us to surmount this magnificent range to reach the territory in which our investigations were to be made. The special aeroplane selected was equipped with radio for both sending and receiving, and was in touch, or could be in touch at all times, with the Signal Service Corps, as well as with the headquarters and branches of the Company.

Owing to clouds in the selected pass, the pilot found it necessary to go one hundred fifty miles out of his course to find one that was clear enough to fly through. Beyond these mountains were vast areas of bare wilderness with no signs of human life. Moose were frequently seen.

Our first objective was to find, if possible, a band of Indians reported to live on Stony River. They had been described as being very primitive. Our pilot, who was well informed about this region, said this was the first time he had even landed in this district.

When we found a group of Indians, they were busy catching and storing the running salmon. After drying the fish they are smoked for a few hours and then stored for winter use. These thrifty people have physical features quite unlike the Indians of central, southern and eastern Alaska. Of the twelve individuals studied here, ten had lived entirely on the native foods or practically so. In their 288 teeth only one tooth was found that had ever been attacked by tooth decay, or 0.3 per cent.

Two had come up from the Kuskokwim River, of which the Stony River is a branch. There, they had received a considerable quantity of the "store grub" that had been shipped up the Kuskokwim from Bethel. Twenty-seven per cent of the teeth of these two had been attacked by dental caries.

We then proceeded to Sleet Mute, on the Kuskokwim River, where three individuals were found who had lived entirely on native foods. None of them had ever had a tooth attacked by tooth decay. Seven others had lived partly on native foods and partly on "store grub," and they had dental caries in 12.2 per cent of their teeth.

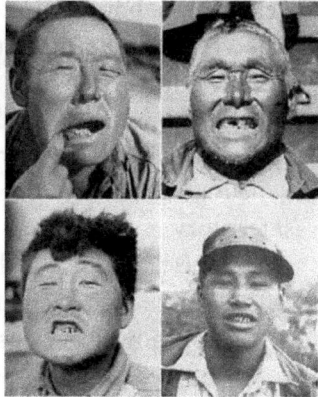

When the primitive Alaskan Eskimos obtain the white man's foods, dental caries become active. Pyorrhea also often becomes severe. In many districts dental service cannot be obtained and suffering is acute and prolonged.

In the various groups in the lower Kuskokwim seventy-two individuals who were living exclusively on native foods had in their 2,138 teeth only two teeth or 0.09 per cent that had ever been attacked by tooth decay. In this district eighty-one individuals were studied who had been living in part or in considerable part on modern foods, and of their 2,254 teeth 394 or 13 per cent had been attacked by dental caries. This represents an increase in dental caries of 144 fold.

It is of interest that while the Eskimos and Indians have lived in accord, they have not intermarried.

An average adult Eskimo man can carry one hundred pounds in each hand and one hundred pounds in his teeth with ease for a considerable distance.

Owing to the bleakness of the winds off the Bering Sea, even in the summer many of the women wear furs. The Eskimo women are both artistic and skillful in needle work. They use fur of different colors for decorating their garments. These women make artistic decorations by carving ivory from walrus teeth. Their teeth are literally "two rows of pearls." It is important to note the width of the arches.

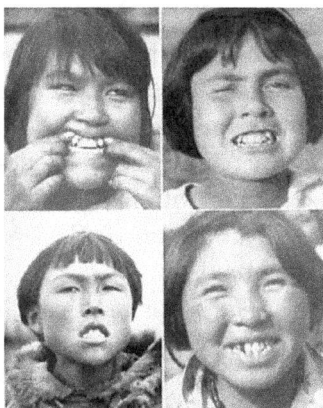

While dental arch deformities or crowded teeth are practically unknown among many of the primitive groups of Eskimos, they occur frequently in the first generation of children born after the parents have adopted the white man's foods. Note the narrow nostrils and changed facial form of these children. This is not due to thumb sucking.

One is continually impressed with the magnificent health of the child life. In our various contacts with them we never heard an Eskimo child crying except when hungry, or frightened by the presence of strangers. The women are characterized by the abundance of breastfood which almost always develops normally and is maintained without difficulty for a year.

> "The human animal is adapted to, and apparently can thrive on, an extraordinary range of different diets, but the Western diet, however you define it, does not seem to be one of them."
> ~ Michael Pollan, In Defense of Food: An Eater's Manifesto

The mothers were completely free of dental caries, and the children of the Eskimos had equally strong teeth.

Since contact with our modern civilization, the Eskimo population for Alaska is very rapidly declining. One authority has quoted the reduction of 50 per cent in population in seventy-five years.

Due to susceptibility to tuberculosis and other diseases the average life span of the Eskimo of Alaska is only 20 years and their race is doomed to extinction within a few generations unless modern medical science comes to their aid.

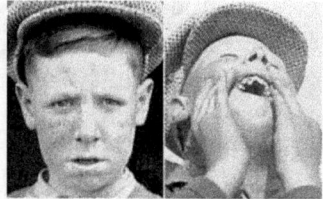

This white boy was born and raised in Alaska on imported foods. His facial deformity includes a lack of development of the air passages, so that he breathes through his mouth. Lack of bone development creates the crowded condition of the teeth. Note his narrow nostrils.

Unless a very radical change is made in the interference with the native supply of game and sea foods, the Eskimo population seems destined to have a rapid decline and an early extinction. Their primitive fish foods have been largely curtailed by the encroachment on their salmon streams made by modern canneries.

Notwithstanding the very inhospitable part of the world in which they reside, with nine or ten months of winter and only two or three of summer, and in spite of the absence for long periods of plant foods and dairy products, the Eskimos were able to provide their bodies with all the mineral and vitamin requirements from sea foods, stored greens and berries and plants from the sea.

44.

Primitive And Modernized North American Indians

Survival In Extreme Climates, With No Possibility Of Dairy Or Agriculture

By Dr. Weston A. Price

That the Indian of today is not in general a counterpart of the native resident at the time of the discovery of America by Columbus is clearly demonstrated both by the skeletal material and by the early records.

Our problem involved the location and study of groups of the original stock, if such were to be found, who were living in accordance with the tradition of their race and as little affected as might be possible by the influence of the white man.

At first thought it might seem impossible that such groups can exist, but as a matter of fact there are still great areas of the American continent inhabited by the original stock living in areas still unexplored.

In order to find Indians as little changed as possible by reason of their contact with the white man, particularly with the white man's foods, I went to northern Canada to the region inside the Rocky Mountain range to study the Indians of Northern British Columbia and the Yukon territory.

Since an aeroplane could not be used, owing to the lack of a base of supplies for fuel for the return trip; and since the MacKenzie water route was impracticable (an expedition could not go up the waterways through Canada on the MacKenzie River and its branches and return the same season), the route selected was that which enters that territory from Alaska on the large waterway of the Stikine River.

This river has cut its channel through the Coast and Cascade Ranges of mountains and has its origin in the high western watershed of the Rockies. It was particularly desirable to reach a group of Indians who could not obtain the animal life of the sea, not even the running salmon. These fish do not enter the waterways draining to the Arctic.

We used a high-powered river transport specially designed for going up rapids on the Stikine River to the end of navigation at Telegraph Creek. At this point large quantities of modern foods are stored during the short open navigation season of the summer to be exchanged for furs during the long winter. A Hudson Bay Post has been established at this point.

Here a truck was chartered which took us over a trail across the Rocky Mountain Divide to the headwaters of the rivers flowing north to the Arctic. At this outpost two guides were engaged and a high powered scow chartered to make the trip down the waterways toward the Arctic on the Diese and Liard Rivers.

This made it possible, in the summer of 1933, to make contact with large bands of Indians who had come out of the Pelly mountain country to exchange their catch of furs at the last outpost of the Hudson Bay Company.

Most of the Indians of Canada are under treaty with the Canadian Government whereby that government gives them an annual per capita bounty. This arrangement induces the Indians in the interior to come out to the designated centers to obtain the bounty. Since it is based on the number in the family, all of the children are brought.

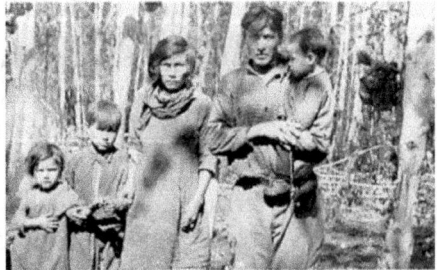

This typical family of forest Indians of Northern Canada presents a picture of superb health.

This treaty, however, was never signed by the Indians of the British Columbia and Yukon Territory. And, accordingly, they have remained as nomadic wandering tribes following the moose and caribou herds in the necessary search to obtain their foods.

The rigorous winters reach seventy degrees below zero. *This precludes the possibility of maintaining dairy animals or growing seed cereals or fruits.* The diet of these Indians is almost entirely limited to the wild animals of the chase. This made a study of them exceedingly important.

The wisdom of these people regarding Nature's laws, and their skill in adapting themselves to the rigorous climate and very limited variety of foods, and these often very hard to obtain, have developed a skill in the art of living comfortably with rugged Nature that has been approached by few other tribes in the world.

The sense of honor among these tribes is so strong that practically all cabins, temporarily unoccupied due to the absence of the Indians on their hunting trip, were entirely unprotected by locks; and the valuables belonging to the Indians were left in plain sight.

The people were remarkably hospitable, and where they had not been taken advantage of were very kind. Many of the women had never seen a white woman until they saw Mrs. Price. Their knowledge of woodcraft as expressed in skill in building their cabins so that they would be kept comfortably warm and protected from the sub-zero weather was remarkable. Their planning ahead for storing

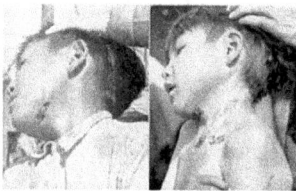

At the point of modernization including the use of the foods of modern commerce, the health problem of the Indians is very different. These modernized Indian children are dying of tuberculosis which seldom kills the primitives.

provisions and firewood strongly emphasized their community spirit. When an Indian and his family moved to a camp site on a lake or river, they always girdled a few more trees than they would use for firewood so that there would be a plentiful supply of dry standing timber for future visitors to the camp.

They lived in a country in which grizzly bears were common. Their pelts were highly prized and they captured many of them with baited pitfalls. Their knowledge of the use of different organs and tissues of the animals for providing a defense against certain of the affections of the body which we speak of as degenerative diseases was surprising.

When I asked an old Indian, through an interpreter, why the Indians did not get scurvy he replied promptly that that was a white man's disease. I asked whether it was possible for the Indians to get scurvy. He replied that it was, but said that the Indians know how to prevent it and the white man does not.

When asked why he did not tell the white man how, his reply was that the white man knew too much to ask the Indian anything. I then asked him if he would tell me. He said he would if the chief said he might.

He went to see the chief and returned in about an hour, saying that the chief said he could tell me because I was a friend of the Indians and had come to tell the Indians not to eat the food in the white man's store.

He took me by the hand and led me to a log where we both sat down. He then described how when the Indian kills a moose he opens it up and at the back of the moose just above the kidney there are what he described as two small balls in the fat. These he said the Indian would take and cut up into as many pieces as there were little and big Indians in the family and each one would eat his piece. They would eat also the walls of the second stomach. By eating these parts of the animal the Indians would keep free from scurvy, which is due to the lack of vitamin C.

The Indians were getting vitamin

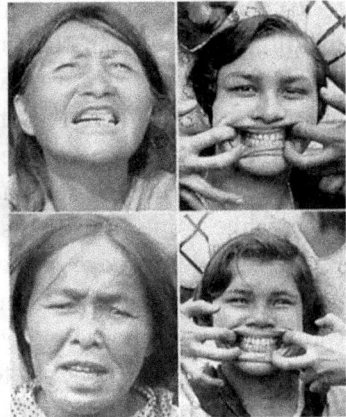

Wherever the Indians were living on their native foods, their physical development including facial and dental arch form was superb with nearly complete immunity to dental caries. These two women and two girls are typical.

C from the adrenal glands and organs. Modern science has very recently discovered that the adrenal glands are the richest sources of vitamin C in all animal or plant tissues. We found these Indians most cooperative in aiding us.

We, of course, had taken presents that we thought would be appreciated by them, and we had no difficulty in making measurements and photographs, nor, indeed, in making a detailed study of the condition of each tooth in the dental arches. I obtained samples of saliva, and of their foods for chemical analysis.

The condition of the teeth, and the shape of the dental arches and the facial form, were superb. Indeed, in several groups examined not a single tooth was found that had ever been attacked by tooth decay.

In an examination of eighty-seven individuals having 2,464 teeth only four teeth were found that had ever been attacked by dental caries. This is equivalent to 0.16 per cent.

As we came back to civilization and studied, successively, different groups with increasing amounts of contact with modern civilization, we found dental caries increased progressively, reaching 25.5 per cent of all of the teeth examined at Telegraph Creek, the point of contact with the white man's foods. As we came down the Stikine River to the Alaskan frontier towns, the dental caries problem increased to 40 per cent of all of the teeth.

Wherever the Indians were living on their native foods, their physical development including facial and dental arch form was superb with nearly complete immunity to dental caries.

A typical mother was studied at her home. She had four children. Her teeth were ravaged by dental caries. She was strictly modern, for she had gold inlays in some of her teeth. The roots of the missing teeth had not been extracted. Twenty of her teeth had active dental caries.

Her little girl, aged four, already

Wherever the Indians had access to the modern foods of commerce the dental conditions were extremely bad. These four individuals are typical.

had twelve very badly carious teeth. Another daughter aged eight had sixteen carious teeth, and her son aged ten had six. The husband was in bed from an acute lung involvement, doubtless tuberculosis.

The children were eating their noon day meal when we arrived, which consisted of a white bread and some stewed vegetables. Milk

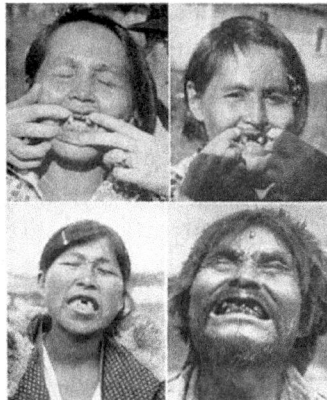

was available for only the small baby in arms. In this Tuscarora group 83 per cent of those examined had dental caries and 38 per cent of all teeth had already been attacked by dental caries.

Every one studied in this reservation was using white-flour products, none were using milk liberally, and only a few in even limited amounts.

I was told that in both reservations a few years ago the Indians grew wheat and kept cows to provide a liberal supply of natural cereal and milk for their families, but of late this practice had been discontinued.

They were now buying their wheat in the form of white flour and their vegetables largely put up in cans. In both reservations they were using commercial vegetable fats, jams and marmalades, sweetened goods, syrups and confections very liberally. It is remarkable how early the child life adopts modern civilization's confections.

The blight of the white man's commerce is seen everywhere in the distorted countenances of even the first generation after the adoption by the parents of the foods of modern commerce. These young people with their deformed dental arches are typical. Note the faulty development of the facial bones as evidenced by the narrow nostrils and crowded teeth.

To find evidence relating to the physical, and particularly to the dental condition of the Indians who inhabited the Pacific slope a thousand or more years ago, a visit was made to the Vancouver Museum at Vancouver which fortunately possesses splendidly preserved specimens of prehistoric periods.

Some of these skulls were uncovered while cutting through a hill for a street extension in the city of Vancouver. Above was a virgin forest of large size green firs and underneath them in the soil there were preserved fallen trunks of other large trees. Several feet below these, burials were uncovered containing skeletons of an early Indian race.

This collection contains also skulls from several places and from prehistoric periods. The teeth are all splendidly formed and free

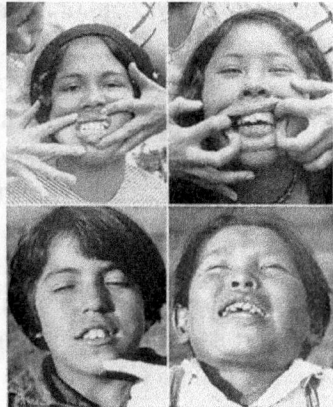

from dental caries. The arches are very symmetrical and the teeth in normal and regular position.

It was important to study the conditions of their successors living in the same general community. Accordingly, we examined the teeth and general physical condition of the Indians in a reservation in North Vancouver, so situated that they have the modern conveniences and modern foods.

In this group of children between eight and fifteen years of age, 36.9 per cent of all the teeth examined had already been attacked by dental caries. No people were found in this group who were living largely on native foods.

Anchorage is the principal city of western Alaska, since it is not only a base for the railroad running north to Fairbanks, but a base for aeroplane companies operating throughout various parts of Alaska. It is accordingly a combination of a coast city with its retail activities and a wholesale base for outfitters for the interior.

It has an excellent government hospital which probably has been built around the life of one man whom many people told us was the most beloved man in all Alaska.

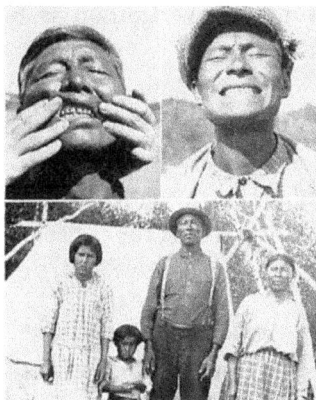

These primitive Indians are in central Canada. The three parents were developed before their district was reached by modern civilization. Note their good physical and facial form in contrast with the pinched nostrils of the two children. The oldest girl has tuberculosis. They are the product of civilization's contact with their primitive parents.

He is Dr. Josef Romig, a surgeon of great skill and with an experience among the Eskimos and Indians, both the primitives and modernized, extending over thirty-six years. I am deeply indebted to him for much information and for assistance in making contacts.

Among the many items of information of great interest furnished by Dr. Romig were facts that fitted well into the modern picture of association of modern degenerative processes with modernization.

He stated that in his thirty-six years of contact with these people he had never seen a case of malignant disease among the truly primitive Eskimos and Indians, although it frequently occurs when they become modernized.

He found similarly that the acute surgical problems requiring operation on internal organs such as the gall bladder, kidney, stomach, and appendix do not tend to occur among the primitive, but are very common problems among the modernized Eskimos and Indians.

Growing out of his experience, in which he had seen large numbers of the modernized Eskimos and Indians attacked with tuberculosis, which tended to be progressive and ultimately fatal as long as the patients stayed under modernized living conditions, he now sends them back when possible to primitive conditions and to a primitive diet, under which the death rate is very much lower than under modernized conditions.

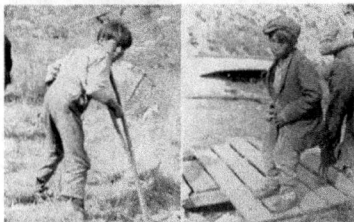

Indeed, he reported that a great majority of the afflicted recover under the primitive type of living and nutrition.

These are typical cripples met at the point of contact of our modern civilization with the primitive Indians. The boy at the left has arthritis in nearly all of his joints. He has several abscessed teeth. The boy at the right has tuberculosis of the spine.

Florida Indians

Using these guides, a study of the Indians of Florida, past and present, permits of comparing the pre-Columbians with those living today in that same territory. We will, accordingly, consider the dental caries problem and that of facial and dental arch form in the Florida Indians by comparing three groups: namely, the pre-Columbian, as evidenced from a study of the skull material in the museums; the tribes of Indians living in as much isolation as is

I was concerned to obtain information from government officials relative to the incidence of tooth decay and the degenerative diseases in various parts of north Scotland. I was advised that in the last fifty years the average height of Scotch men in some parts decreased four inches.
~ Dr. Weston A. Price

possible in the Everglades and Cypress Swamps; and the Indians of the same stock that are living in contact with the foods of modern civilization.

This latter group lives along the Tamiami trail and near Miami. In a study of several hundred skulls taken from the burial mounds of southern Florida, the incidence of tooth decay was so low as to constitute an immunity of apparently one hundred per cent, since in several hundred skulls not a single tooth was found to have been attacked by tooth decay.

Dental arch deformity and the typical change in facial form due to an inadequate nutrition were also completely absent, all dental arches having a form and interdental relationship such as to bring them into the classification of normal.

Skulls of primitive Indians showed superb dental arches typical of Nature's normal plan. The splendid position of the third molars was worth noting which are so frequently defective in position and quality in our modern white civilization.

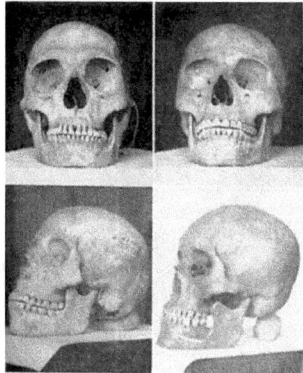

The Indian skulls that have been uncovered in many parts of the United States and Canada show a degree of excellence comparable to those seen in this Figure. These levels of excellence were the rule with them, not the exception as with us. The parents of these individuals knew what they and their children should eat!

The Indian skulls that have been uncovered in many parts of the United States and Canada show a degree of excellence. These levels of excellence were the rule with them, not the exception as with us. The parents of these individuals knew what they and their children should eat!

It is of interest that the quality of the skeletal material that is taken from the mounds showed unusually fine physical development and freedom from diseases of the joints. In contrast with this, many of the individuals of the modernized group were suffering from advanced deformities of the skeleton due to arthritic processes.

Another striking feature was the greater thickness of these skulls when compared to modern skulls.

For the study of a group of Indians now living in a high western state, Albuquerque, New Mexico, was visited.

Several other Indian studies have been made including studies of

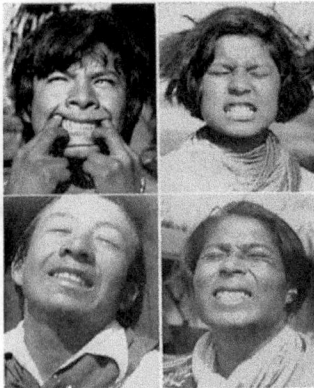

living groups, recently opened burials and museum collections, all of which support the findings recorded here. I am indebted to the directors and to the staffs of these institutions for their assistance.

Notwithstanding the wide range of physical and climatic conditions under which primitive Indians had been living, their incidence of tooth decay while on their native foods was always near zero; whereas, the modernized Indians of these groups showed very high incidence of dental caries.

The Seminole Indians living today in southern Florida largely beyond contact with the white civilization still produce magnificent teeth and dental arches of which these are typical. They live in the Everglade forest and still obtain the native foods.

A summary of percentages follows: *Primitive Indians*: Pelly Mountain, 0.16 per cent; Juneau, 0.00 per cent; Florida Pre-Columbian, 0.00 per cent; Florida Seminoles, 4.0 per cent.

Modernized Indians: Telegraph Creek, 25.5 per cent; Alaska Frontier, 40.0 per cent; Mohawk Institute, 17 per cent; Brantford Reservation Public School, 28.5 per cent; Brantford Reservation Hospital, 23.2 per cent, Tuscarora Reservation, 38.0 per cent; Winnipeg Lake Reservation, 39.1 per cent.

The foods used by the primitives varies according to location and climate. The foods of the modernized groups in all cases were the typical white man's foods of commerce.

The Indians like several primitive races I have studied are aware of the fact that their degeneration is in some way brought about by their contact with the white man. The dislike of the American Indian for the modern white civilization has been emphasized by many writers.

In my studies among the Seminole Indians of Florida I found great difficulty in communicating with or making examination of the isolated Seminoles living deep in the Everglades and Cypress Swamp.

Fortunately, I had the able assistance of one of their own tribe, a government nurse who had been very helpful to them and also a white man who had befriended them and whom they trusted. With their assistance I was able to carry out very detailed studies.

It was of interest, however, that when we arrived at a settlement in the bush we practically always found it uninhabited. Our Indian guide would go into the surrounding scrub and call to the people assuring them it was to their advantage to come out, which they finally did.

I was told that this attitude had grown out of the belief on their part that their treaties had been violated. These isolated Seminole Indian women had the reputation of turning their backs on all white men.

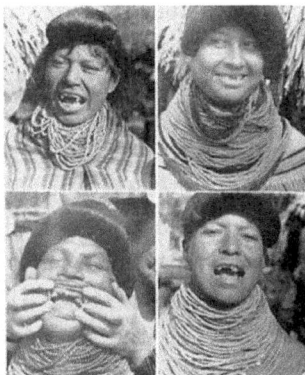

Seminole Indians. Apart from dental caries, note the change in facial and dental arch form in the children of this modernized group. They have a marked lack of development of the facial bones with a narrowing of the nostrils and dental arches with crowding of the teeth. Their faces are stamped with the blight which so many often think of as normal because it is so common with us.

A United States Press report provides an article (Cleveland Press, June 19, 1938) with the heading "Tribes 'Fed Up' Seek Solitude, Indians Dislike Civilization, Ask Land Barred to White Men." The article continues:

The Bureau of Indian Affairs revealed today that five Indian tribes in Oklahoma are "fed up" with white civilization and want new, secluded tribal lands.

So widespread is the discontent among the 100,000 Indians living in Oklahoma, officials said, that serious study is being given to the possibility of providing new lands where the redman may hunt and fish as his ancestors did.

Dissatisfaction has been brewing for a long time as a result of an increasing Indian population, decreasing Indian lands and unsatisfactory economic conditions. It was brought officially to the notice of bureau officials several days ago when a delegation, headed by Jack Gouge, a Creek Indian from Hanna, Okla., told Indian Commissioner John Collier that most of the Oklahoma Indians wanted new tribal lands away from white civilization.

So anxious are his people to escape from the white man and his influences, Jack Gouge said, that an organization of about 1000 Indians has been formed to press the demands. It is known as the "Four Mothers," apparently representing four of the "civilized tribes"— the Creeks, Choctaws, Cherokees and Chickasaws.

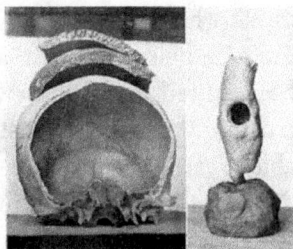

The fifth civilized tribe, the Seminoles of Oklahoma, are negotiating with the Mexican government for tribal lands in that country.

These tribes are described as "civilized" because of the high degree of culture they attained in their original tribal lands along the eastern coast. As their eastern lands became valuable the Indians were moved to the area which is now Oklahoma.

Example of greater thickness of pre-Columbian Indian skulls in Florida than modern skulls. Right: Illustration of bone surgery of ancient Florida Indians. Note healing of margins of trephined opening into a cyst, of the lower jaw. This is typical of the advanced surgery of the Peruvian Indians.

At the turn of the century, however, with the discovery of oil there the new tribal lands were broken up. The Indians were forcibly removed to small tracts despite their desire to remain together.

Indian Bureau officials do not conceal their bitterness over the white man's "treachery." One official pointed out that about 300 treaties have been signed with the Indians and that practically every one has been violated.

It will be most fortunate if in the interest of science and human betterment such a program as this will be carried out in order to permit these Indians to live in accordance with the accumulated wisdom of their various tribes. Their preservation in isolation would preserve their culture. The greatest heritage of the white man today is the accumulated wisdom of the human race.

45.

Isolated And Modernized Melanesians

By Dr. Weston A. Price

If the causative factors for the physical degeneration of mankind are practically the same everywhere, it should be possible to find a common cause operating, regardless of climate, race, or environment.

Melanesians are an ethnic group from Melanesia, an island around Australia. Melanesia is a subregion of Oceania extending from the western end of the Pacific Ocean to the Arafura Sea, and eastward to Fiji.

On reaching the isolated groups our greetings and the purpose of the mission were conveyed by our interpreters to the chiefs. Much time was often lost in going through necessary ceremonials and feasting. In every instance we received a very cordial reception and excellent cooperation. In no instance was there antagonism.

Through the underground telegraph they always seemed to know we were coming and had prepared for us.

When these formalities were once over and our wishes made known, the

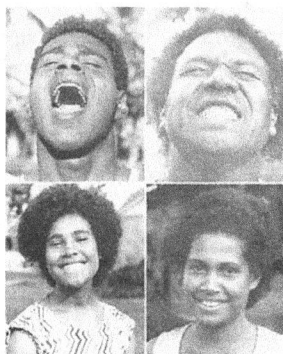

The development of the facial bones determines the size and shape of the palate and the size of the nasal air passages. Note the strength of the neck of the men above and the well proportioned faces of the girls below. Such faces are usually associated with properly proportioned bodies. Tooth decay is rare in these mouths so long as they use an adequate selection of the native foods.

chiefs instructed the members of their tribes to carry out our program for making examinations, recording personal data, making photographs, and collecting samples of foods for chemical analysis. The food samples were either dried or preserved in formalin.

In many instances the only contact with civilization had consisted of the call of a small trading ship once or twice a year to gather up the copra or dried coconut, sea shells and such other products as the natives had accumulated for exchange. Payment for these products was usually made in trade goods and not in money.

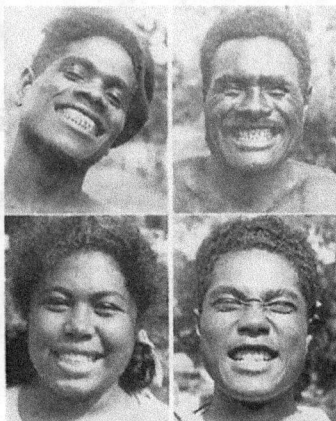

These Melanesians are typical in general physical build and facial and dental arch form of their race which is spread over a wide area of Islands in the southeastern Pacific. The nutrition of all is adequate for them to develop and maintain their racial pattern.

The following articles consisted nearly always of 90 per cent of the total value: white flour and sugar. Ten per cent consisted of wearing apparel or material for that apparel.

While the missionaries have encouraged the people to adopt habits of modern civilization, in the isolated districts the tribes were not able to depart much from their native foods because of the infrequency of the call of the trader ship. Effort had been made in almost all of the islands to induce the natives to cover their bodies, especially when in sight of strangers.

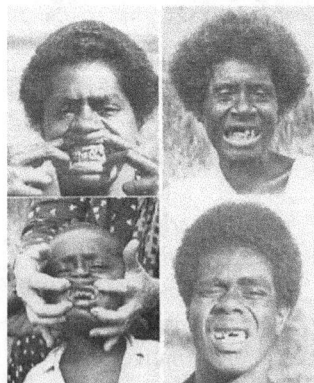

These natives of the Fiji Islands illustrate the effect of changing from the native food to the imported foods of commerce. Tooth decay becomes rampant and with it is lost the ability to properly masticate the food. Growing children and child bearing mothers suffer most severely from dental caries.

In several islands regulatory measures had been adopted requiring the covering of the body. This regulation had greatly reduced the primitive practice of coating the surface of the body with coconut oil, which had the effect of absorbing the ultra-violet rays thus preventing injury from the tropical sun.

This coating of oil enabled them to shed the rain which was frequently torrential though of short duration. The irradiation of the coconut oil was considered by the natives to provide, in addition, an important source of nutrition. Their newly acquired wet garments became a serious menace to the comfort and health of the wearers.

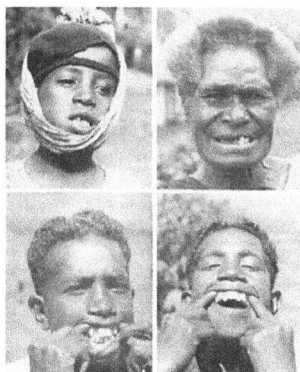

The early navigators who visited these South Sea Islands reported the people as being exceedingly strong, vigorously built, beautiful in body and kindly disposed. There were formerly dense populations on most of the inhabitable islands.

In contrast with this, one now finds that on many of the islands the death rate has come to so far exceed the birth rate that the very existence of these racial groups is often seriously threatened.

No dentists or physicians are available on most of these islands. Toothache is the only cause of suicide. The new generation born after the parents adopt the imported modern foods often have a change in the shape of the face and dental arches. The teeth are crowded as shown above.

My guide told me that it had always been essential, as it is today, for the people of the interior to obtain some food from the sea, and that even during the times of most bitter warfare between the inland or hill tribes and the coast tribes, those of the interior would bring down during the night choice plant foods from the mountain areas and place them in caches and return the following night and obtain the sea foods that had been placed in those depositories by the shore tribes.

The individuals who carried these foods were never molested, not even during active warfare.

(Author's Note: It's true that human beings require some foods of animal origin for optimum nutrition. In civilized societies, this nutrition should be provided by the dairy enterprise. Constitution of milk is very similar to blood. Milk is a civilized or humane way to obtain animal proteins.

Aborigines who have no concept of growing food or milking animals, can be justified in killing animals for food.

In fact, agriculture and dairy are more than adequate to supply all our nutritional needs. This is evidenced by highly developed martial races of Indian sub-continent and other places.

Most of these races have followed a locto-vegetarian program since time immemorial. Meat, if at all, was consumed only in ritualistic sacrifices on special occasions. Meat was never the dietary mainstay of these people.

India was home to the highest number of martial races and the British expanded their empire by recruiting them in large numbers.

Vaisya means produce food grain, krsi, agriculture, not produce food in the slaughterhouse. No. Slaughterhouse, even the sixth-class, seventh-class men... They did not know how to produce food, how to live. That means the aborigines in the jungle. They were hunting one animal, then eating, not that civilized nation, organized slaughterhouse. Oh, how horrible it is. If you want to eat an animal, then you go to the jungle, kill one animal, and eat. The government is not going to maintain a slaughterhouse for you. You see? This is the civilization. So our eatables should be food grains -- krsi-go-raksya -- and milk. Krsi means by agriculture process you can produce fruits, flower, vegetables, then rice, wheat, and pulses, and you have got milk. Then where is your want, scarcity? This is civilization. Meat-eating is meant for the sixth-class, seventh-class men who does not know, who remain naked, and they can neither produce food neither cloth in the jungle. It is for them. They also were not very much expert to maintain a slaughterhouse. When you need, you can kill one lower animal, not cow. The cow is not available in the jungle. You can have some deer or some boar. So these unimportant animals were killed by them.

~ Srila Prabhupada (Lecture, Srimad-Bhagavatam 6.1.22 -- Chicago, July 6, 1975)

These soldiers fought in World War II on all Allied fronts. The concept already had a precedent in Indian culture as one of the four orders (varnas) in the Vedic-Hindu social system are known as the Kshatriya, literally "warriors."

Some of the principal martial races identified by the British on Indian subcontinent were: Ahirs/Yadavs, Awans, Bhumihar, Bunts, Dhangars (Hatkar), Dhund Abbasis, Khatris, Dogra, Gakhars, Garhwalis, Ghumman, Gujjar, Gurkhas, Janjua, Jats, Kamboj/ Kamboh, Khokhar, Kodava (Coorgs), Kumaoni/Kumaunis, Mahars, Marathas, Mohyals, Nairs, Pashtuns, Qaimkhanis, Rors, Reddys, Rajputs, Sainis, Sikhs, Sudhan, Tanolis, Tarkhans.

A lacto vegetarian diet is a vegetarian diet that includes dairy products such as milk, cheese, yogurt, butter, ghee, cream, and kefir, but excludes eggs. Apart from Indian sub-continent, also residents of the classical Mediterranean such as the Pythagoreans, are or were lacto-vegetarians.)

46.

Isolated And Modernized Polynesians

By Dr. Weston A. Price

Polynesia is a subregion of Oceania, made up of over 1,000 islands scattered over the central and southern Pacific Ocean. The characteristics of the Polynesian race included straight hair, oval features, happy, buoyant dispositions and splendid physiques.

The first group studied was made up of the people of the Marquesas Islands which are situated 9 degrees south latitude and 140 degrees west longitude, about 4,000 miles due west of Peru. Few, if any, of the primitive racial stocks of the South Sea Islands were so enthusiastically extolled for their beauty and excellence of physical development by the early navigators. Much tooth decay prevails today. They reported the Marquesans as vivacious, happy people numbering over a hundred thousand on the seven principal islands of this group.

Probably in few places in the world can so distressing a picture be seen today as is found there. A French government official told me that the native population had decreased to about two thousand, chiefly as a result of the ravages of tuberculosis. Serious epidemics of small-pox and measles have at times taken a heavy toll. In a

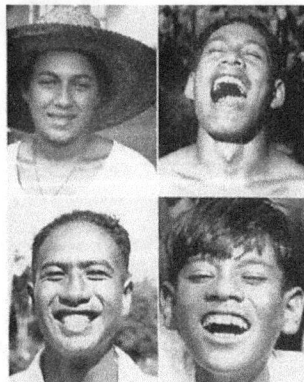

Polynesians are a beautiful race and physically sturdy. They have straight hair and their color is often that of a sun tanned European. They have perfect dental arches.

group of approximately one hundred adults and children I counted ten who were emaciated and coughing with typical signs of tuberculosis. Many were waiting for treatment at a dispensary eight hours before the hour it opened.

In the past some of the natives have had splendid physiques, fine countenances, and some of the women have had beautiful features. They are now a sick and dying primitive group. A trader ship was in port exchanging white flour and sugar for their copra (dry coconut).

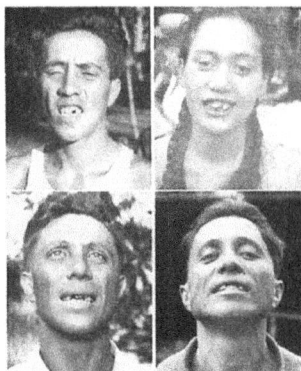

Wherever the native foods have been displaced by the imported foods, dental caries becomes rampant. These are typical modernized Tahitians.

Tooth decay was rampant. At the time of the examination, 36.9 per cent of the teeth of the people using trade food in conjunction with the available local food had been attacked by tooth decay. The individuals living entirely on native foods were few.

Some early navigators were so highly impressed with the beauty and health of these people that they reported the Marquesas Islands as the Garden of Eden.

Tahiti is the principal island of the Society group. It is situated 17 degrees south of the equator, 149 degrees west longitude. Fortunately degeneration has not been so rapid nor so severe here. The Tahitian population, however, has reduced from over two

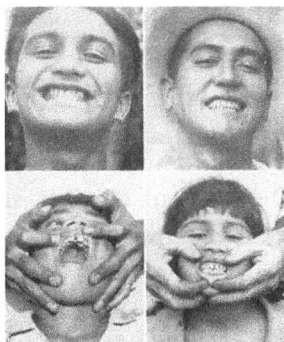

These Polynesians live on the island of Rarotonga. At the top are two examples of typically fine faces and teeth. Below, at left, is seen a full blood Polynesian child with the dental arch so small that the permanent laterals are developing inside the arch. His parents used imported food. At the right below is a mixed blood of white and Polynesian. Note the normal spacing of the temporary teeth before the permanent set appears. Parents used native foods.

hundred thousand as early estimated, to a present native population estimated at about ten thousand.

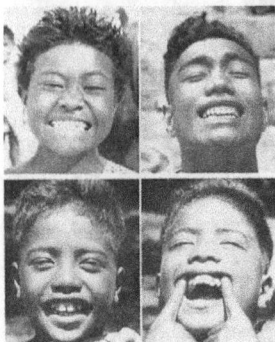

Note the marked difference in facial and dental arch form of the two Samoan primitives above and the two modernized below. The face bones are underdeveloped below causing a marked constriction of the arches with crowding of the teeth. This is a typical expression of inadequate nutrition of the parents.

These islands are also a part of French Oceania. Many of the able bodied men were taken from these French Islands to France to fight in the World War. Only a small percentage, however, returned, and they were mostly crippled and maimed.

The Tahitians are a buoyant, light-hearted race, fully conscious, however, of their rapid decline in numbers and health. Many of the more primitive are very fine looking and have excellent dental arches.

It is a matter of great importance that the inhabitants of these South Sea Islands were skillful navigators and boat builders. It was a common occurrence for expeditions both peaceful and aggressive to make journeys of one and two thousand miles in crafts propelled by man power and wind and carrying in addition an adequate supply of water and food for their journey.

If one will picture a community of several thousand people with an average of 30 per cent of all the teeth attacked by dental caries and not a single dentist or dental instrument available for assistance of the entire group, a slight realization is had of the mass suffering that has to be endured.

Commerce and trade for profit blaze the way in breaking down isolation's barriers, far in advance of the development of health agencies and emergency relief unwittingly made necessary by the trade contact.

In American Samoa through the cooperation of the educational authorities and the Director of the Department of Health, Commander Stephenson, and under the direct supervision of Lieutenant Commander Lowry, the dental surgeon, a group of four young men of the native teaching staff was selected and given instructions for the removal of the deposits. Equipment in the form of instruments has since been provided, in part through the kindness and generosity of some dental manufacturers. This probably constitutes the only native dental service that has ever been available in any of the Pacific Island groups.

The intelligence and aptness with which these men were able to learn the fundamental principles, and their skill in carrying out a highly commendable prophylactic operation was indeed remarkable.

I gave them pieces of soap and asked them to carve a reproduction of an extracted tooth which was given as a model and in which they were required to increase all diameters to a given amount. Their work would probably equal if not exceed in excellence that of the first effort of 90 per cent of American dental students. Many of these natives are very dexterous with their fingers and are skilled artists in carving wood and other material.

A great service could be rendered to these people who are in the process of modernization, but who have no opportunity for dental assistance, by teaching some of the bright young men certain of the procedures for rendering

Wherever the Polynesians are being modernized a change is occurring in facial form which is progressively more severe in the younger members of the family. These girls of an Hawaiian family demonstrate this. Note the change in facial form in the sister to the right. The face is longer and narrower, the nostrils pinched and the chin is receding. The tribal facial pattern is lost.

first aid. They could be compensated by contributions of native foods and native wares much as our itinerant dentists were in earlier days. The people would not have money to pay an American or European dentist for his service until trade is carried on with currency.

Nearly all these racial stocks are magnificent singers for which Nature has well-equipped them physically. Their artistry can be judged by the fact that they sing very difficult music unaccompanied

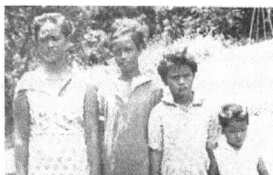

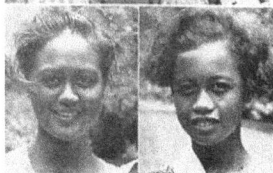

and undirected. A large native chorus at Nukualofa, in the Tongan Group, sang without accompaniment "The Hallelujah Chorus" from Handel's Messiah with all the parts and with phenominal volume and modulation. Much of their work, such as rowing their largest boats, and many of their sports are carried out to the rhythm of hilarious music.

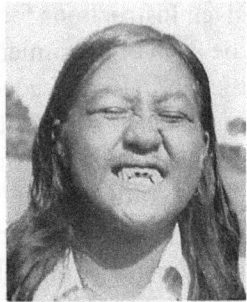

The Polynesian race is rapidly disappearing with modernization. Tooth decay becomes extreme as shown in the girl above. This girl has tuberculosis, one of the physical injuries which accompany modernization.

Many of the island groups recognize that their races are doomed since they are melting away with degenerative diseases, chiefly tuberculosis. Their one overwhelming desire is that their race shall not die out. They know that something serious has happened since they have been touched by civilization. Surely our civilization is on trial both at home and abroad.

47.

Isolated And Modernized African Tribes

By Dr. Weston A. Price

A frica has been the last of the large continents to be invaded and explored by our modern civilization. It has one of the largest native populations still living in accordance with inherited traditions. Accordingly, it provides a particularly favorable field for studying primitive racial stocks.

This study of primitive racial stocks, with the exception of some Indian groups, has been largely concerned with people living under physical conditions quite different from those which obtain in the central area of a large continent.

Considering that the most universal scourge of modern civilization is dental caries, though it is only one of its many degenerative processes, it is important that we study these people to note how they have solved the major problems of living in so severe and disciplining an environment as provided in Africa.

This was done during the summer of 1935. Our route took us through the Red Sea and down the Indian Ocean to enter the African continent at Mombasa below the equator and then across Kenya and Uganda into Eastern Belgian Congo, and thence about 4,000 miles down the long stretch of the Nile through Sudan to the modernized civilization of Egypt.

This journey covered most of the country around Ethiopia and gave us contact with several of the most primitive racial stocks of that country. These people are accordingly the neighbors of the Abyssinians or Ethiopians.

Since the various tribes speak different languages and are under different governments, it was necessary to organize our safari in connection with the local government officials in the different districts.

During these journeys in Africa which covered about 6,000 miles, we came in contact with about thirty different tribes. Special attention was given to the foods, samples of which were obtained for chemical analysis. Over 2,500 negatives were made and developed in the field.

If any one impression of our experiences were to be selected as particularly vivid, it would be the contrast between the health and ruggedness of the primitives in general and that of the foreigners who have entered their country. That their superior ruggedness was not racial became evident when through contact with modern civilizations degenerative processes developed.

Very few of the many Europeans with whom we came in contact had lived in central Africa for as much as two years without serious illness or distinct evidence of physical stress. That the cause was not the severity of the climate, but something related to the methods of living, was soon apparent.

In all the districts it was recognized and expected that the foreigners must plan to spend a portion of every few years or every year outside that environment if they would keep well. Children born in that country to Europeans were generally expected to spend several of their growing years in Europe or America if they would build even relatively normal bodies.

One exacting condition of the environment that we encountered was the constant exposure to disease. Dysentery epidemics were so severe and frequent that we scarcely allowed ourselves to eat any food that had not been cooked or that we had not peeled ourselves. In general, it was necessary to boil all drinking water.

We dared not allow our bare feet to touch a floor of the ground for fear of jiggers which burrow into the skin of the feet. Scarcely ever when below 6,000 feet were we safe after sundown to step from behind mosquito netting or to go out without thorough protection against the malaria pests. These malaria mosquitoes which include many varieties are largely night feeders. They were thought to come out soon after sundown.

We were advised that the most dangerous places for becoming infected were the public eating houses, since the mosquitoes hide under the tables and attack the diner's ankles if they are not adequately protected. We rigidly followed the precaution of providing adequate protection against these pests.

Disease-carrying ticks were so abundant in the grass and shrubbery that we had to be on guard constantly to remove them from our clothing before they buried themselves in our flesh. They were often carriers of very severe fevers.

We had to be most careful not to touch the hides with which the natives protected their bodies from the cold at night and from the sun in the daytime without thorough sterilization following any contact. There was grave danger from the lice that infected the hair of the hides.

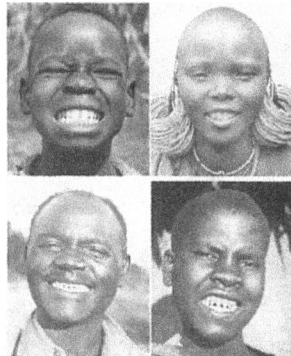

We dared not enter several districts because of the dreaded tsetse fly and the sleeping sickness it carries.

One wonders at the apparent health of the natives until he learns of the unique immunity they have developed and which is largely transmitted to the offspring. In several districts we were told that practically every living native had had typhus fever and was immune, though the lice from their bodies could transmit the disease.

The development of the faces and dental arches in many African tribes is superb. The girl at the upper right is wearing several earrings in the lobe of each ear. The Wakamba tribe points the teeth as shown here. This does not cause tooth decay while they live on their native food.

One also wonders why people with such resistance to disease are not able to combat the degenerative diseases of modern civilization. When they adopt modern civilization they then become susceptible to several of our modern degenerative processes, including tooth decay.

Dr. Anderson who is in charge of a splendid government hospital in Kenya, assured me that in several years of service among the primitive people of that district he had observed that they did not suffer from appendicitis, gall bladder trouble, cystitis and duodenal ulcer. Malignancy was also very rare among the primitives.

It is of great significance that we studied six tribes in which there appeared to be not a single tooth attacked by dental caries nor a single malformed dental arch. Several other tribes were found with nearly complete immunity to dental caries. In thirteen tribes we did not meet a single individual with irregular teeth.

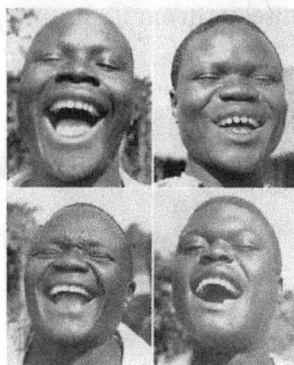

Where the members of these same tribes had adopted modern civilization many cases of tooth decay were found. In the next generation following the adoption of the European dietaries dental arch deformities frequently developed.

In this bird's eye view we are observing changes that have been in progress during many hundreds or thousands of years. The Arabs have been the principal slave dealers working in from the east coast of Africa. They have maintained their individuality without much blending except on the coast. They have not become an important part of the native stock of the interior.

The reward of obeying nature's laws of nutrition is illustrated in this west Nile tribe in Belgian Congo. Note the breadth of the dental arches and the finely proportioned features. Their bodies are as well built as their heads. Exceedingly few teeth have been attacked by dental caries while on their native foods.

These primitive native stocks can be largely identified on the basis of their habits and methods of living. The Nilotic tribes have been chiefly herders of cattle and goats and have lived primarily on dairy products, including milk, with occasional blood and meat, and with a varying percentage of vegetable foods.

It was most interesting to observe that in every instance these cattle people dominated the surrounding tribes. They were characterized by superb physical development, great bravery and a mental acumen that made it possible for them to dominate because of their superior intelligence. Among these Nilotic tribes the Masai forced their way farthest south and occupy a position between two of the great Bantu tribes, the Kikuyu and the Wakamba. Both of these latter tribes are primarily agricultural people.

Masai Tribe

The Masai are tall and strong. Typically these men and women were much taller than our six-foot guide. It is interesting to study the methods of living and observe the accumulated wisdom of the Masai.

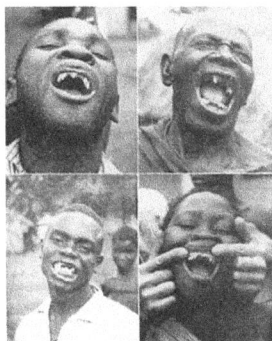

They are reported to have known for over two hundred years that malaria was carried by mosquitoes, and further they have practiced exposing the members of their tribes who had been infected with syphilis by the Arabs to malaria to prevent the serious injuries resulting from the spirochetal infection.

Yet modern medicine boasts of being the discoverers of this great principle of using malaria to prevent or relieve syphilitic infections of the spinal cord and brain.

These people stood against slavery and lived alongside most wild animals with an aversion to eating game and birds. Maasai land now has East Africa's finest game areas. Maasai society never condoned traffic of human beings, and outsiders looking for people to enslave avoided the Masai.

Wherever the Africans have aidopted the foods of modern commerce, dental caries was active, thus destroying large numbers of the teeth and causing great suffering. The cases shown here are typical of workers on plantations which largely use imported foods.

These members of the Masai tribe illustrate the splendid nutrition provided by their diet of cattle products namely: milk, butter and very occasional blood and meat. The chief was also well over six feet. Masai ladies wear the customary decorations of coils of copper wire bracelets and anklets which largely constitute the attire of the girls.

I saw the native Masai operating on their cattle with skill and knowledge. The Masai have no currency and all their transactions are made with cows or goats.

A valuable cow was not eating properly, and I observed them taking a thorn out of the inside of her mouth. The surgical operation was done with a knife of their own making and tempered by pounding. The wound was treated by rubbing it with the ashes of a plant that acted as a very powerful styptic.

Their knowledge of veterinary science is quite remarkable. I saw them treating a young cow that had failed to conceive. They apparently knew the cause and proceeded to treat her as modern veterinaries might do in order to overcome her difficulties.

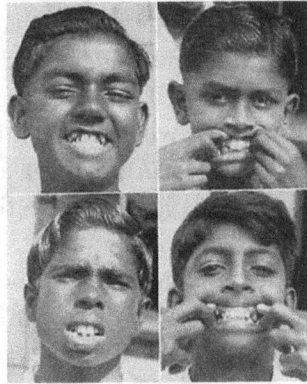

For their food throughout the centuries they have depended very largely on milk, reinforced with vegetables and fruits and occasional blood and meat. Their diet has largely been free from meat which helped the wildlife to flourish in their areas. Former Masai lands are now the world's biggest wildlife reserves. They have been the protectors of nature.

They milk the cows daily. They bleed the steers occasionally, especially during the drought period but never more than once a month. In one such instance, a torque was placed around the neck before the puncture was made. The animals did not even flinch when struck by the arrow, the operation was done so quickly and skillfully. When sufficient blood was

In Cairo, in the new generations, born after the parents had adopted typical modernized diets of Europeans, there was a marked change in the facial and dental arch forms of the adolescent children. Note the narrowing of the nostrils and dental arches and the crowding of the teeth in these four typical young men.

drawn, the torque was removed and the blood immediately stopped flowing. A styptic made of ashes referred to above was used. This serves also to protect the wound from infection.

Their estimate of a desirable dairy stock is based on quality not quantity. They judge the value of a cow for keeping in their herd by the length of time it takes her calf to stand on its feet and run after it is born, which is only a very few minutes.

This is in striking contrast with the practice of our modern dairymen who are chiefly concerned with the quantity of milk and quantity of butter fat rather than with its value as a source of special factors for nutrition.

Many of the calves of the modern high-production cows of civilized countries are not able to stand for many hours after birth, frequently twenty-four. This ability to stand is very important in a country infested with predatory animals; such as lions, leopards, hyenas, jackals and vultures.

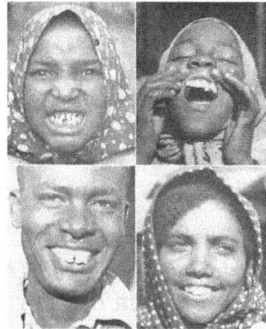

Disturbed nature may present a variety of deformity patterns. In the upper left the upper arch is much too small for the lower and nearly goes inside it. The upper right is narrowed with crowding of the teeth. Both lower cases demonstrate an underdevelopment of the mandible of the lower jaw. (In Khartoum)

This reminded me of my experience in Alaska in studying the reindeer of the Eskimos. I was told that a reindeer calf could be dropped in a foot of snow and almost immediately it could run with such speed that the predatory animals, including wolves, could not catch it. And, moreover, that these fawns would go almost immediately after their birth with a herd on a stampede and never be knocked down.

The problem of combating the predatory animals, particularly the lions, calls for greater skill and bravery than is required by other tribes in Africa. The lions live on the large grazing animals, particularly the cattle, from which they select the strongest. In driving over the rural areas, we frequently saw one or two men or boys guarding an entire herd with only their spears.

Their skill in killing a lion with a spear is one of the most superb of human achievements. I was interested to learn that they much prefer their locally made spears to those that are manufactured outside and brought in, because of their certainty that they will not break, will withstand straightening regardless of how much they are bent and because due to the process of manufacture will take a very sharp edge.

On one occasion, after we had been kept awake much of the night by the roaring of the lions and neighing of the zebras that were being attacked by the lions, we visited a Masai manyata nearby in the morning to learn that when they let their cattle and goats out of the corral of acacia thorns, three or four spearsmen went ahead in search of the lions that might be waiting to ambush the cattle. They apparently did not have the slightest fear. The lions evidentally had made a kill nearby. This the natives determined by the number of coyotes.

The heart and courage of these people has been largely broken by the action of the government in taking away their shields in order to prevent them fighting with the surrounding native tribes as formerly. They depended upon their shields to protect them from the arrows of the other tribes. The efforts to make agriculturists of these Masai people are not promising.

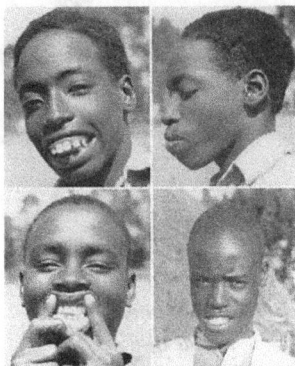

Africa6.jpgAs in our civilization, even the first generation, after the adoption of modernized foods may show gross deformities. Note the extreme protrusion of the upper teeth with shortening of the lower jaw in the upper pictures and the marked narrowing with lengthening of the face in the lower views. The injury is not limited to the visible structures.

In a typical manyata the chief has several wives. Each one has a separate dwelling. Timber and shrubbery are so scarce in this vicinity that the dwellings are built of clay mixed with cow dung which is plastered over a framework of twigs. Many chiefs are over six feet in height.

The Masai live in a very extensive game preserve in which hundreds of thousands of grazing animals enjoy an existence protected from man since even the natives are not allowed to kill the animals.

They seemed to be preserved for the numerous lions which occasionally become very bold since they have an abundance of food and no enemies. Recently the local government authorities found it necessary to shoot off eighty of the lions in a particular district because of their aggressiveness.

In the Masai tribe, a study of 2,516 teeth in eighty-eight individuals distributed through several widely separated manyatas showed only four individuals with caries. These had a total of ten carious teeth, or only 0.4 per cent of the teeth attacked by tooth decay.

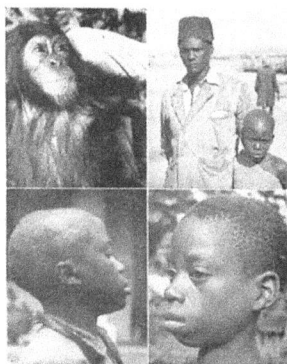

Kikuyu Tribe, Kenya.

In contrast with the Masai, the Kikuyu tribe, which inhabits a district to the west and north of the Masai, are characterized by being primarily an agricultural people. Their chief articles of diet are sweet potatoes, corn, beans, and some bananas, millet, and Kafir corn, a variety of Indian millet.

A very frequent injury appearing in the offspring after the adoption of less efficient foods often involves a marked depression of the middle third of the face as illustrated in the three boys in this view. Note the comparison with the chimpanzee face.

The women use special diets during gestation and lactation. The girls in this tribe, as in several others, are placed on a special diet for six months prior to marriage. They nurse their children for three harvests and precede each pregnancy with special feeding.

The Kikuyus are not as tall as the Masai and physically they are much less rugged. One of the striking tribal customs is the making of large perforations in the ears in which they carry many metal ornaments.

The development of the faces and dental arches in many African tribes is superb.

Muhima Tribe, Uganda

This tribe resides in southern Uganda. They, like the Masai, are primarily a cattle raising people and live on milk with occasional blood and meat. The district in which they live is to the east of Lake Edward and the Mountains of the Moon. They constitute one of the very primitive and undisturbed groups.

While the Masai raise chiefly the hump-backed cattle, the herds of this Muhima or Anchola tribe are characterized by their large wide-spread horns. Like the Masai, they are tall and courageous. They defend their herds and their families from lions and leopards with their primitive spears.

Like the other primitive cattle people, they dominate the adjoining tribes. In a study of 1,040 teeth of thirty-seven individuals, not a single tooth was found with dental caries. This tribe makes their huts of grass and sticks.

Watusi Tribe

This is a very interesting tribe living on the east of Lake Kivu, one of the headwaters of the West Nile in Ruanda which is a Belgian Protectorate. They are tall and athletic. Their faces differ markedly from those of other tribes, and they boast a very noble inheritance.

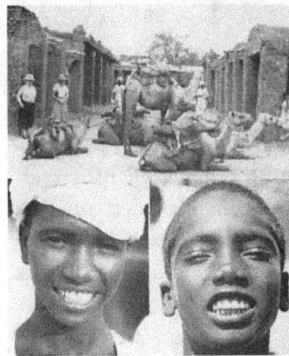

According to legend, a Roman military expedition penetrated into central Africa at the time of Anthony and Cleopatra. A phalanx remained, refusing to return with the expedition. They took wives from the native tribes and passed laws that thereafter no marriage could take place outside their group. They have magnificent physiques. Many stand over six feet without shoes.

In the hot desert countries of Asia and Africa camel's milk is an important item of human nutrition. The teeth of the Arabs, as illustrated below, are excellent. Large areas could not maintain human life without the camel and its milk.

The Government of Kenya has for several years sponsored an athletic contest among the various tribes, the test being one of strength for which they use a tug-of-war. One particular tribe has carried off the trophy repeatedly. This tribe resides on the east coast of Lake Victoria. The members are powerful athletes and wonderful swimmers.

They are said not to have been conquered in warfare when they could take the warfare to the water. One of their methods is to swim under water to the enemy's fleet and scuttle their boats. They fight with spears under water with marvelous skill. Their physiques are magnificent. In a group of 190 boys who had been gathered into a government school near the east coast of Lake Victoria only one boy was found with dental caries, and two of his teeth had been affected.

As one travels down the West Nile and later along the western border of Ethiopia many unique tribes are met. Members of these tribes wear little or no clothing. They have splendid physiques and high immunity to dental caries.

The reward of obeying nature's laws of nutrition is illustrated in these tribes. Breadth of the dental arches and the finely proportioned features are worth noting. Their bodies are as well built as their heads. Exceedingly few teeth have been attacked by dental caries while on their native foods.

Bogora Mission, Belgian Congo

This mission is located west of Lake Albert and includes members of the Bahema and Balendu tribes. While the Bahema tribe originally lived very largely on cattle products, milk with occasional blood and meat, in this district, the herds were small and they were using a considerable quantity of cereals, chiefly corn and beans, some sweet potatoes and bananas. These latter were the chief foods of the other tribes, in addition to goats' milk.

Baitu Tribe, Nyunge, Ruanda, Belgian Protectorate

This district lies south of Uganda and east of Belgian Congo proper, northwest of Tanganyika. It lies just east of Lake Kivu. When we learn that Lake Kivu was only discovered in 1894, even though it is one of the important sources of the Nile waters, we realize the primitiveness of the people of this and adjoining districts. This group lives largely on dairy products from cattle and goats, together with sweet potatoes, cereals and bananas.

In a study of 364 teeth of thirteen individuals, not a single tooth was found to have been attacked by dental caries.

Native Hotel Staff at Goina, Belgian Congo

This group consisted of the inside and outside servants of a tourist hotel on Lake Kivu.

An examination of 320 teeth of ten individuals revealed twenty teeth with caries, or 6.3 per cent. It is significant that all of these carious teeth were in the mouth of one individual, the cook. The others all boarded themselves and lived on native diets. The cook used European foods.

Where the members of the African tribes had attached themselves to coffee plantations and were provided with the imported foods of white flour, sugar, polished rice and canned goods, tooth decay became rampant.

Wherever the Africans have adopted the foods of modern commerce, dental caries was active, thus destroying large numbers of the teeth and causing great suffering.

Anglo-Egyptian Sudan has an area approximately one-third that of the United States. It is traversed throughout its length from south to north by the Nile. There are several tribes living along this great waterway, which are of special interest now owing to their close proximity to Ethiopia.

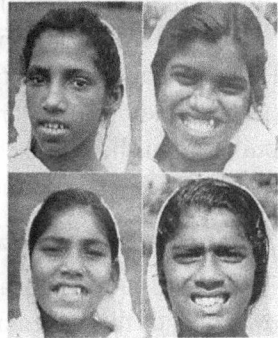

Both girls and boys in the modernized colonies in Cairo showed typical deformity patterns in faces and dental arches. The health of these groups is not comparable to that of those living on the native

There are wonderful hunters and warriors among them. In hunting they use their long-bladed spears almost entirely. The shores of the Nile for nearly a thousand miles in this district are lined with papyrus and other water plants to a depth of from several hundred yards to a few miles.

Back of this area the land rises and provides excellent pasturage for the grazing cattle. Some of the tribes are very tall, particularly the Neurs. The women are often six feet or over, and the men seven feet, some of them reaching seven and a half feet in height.

I was particularly interested in their food habits both because of their high immunity to dental caries which approximated one hundred per cent, and because of their physical development.

Many of these tribes, like the Neurs, wear no clothing and decorate their bodies with various designs, some of them representing strings of beads produced by putting foreign substances under the skin in definite order.

They have maintained a particularly bitter warfare against the Arab slave dealers who have come across from the Red Sea coast to carry off the women and children. In isolated districts even to this day they are suspicious of foreigners. We were told that in one district adjoining Ethiopia all light skinned people are in danger and cannot safely enter that territory without a military escort.

Neurs, Malakal, Sudan.

The Neurs at Malakal on the Nile River are a unique tribe because of their remarkable stature. Many of the women are six feet tall and the men range from six feet to seven and a half feet in height. They also make extensive use of dairy products in their diet. A study of 1,268 teeth of thirty-nine individuals revealed only six teeth with dental caries, or 0.5 per cent. Only three individuals had caries, or 7.7 per cent.

It is of interest that of the two boys in the Arab school at Omdurman with dental caries one was the son of a rich merchant and used liberally sweets and European foods.

The Arabs in several districts use camels' milk extensively. It is nutritious, and in much of the desert country constitutes the mainstay of the nomads for months at a time. The primitive Arabs studied had fine dental arches with very little deformity.

Even the horses ridden by the Arab chiefs in moving their camel herds across the desert are often dependent, sometimes for as long as three months, upon the milk of the camels for their nutrition.

The primitive Arab girls have splendidly developed faces and fine dental arches. Their natural beauty, however, is rapidly lost with modernization.

In the hot desert countries of Asia and Africa camel's milk is an important item of human nutrition. The teeth of the Arabs are excellent. Large areas could not maintain human life without the camel and its milk.

Both girls and boys in the modernized colonies in Cairo showed typical deformity patterns in faces and dental arches. The health of these groups is not comparable to that of those living on the native dietaries. Reproductive efficiency in these generations is greatly reduced.

While slavery of the old form no longer exists in the so-called civilized countries, in its new form it is a most tragic reality for many of the people. Taxes and the new order of living make many demands. For many of these primitive tribes a new suit of clothes could formerly be had every day with no more trouble than cutting a new banana leaf.

With the new order they are requested to cover their bodies with clothing. Cloth of all kinds including the poorest cotton has to be imported. They must pay an excessive charge due to the long transportation cost for the imported goods, a charge which often exceeds the original cost in the European or American markets by several fold.

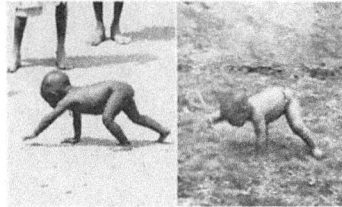

In order to pay their head tax they are frequently required to carry such products as can be used by the government officials, chiefly foods, over long distances and for part of each year. These foods are often those which not only *These two native African children scooted around on all fours so swiftly that it was difficult to take their pictures. We did not see them stand up. They behaved very much like tame chimpanzees.* the adults, but particularly the growing children sorely need for providing body growth and repair. This naturally has produced a current of acute unrest and a chafing under the foreign domination.

As we encircled Ethiopia we found the natives not only aware of what was going on in that border country, but deeply concerned regarding the outcome. From their temper and sympathetic attitude for the oppressed Ethiopians, it would not be surprising if sympathizers pass over the border into that country to support their crushed neighbors.

The problem is accordingly very much larger than the interest of some particular foreign power. It deals directly with the future course of events and the attitude of the African natives in general toward foreign domination.

The native African is not only chafing under the taxation by foreign overlords, but is conscious that his race becomes blighted when met by our modern civilization. I found them well aware of the fact that those of their tribes who had adopted European methods of living and foods not only developed rampant tooth decay, but other degenerative processes.

In one of the most efficiently organized mission schools that we found in Africa, the principal asked me to help them solve a serious problem. He said there was no single question asked them so often by the native boys in their school as why it is that those families that have grown up in the mission or government schools were physically not so strong as those families who had never been in contact with the mission or government schools.

The happiness of the people in their homes and community life is everywhere very striking. A mining prospector who had spent two decades studying the mineral deposits of Uganda was quoted to me as stating that if he could have the heaven of his choice, it would be to live in Uganda as the natives of Uganda had lived before modern civilization came to it.

While inter-tribal warfare has largely ceased, a new scourge is upon them, namely the scourge which comes with modern civilization. As in the primitive racial stocks previously studied and reported, we found that modernizing forces were often associated with a very marked increase of the death rate over the birth rate.

In some districts in Africa a marked degeneration is taking place. Geoffrey Gorer in his book, "Africa Dances," which was written after making studies in West Africa, discusses this problem at length.

He quotes figures given by Marcel Sauvage in his article on French Equatorial Africa: "In 1911 French Equatorial Africa had

"But have people really become healthier or happier by developing such a high-tech, dependent, urbanized life-style? Has the quality of life really improved? Has it been a fair trade, fresh water for the recycled chemicals and sewage called city water? Or clean air for the manmade gaseous substances now substituting for air? Or fresh fruits, vegetables, and milk for the canned, preserved, frozen, flavorless, watered-down products sold as eatables in the markets?

~ Rupanuga dasa, (Krishna's Bread-and-Butter Economics)

twenty million negro inhabitants; in 1921 there were seven and a half million; in 1931 there were two and a half million."

Major Browne, a high official of the British Government Administrative Department of Kenya, with long experience, states in the closing paragraph of his book entitled, "The Vanishing Tribes of Kenya," the following:

It must also be remembered that the "blessings of civilization" are not in practice by any means as obvious as some simple-minded folk would like to believe. It can be said with fair accuracy that among the tribes with which we have been dealing there is, in their uncontaminated society, no pauperism, no paid prostitution, very little drunkenness, and on the whole astonishingly little crime; while practically everyone has enough to eat, sufficient clothing, and an adequate dwelling, according to the primitive native standard. Of what civilized community can as much be said?

Civilizations have been rising and falling not only through all the period of recorded history, but long before as evidenced by archeological findings. If we think of Nature's calendar as one in which centuries are days and civilizations are years, the part current events are playing in the history of a great continent like Africa may be mere incidents.

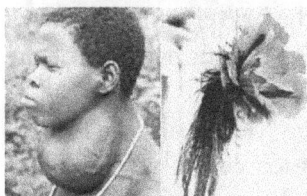

This African woman with goiter has come down from the 9000 foot level in the mountains in Belgian Congo near the source of the Nile to a 6000 foot level to gather special plants for burning to carry the ashes up to her family to prevent goiter in her children. Right, a Nile plant, a water hyacinth burned for its ashes.

This much we do know that throughout the world some remnants of several primitive racial stocks have persisted to this day even in very exacting environments and only by such could they have been protected.

In my studies of these several racial stocks I find that it is not accident but accumulated wisdom regarding foods that lies behind their physical excellence and freedom from our modern degenerative processes, and further, that on various sides of our world the primitive people know many of the things that are essential for life-things that our modern civilizations apparently do not know. These are the fundamental truths of life that have put them in harmony with Nature through obeying her nutritional laws.

Whence this wisdom? *Was there in the distant past a world civilization that was better attuned to Nature's laws and have these remnants retained that knowledge?* If this is not the explanation, it must be that these various primitive racial stocks have been able through a superior skill in interpreting cause and effect, to determine for themselves what foods in their environment are best for producing human bodies with a maximum of physical fitness and resistance to degeneration.

To conclude, primitive native races of eastern and central Africa have in their native state a very high immunity to dental caries, ranging from 0 to less than 1 per cent of the teeth affected for many of the tribes. Where modernized, however, the incidence increased to 12.1 per cent.

In the matter of facial deformity thirteen tribes out of twenty-seven studied presented so high a standard of excellence that not a single individual in the group was found with deformed dental arches.

Their nutrition varied according to their location, but always provided an adequate quantity of body-building and repairing material, even though much effort was required to obtain some of the essential food factors.

Many tribes practiced feeding girls special foods for an extended period before marriage. Spacing of children was provided by a system of plural wives.

48.

Isolated And Modernized Australian Aborigines

By Dr. Weston A. Price

Our problem of throwing light upon the cause of the physical breakdown of our modern civilization, with special consideration of tooth decay and facial deformity, requires a critical examination of individuals living in as wide a range of physical conditions as may be possible.

This requires that the Aborigines of Australia be included in this examination of human reactions to physical environments. These were studied in 1936.

In selecting the individuals in the various groups special effort was made to include children between the ages of ten and sixteen years in order to have an opportunity to observe and record the condition of the dental arches after the permanent teeth had erupted.

This was necessary because the deciduous dentition or first set of teeth may be in normal position in the arches with a correct relationship between the arches, and the permanent dentition show marked irregularity.

The shape of the dental arches of the infant at birth and the teeth that are to take their place in the arches have considerable of their calcification at birth. The development of the adult face, however, does not occur until the permanent teeth have erupted. The general shape or pattern is largely influenced by the position and direction of the eruption of the permanent teeth. These studies, accordingly, have included a careful, detailed record of the shape of the dental arch of each individual.

The Australian Aborigines constitute one of the most unique primitive races that have come out of the past into our modern times. We are particularly concerned with those qualities that have made possible their survival and cultural development.

The Aborigines are of special interest because they have come out of a very distant past and are associated with animal life which is unique in being characterized as a living museum preserved from the dawn of animal life on the earth.

Many of the animal species that are abundant in Australia are found only in fossil form on other continents.

The Aborigines are credited with having the most primitive type of skeletal development of any race living today. The eyes are very deep set, the brows very prominent giving them an expression that identifies them as a distinct racial type.

Their skill in tracking and outwitting the fleet and very cunning animal life of their land is so remarkable that they have been accredited with a sixth sense. They have been able to build good bodies and maintain them in excellent condition in a country in which the plant life, and consequently the lower animal life can be maintained at only a very low level because of the absence of rain.

Over half of Australia has less than ten inches of rain a year. It is significant that the natives have maintained a vigorous existence in districts in which the white population which expelled them is unable to continue to live. Among the white race there, the death rate approaches or exceeds the birth rate.

They are very fond of decorations on their bodies. Little baldness was seen even in the very old.

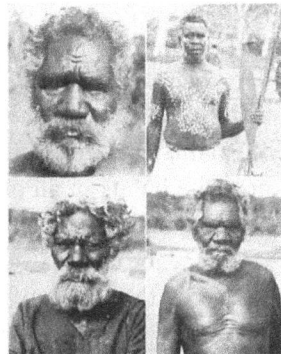

The Aborigines of Australia are recognized to be one of the oldest living race of mankind. Note the prominent eyebrows and deep set eyes. The man at the upper right is holding his spears and wamara, or spear thrower. They are very fond of decorations on their bodies. Little baldness was seen even in the very old.

They have developed a device for throwing spears, which makes them more deadly than any in the world. I witnessed a group of the present-day natives throwing their spears at a target which consisted of a banana stalk much smaller than a man's body. They threw the spears from a distance which I estimated to be seventy-five yards. About thirty spears were thrown and several pierced the banana stalk and the others were stuck in the ground close around it.

This was accomplished by means of a wamara or throwing stick approximately as long as the arm, with a strong hand grip at one end and a device on the other end for engaging in a depression in the butt of the spear. This was thrown by poising the spear about the level of the shoulder, the spear supported by the fingers of the hand which swung the throwing stick. The latter extended back over the shoulder. The impact of their spears has often been demonstrated to be sufficient to completely penetrate a man's body. Their method of tempering wood for the points of the spears was such that the spearheads offered great resistance.

These natives decorate their bodies with paints for dances and sports. They know the habits of all of the animals and insects so well that they are able to reproduce the calls of the animals and thus decoy them into traps.

Some of the water birds maintain sentinels at lookout points to guard those in the water. The Aborigines are able to decoy these birds by most ingenious methods. They travel with their bodies disguised by grass and shrubbery and enter the water with a headgear made from feathers of one of the birds.

Once in the water, they then maneuver in a manner similar to that of the birds and go among the flock of wild ducks or swans. Working entirely under water, they draw the birds under

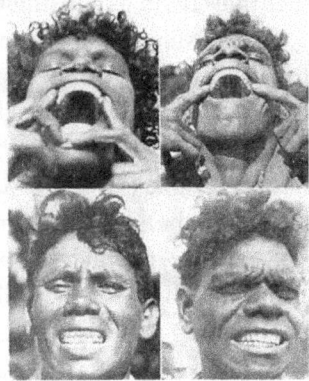

Very few primitive races seem to deserve so much credit for skill in obeying nature's laws as these primitive Aborigines because of the perpetual drought hazards of much of the land they live in. Half of Australia has less than ten inches of rain per year. Note the magnificent dental arches and beautiful teeth of these primitives. Tooth decay was almost unknown in many districts.

one by one and take load after load to shore without raising the suspicion of the flock.

When working among the kangaroos they are so skilled in preparing movable blinds that they can kill many in a grazing wild pack without alarming the rest.

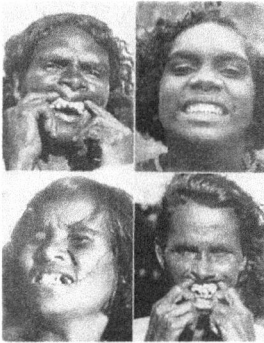

Wherever the primitive Aborigines have been placed in reservations and fed on the white man's foods of commerce dental caries has become rampant. This destroys their beauty, prevents mastication, and provides infection for seriously injuring their bodies. Note the contrast between the primitive woman in the upper right and the three modernized women.

Their skill at fishing probably exceeds that of any other race. They are so highly trained in the knowledge of the habits of the fish and the type of movement that the fish transmits to the water and to the reeds in the water, that one of their important contests between tribes is to see how many fish can be struck in succession with a spear, the fish never being seen, their only information as to its whereabouts being the change in the surface of the water and movement of grasses that are growing in the water as the fish moves. The fish are startled by the umpire's striking the water. The experts bring up a fish six times out of eight. These fishing contests are held along the banks of lakes and rivers where the water is deep enough for some of the reeds and grasses to come to the surface. The contestants travel in canoes.

The native canoe is cut in one piece from the side of a tree, the cutting being done with stone axes. The canoe offers an exceedingly treacherous platform from which a standing man must throw his spear. For some of the contests the canoe carries a paddler, but in the most exacting contests the spear man must manage his own flat-bottomed canoe.

The skill of the Aborigines in tracking is so phenomenal that practically every large modern town or city in Australia has one or more of these men on its police staff today to track criminals.

For weeks, they carry the detailed information about the characteristics of the prisoner's foot across the desert, and when they come across the man's foot print they recognize it among all others in the same path. Every leaf that is turned over or grain of sand on bare rocks has meaning for them.

Their social organization is such that almost every person who had been in intimate contact with them, testified that they had never known any of the Aborigines to be guilty of the theft of anything. Even where partly modernized, as they are in the large government reservations they are trustworthy.

A nurse in an emergency hospital told me that she continually left her money, jewelry and other objects of personal property freely exposed and available where many of the hundreds of primitives passing could pick them up, and that she had never known them to take anything. The other nurses had had the same experience.

Every boy and girl among these Aborigines must pass many examinations. Their early schooling includes the tracking of small animals and insects. The small boys begin throwing spears almost as soon as they can stand up straight.

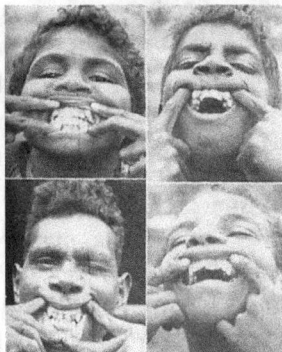

No young man can even witness a meeting of the council, let alone become a member of it, until he has passed three supreme tests of manhood.

First, he is tested for his ability to withstand hunger without complaint. The test for this is to go on a march for two or three days over the hot desert and assist in preparing the meals and not partake of any himself. He must not complain. If he becomes too weak, he is given a small portion.

There are tests for fear in which he is placed under the most trying ordeals without knowing that it is part of his examination, and he must demonstrate that he will accept death rather than flee.

It is remarkable that regardless of race or color the new generations born after the adoption by primitives of deficient foods develop in general the same facial and dental arch deformities and skeletal defects. Note the characteristic narrowing of the dental arches and crowding of the teeth of this modernized generation of Aborigines and their similarity to the facial patterns of modern whites.

No member of their society would be allowed to continue to live with the tribe if he had defied the ideals of the group. Immorality is cause for immediate death.

The growing boys among the Aborigines are taught deference and esteem for their elders in many impressive ways. A boy may not kill or capture a slow moving animal. That is left for the older men. He must limit his hunting primarily to the fast fleeing kangaroos and wallabies, whom even a man on horseback cannot outdistance. Racketeers and such unsocial beings could not exist in this type of civilization.

Marriages are arranged according to very distinct tribal patterns and every girl is provided with a husband at a time decided by the council.

Their code of ethics is built around the conception of a powerful Supreme Force that is related to the sun. They believe that there is an after-existence in which the myriads of stars represent the spirits of the Aborigines that lived before.

The boys and girls are taught the names of the great characters that make up the different constellations. These were individuals who had conquered all of the temptations of life and had lived so completely in the interest of others that they had fulfilled the great motivating principle of their religion, which is that life consists in serving others as one would wish to be served. The seven stars of Pleiades were seven beautiful maidens that had surpassed most other girls in their devotion and service in the interest of their tribe.

A part of a young men's examination to determine his ability to withstand pain and his power of self-control consists in performing an operation at the time of his graduation. This operation is at the same time calculated to provide him with his badge of attainment.

It consists of the boy's lying on his back and allowing the appointed operator to knock out one of his front upper teeth. This is done by putting a peg against the tooth and hitting it a series of sharp blows with a stone. He must endure this without flinching. We saw scores that carried this diploma. Prior to this, other very severe tests of physical endurance had been successfully completed.

The marvelous vision of these primitive people is illustrated by the fact that they can see many stars that our race cannot see. In this connection it is authoritatively recorded regarding the Maori of New Zealand that they can see the satellites of Jupiter which are only visible to the white man's eye with the aid of telescopes.

These people prove that they can see the satellites by telling the man at the telescope when the eclipse of one of the stars occurs. It is said of these primitive Aborigines of Australia that they can see animals moving at a distance of a mile which ordinary white people can not see at all.

While these evidences of superior physical development command our most profound admiration, their ability to build superb bodies and maintain them in excellent condition in so difficult an environment commands our genuine respect. It is a supreme test of human efficiency.

It is doubtful if many places in the world can demonstrate so great a contrast in physical development and perfection of body as that which exists between the primitive Aborigines of Australia who have been the sole arbiters of their fate, and those Aborigines who have been under the influence of the white man.

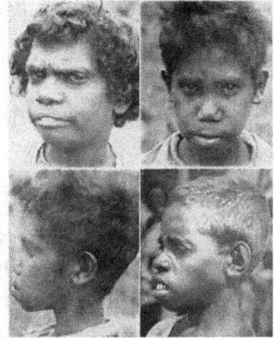

Deformity patterns produced in the modernized Aborigines of Australia by white men's food. Note the undershot mandible, upper left, the pinched nostrils and facial deformity of all four.

The white man has deprived them of their original habitats and is now feeding them in reservations while using them as laborers in modern industrial pursuits.

This contrast between the primitive Aborigines as they still exist in isolated communities in Australia and the modern members of the clans is not, however, much greater than that between these excellent primitives and the whites, near whom they are living.

In my comparative study of primitive races in different parts of the world, of modernized members of their groups and of whites who have displaced them, as well as in my study of our typical modern social organization, I have seldom, if ever, found whites suffering so tragically from evidence of physical degeneration, as expressed in tooth decay and change in facial form, as are the whites of eastern Australia.

This has occurred on the very best of the land that these primitives formerly occupied and becomes at once a monument to the wisdom of the primitive Aborigines and a signboard of warning to the modern civilization that has supplanted them. Their superb physical excellence is demonstrated in every isolated group in the primitive stocks with which we came in contact.

When living in the Bush they are largely without clothing. Where they are congregated in the reservations they are required to wear clothing. It is important to note in these people the splendid proportions of the faces, all of which are broad, with the dental arches wide and well contoured. This is Nature's normal form for all humans. Tooth decay was almost unknown in many districts.

Very few primitive races seem to deserve so much credit for skill in obeying nature's laws as these primitive aborigines because of the perpetual drought hazards of much of the land they live in. Half of Australia has less than ten inches of rain per year.

Wherever the primitive Aborigines have been placed in reservations and fed on the white man's foods of commerce dental caries has become rampant. This destroys their beauty, prevents mastication, and provides infection for seriously injuring their bodies.

Various factors in the changed environment were studied critically. Samples of foods were gathered for chemical analysis; and the changes in the modern diet from that which was characteristic of the primitives were studied. When the teeth of the primitives and the teeth found in the skulls that had been assembled in the museums were examined, it was found that dental caries or tooth decay was exceedingly rare among the isolated groups.

Those individuals, however, who had adopted the foods of the white man suffered extremely from tooth decay as did the whites. Where they had no opportunity to get native food to combine with the white man's food their condition was desperate and extreme.

It is quite impossible to imagine the suffering that these people were compelled to endure due to abscessing teeth resulting from rampant tooth decay. As we had found in some of the modernized islands of the Pacific, we discovered that here too, discouragement and a longing for death had taken the place of a joy in living in many. Few souls in the world have experienced this discouragement and this longing to a greater degree.

One of the most important phases of our special quest was to get information that would throw light on the degeneration of the facial pattern that occurs so often in our modern civilization. This has its expression in the narrowing and lengthening of the face and the development of crooked teeth.

It is most remarkable and should be one of the most challenging facts that can come to our modern civilization that such primitive races as the Aborigines of Australia, have reproduced for generation after generation through many centuries-no one knows for how many thousands of years-without the development of a conspicuous number of irregularities of the dental arches.

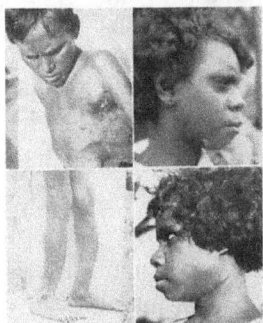

Yet, in the next generation after these people adopt the foods of the white man, a large percentage of the children developed irregularities of the dental arches with conspicuous facial deformities. Severe deformities of the face were frequently seen in the modernized groups.

The disturbance in facial growth is often so serious as to make normal breathing through the nose very difficult. This is primarily due to faulty development of the maxillary bones.

Aborigines in Australia living on a reservation. The boy at the upper left has suppurating tubercular axillary glands. The girl at the upper right has pus running to the outside of her face from an abscessed tooth. The boy whose legs are shown at the lower left has a badly deformed body from malnutrition. The girl at the lower right has tubercular glands of the neck.

The data obtained from a study of the native Australians who are located in a reservation near Sydney, at LeParouse, revealed that among the Aborigines 47.5 per cent of the teeth had been attacked by dental caries, and 40 per cent of the individuals had abnormal dental arches.

For the women of this group, 81.3 per cent of all the teeth had been attacked by dental caries, and for the men, 60.4 per cent, and for the children, 16.5 per cent. In this group 100 per cent of the individuals were affected by dental caries.

Palm Island is a government reservation situated in the ocean about fifty miles from the mainland, off the east coast of Australia, about two-thirds of the way up the coast. It was reached by a government launch.

Included in the population of this reservation are a large number of adults who have been moved from various districts on the mainland of Central and Eastern Australia and many children who were born either before or after their parents were moved to this reservation. The food available on the Island is almost entirely that provided by the government.

Of ninety-eight individuals examined and measured, 53.1 per cent of them had dental caries. For the group as a whole, 8.9 per cent of all of the teeth were affected; for the women, 21.2 per cent; for the men, 14.2 per cent; and for the children, 5.8 per cent. Fifty per cent of the children had deformed dental arches, which occurred in only 11 per cent of the adults.

Cape Bedford is situated about three-fourths of the way up the east coast and is so isolated that it was necessary for us to use a special aeroplane to reach it. Landing was made on the beach.

This group of people is under the management of a German Lutheran missionary. They are dependent almost entirely on the food provided by the mission and the government. The official in charge had spent fifty years in devoted service to these native people. We found him exceedingly sad because of the very rapid breakdown that was in progress among the natives in his care.

The dental caries for the group of eighty-three individuals studied was 12.4 per cent of their 2,176 teeth examined. For the women, this amounted to 37.2 per cent of the teeth; for the men, 8.4 per cent; and for the children, 6.1 per cent. Of the eighty-three individuals, 48.1 per cent had been affected by dental caries.

Many of the adults in this group had been born on plantations under the influence of the modern nutrition, and many of the children had been born in the mission. For the adults, 46 per cent had abnormally formed dental arches, and for the children, 41.6 per cent. We were advised that deaths occurred very frequently from tuberculosis. These people are fully dependent on the imported foods supplied by the officials.

Our next stop, using the special aeroplane, was at Lockhart River, which is about four-fifths of the way up the east coast of Australia. Here again we were able to land on the beach near a large group of primitive Aborigines. The isolation here is so nearly complete that they are dependent upon the sea and the land for their foods.

This part of Australia, namely, the York Peninsula, is still so primitive that there has been very little encroachment by the white population. It will be remembered that in this area there are no roads, the country being a primitive wilderness.

Of fifty-eight individuals examined, their 1,784 teeth revealed that only 4.3 per cent had been attacked by dental caries. Some of these men had at some time worked on cattle ranches for the white men.

A reservation called Cowall Creek on the west side of York Peninsula situated on the Gulf of Carpenteria, was reached by flying our special plane to Horn Island in the Torres Strait north of Australia and proceeding from there by boat to Thursday Island, and on, by boat, to Cowall Creek.

In this reservation thirty-five individuals were studied and found to be in a very pathetic condition. We were told that deaths occurred frequently. Of the 976 teeth examined, 24.6 per cent had been attacked by tooth decay. Many of these adults had been raised in the bush. Of the individuals studied, 68.6 per cent had had dental caries.

One can scarcely visualize, without observing it, the distress of a group of primitive people situated as these people are, compelled to live in a very restricted area, forced to live on processed food provided by the government, while they are conscious that if they could return to their normal habits of life they would regain their health.

Many individuals were seen with abscessing teeth. One girl was seen with a fistula exuding pus on the outside of her face. Another girl had tubercular glands of the neck.

In their native life where they could get the foods that keep them well and preserve their teeth, they had no need for dentists. Now they have need, but have no dentists.

It is easy to chide and blame the officials who provide them with the modernized foods under which they are breaking, but it must be remembered that practically all modern civilizations are more or less in the same plight themselves.

An opportunity was provided for examining a group of the native Aborigines of Australia who made up the crew of eighteen for a pearl-fishing boat. These individuals could be readily divided into two groups; namely, those who had been raised in the Bush and those who had been raised in missions.

For the thirteen raised in the Bush, not a single tooth of their 364 teeth had ever been attacked by tooth decay and not a single individual had deformed dental arches. In contrast with this, of the five raised in the mission, 19.3 per cent of their 140 teeth had been attacked by tooth decay and 40 per cent of these individuals had abnormal dental arches.

The cook on the government boat was an aboriginal Australian from Northern Australia. He had been trained on a military craft as a dietitian. Nearly all his teeth were lost. It is of interest that while the native Aborigines had relatively perfect teeth, this man who was a trained dietitian for the whites had lost nearly all his teeth from tooth decay and pyorrhea.

An interesting incident was brought to my attention in one of the Australian reservations where the food was practically all supplied by the government. I was told by the director in charge, and in further detail by the other officials, that a number of native babies had become ill while nursing from their mothers. Some had died.

By changing the nutrition to a condensed whole milk product, the babies recovered. When placed back on their mother's breast food they again became ill. The problem was: Why was not their mothers' milk adequate?

I was later told by the director of a condition that had developed in the pen of the reservation's hogs which were kept to use up the scraps and garbage from the reservation's kitchens. He reported that one after another the hogs went down with a type of paralysis and could not get up. The symptoms were suggestively like vitamin A deficiency in both the babies and the hogs, and indicated the treatment.

The rapid degeneration of the Australian Aborigines after the adoption of the government's modern foods provides a demonstration that should be infinitely more convincing than animal experimentation. It should be a matter not only of concern but deep alarm that human beings can degenerate physically so rapidly by the use of a certain type of nutrition, particularly the dietary products used so generally by modern civilization.

The child life among the Aborigines of Australia proved to be exceedingly interesting. Children develop independence very young and learn very early to take care of themselves. Mothers are very affectionate and show great concern when their children are not thriving. These children were keenly interested in everything that I did, but were not alarmed or frightened.

The wonderful wisdom of these primitive people was attested by the principal of the public school at Palm Island. A mother died and her nursing infant was taken care of by its maternal grandmother, who had not recently given birth to a child. She proceeded to carry out the primitive formula for providing breast food by artificial means.

Her method was to make an ointment of the fresh bodies of an insect which made its nest in the leaves of a certain tree. This she rubbed on her breast and in a short time produced milk liberally for this foster child.

I was shown the type of insect, photographed its nest and the colony inside when the nest was opened. The people who vouched for this circumstance declared that they had seen the entire procedure and knew the facts to be as stated. They further stated that this was common knowledge among the Aborigines.

Another important source of information regarding the Aborigines of Australia was provided by a study of the skeletal material and skulls in the museums at Sydney and Canberra, particularly the former. I do not know the number of skulls that are available there for study, but it is very large.

I examined many and found them remarkably uniform in design and quality. The dental arches were splendidly formed. The teeth were in excellent condition with exceedingly little dental caries. It was of interest to note the very heavy orbital ridges which characterize this race.

The buried skulls throughout Australia provide a dependable record of their physical excellence and splendid facial and dental arch forms.

It is a matter of concern that if a scale were extended a mile long and the decades represented by inches, there would apparently be more degeneration in the last few inches than in the preceding mile. This gives some idea of the virulence of the blight contributed by our modern civilization.

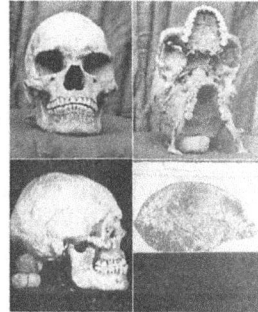

The foods available to these people in their natural habitat are exceedingly limited in variety and quantity, due to the absence of rains, and unfertility of the soil. For plant foods they used roots, stems, leaves, berries and seeds of grasses and a native pea eaten with tissues of large and small animals. They are able to balance their rations to provide the requisites for splendid body building and body repair.

In several parts of Australia, which originally supported a large population of the primitives, none are left except a few

The buried skulls throughout Australia provide a dependable record of their physical excellence and splendid facial and dental arch forms.

score in reservations. These also are rapidly disappearing. Their fertility has been so greatly reduced that the death rate far exceeds the birth rate.

This group provides evidence of exceptional efficiency in obeying the laws of Nature through thousands of years, even in a parched land that is exceedingly inhospitable because of the scant plant foods for either men or animals.

In Hammond Island, after examining the children at the mission school, I inquired whether there were not families on the island that were living entirely isolated from contact with modern influences.

I was taken to the far side of the island to an isolated family. This family had continued to live on their own resources. They were raising vegetables including bananas, pumpkins, and pawpaws. In the cases of the three girls in the family, one with a child five months of age, only six of their eighty-four teeth had been attacked by tooth decay, or 7.1 per cent, as compared with 16.5 per cent for the entire group on this island. These three girls all had normally developed dental arches and normal features.

The Catholic priest who had charge of the mission on this island told me that this family practically never asked for assistance of any kind, and was always in a position to help others. They were happy and well nourished. It is important to note that the progressive degeneration in facial form which occurred in many of the families on the other islands was not found in this family.

In the Torres Strait Islands, physical characteristics of the residents, regardless of their tribal group, were, sturdy development throughout their bodies, broad dental arches, and for all of those who had always lived only on their native food, a close proximity to one hundred per cent immunity to dental caries.

These men are natural mariners. They do not hesitate to make long trips even in rough seas in their homemade crafts. They have an uncanny skill in determining the location of invisible coral reefs. They relate the height of the swell as it rolls over the reef to particular color tones in the water, all of which were too vague for me to see even when they were pointed out.

It would be difficult to find a more happy and contented people than the primitives in the Torres Strait Islands as they lived without contact with modern civilization. Indeed, they seem to resent very acutely the modern intrusion.

They not only have nearly perfect bodies, but an associated personality and character of a high degree of excellence. One is continually impressed with happiness, peace and health while in their congenial presence.

These people are not lazy, but they do not struggle over hard to obtain food. Necessities that are not readily at hand they do not have. Their home life reaches a very high ideal and among them there is practically no crime.

In their native state they have exceedingly little disease. Dr. J. R. Nimmo, the government physician in charge of the supervision of this group, told me in his thirteen years with them he had not seen a single case of malignancy, and had seen only one that he had suspected might be malignancy among the entire four thousand native population.

He stated that during this same period he had operated several dozen malignancies for the white population, which numbers about three hundred. He reported that among the primitive stock other affections requiring surgical interference were rare.

49.

Isolated And Modernized New Zealand Maori

Dr. Weston A. Price

Because of the fine reputation of the racial stock in its primitive condition, it was with particular interest that studies were made in New Zealand. Pickerill, in his book The Prevention of Dental Caries and Oral Sepsis, has made a very extensive study of the New Zealand Maori, both by examination of the skulls and by examination of the relatively primitive living Maori. He states:

In an examination of 250 Maori skulls—all from an uncivilized age—I found carious teeth present in only two skulls or 0.76 per cent. By taking the average of Mummery's and my own investigations, the incidence of caries in the Maori is found to be 1.2 per cent in a total of 326 skulls. This is lower even than the Esquimaux, and shows the Maori to have been the most immune race to caries, for which statistics are available.

Comparing these figures with those applicable to the present time, we find that the descendants of the Britons and Anglo-Saxons are afflicted with dental caries to the extent of 86 per cent to 98 per cent; and after examining fifty Maori school children living under European conditions entirely, I found that 95 per cent of them had decayed teeth.

The reputation of the Maori people for splendid physiques has placed them on a pedestal of perfection. Much of this has been lost in modernization. However, through the assistance of the government, I was able to see many excellent physical specimens.

A young Maori man who stands about six feet four inches and weighs 230 pounds was examined. The Maori men have great physical endurance and good minds. Many fine lawyers and government executives are Maori.

The breakdown of these people comes when they depart from their native foods to the foods of modern civilization, foods consisting largely of white flour, sweetened goods, syrup and canned goods. The effect is similar to that experienced by other races after using foods of modern civilization.

Only about one tooth per thousand teeth had been attacked by tooth decay before they came under the influence of the white man.

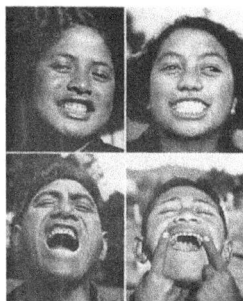

Since the discovery of New Zealand the primitive natives, the Mann, have had the reputation of having one of the finest teeth and one of the finest bodies in the world. These faces are typical. Only about one tooth per thousand teeth had been attacked by tooth decay before they came under the influence of the white man.

With the advent of the white man in New Zealand tooth decay has become rampant. The suffering from dental caries and abscessed teeth is very great in the most modernized Maori.

Whereas the original primitive Maori had reportedly the finest teeth in the world, the whites now in New Zealand are claimed to have the poorest teeth in the world. An analysis of the two types of food reveals the reason.

In striking contrast with the beautiful faces of the primitive Maori those born since the adoption of deficient modernized foods are grossly deformed. There was marked underdevelopment of the facial bones, one of the results being narrowing of the dental arches with crowding of the teeth and an underdevelopment of the air passages.

Through the kindness of the director of the Maori Museum at Auckland, I was able to examine many Maori skulls. The skulls belonged to the pre-Columbian period. Splendid design of the face and dental arches and high perfection of the teeth was worth noting.

One of the most important developments to come out of these investigations of primitive races is the evidence of a rapid decline in maternal reproductive efficiency after an abandonment of the native foods.

It was particularly instructive to observe the diligence with which some of the isolated Maori near the coast sought out certain types of food in accordance with the tradition and accumulated wisdom of their tribes.

Apart from seafood, they make abundant use of edible kelp, as do many sea bordering races. They also use large quantities of fern root which grows abundantly and is very nutritious. It is much easier for the moderns to exchange their labor for the palate tickling devitalized foods of commerce than to obtain the native foods of land and sea.

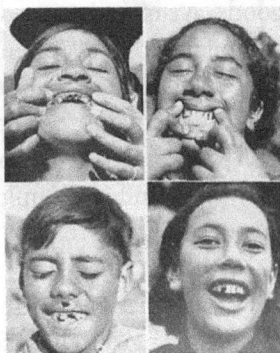

Probably few primitive races have developed calisthenics and systematic physical exercise to so high a point as the primitive Maori. On arising early in the morning, the chief of the village starts singing a song which is accompanied by a rhythmic dance. This is taken up not

With the advent of the white man in New Zealand tooth decay has become rampant. The suffering from dental caries and abscessed teeth is very great in the most modernized Maori.

only by the members of his household, but by all in the adjoining households until the entire village is swaying in unison to the same tempo.

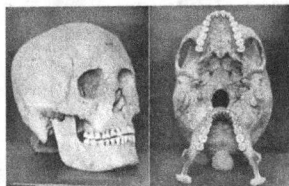

The large collections of skulls of the ancient Mann of New Zealand attest to their superb physical development and to the excellence of their dental arches.

This has a remarkably beneficial effect in not only developing deep breathing, but in developing the muscles of the body, particularly those of the abdomen, with the result that these people maintain excellent figures to old age.

Sir Arbuthnot Lane said of this practice the following:

As to daily exercise, it is shown here that every person capable of movement can benefit by it, and I am certain that the only natural and really beneficial system of exercise is that developed through long ages by the New Zealand Maori and their race-brothers in other lands.

The Maori race developed a knowledge of Nature's laws and adopted a system of living in harmony with those laws to a very high degree. They accomplished this largely through diet and a system of social organization designed to provide a high degree of perfection in their offspring.

The fact that they were able to maintain an immunity to dental caries so high that only one tooth in two thousand had been attacked by tooth decay (which is probably as high a degree of immunity as that of any contemporary race) is a strong argument in favor of their plan of life.

50.

Ancient Civilizations Of Peru

Dr. Weston A. Price

A t the time the Spanish Conquistadors arrived in Peru one of the most unique of the ancient cultures held sway over both the mountain plateaus and the coastal plains from Santiago of Chile northward to Quito, Equador, a distance of about 1200 miles. This culture took its name from the ruling emperors called Incas. The capital of their, great kingdom was Cuzco, a city located between the East and West Cordillera Ranges of the Andes.

These parallel ranges are from fifty to two hundred miles apart. Between them is situated a great plateau ranging from 10,000 to 13,000 feet above the sea. The mountain ranges are snow-capped and include in Peru alone fifty peaks that are over 18,000 feet in altitude, ranging up to 22,185 feet in Mount Huascaran. Only Mount Aconcagua in Chile is higher. It is 23,075 feet—the highest mountain in the Americas.

The air drift is across South America from east to west, carrying vast quantities of water received by evaporation from the Atlantic Ocean. This moisture is precipitated rapidly when the clouds are forced into the chill of the higher Andes. In the rainy season the great plateau area is frequently well watered, though not in sufficient quantity to meet the needs of agriculture for much of the territory.

In the past the precipitation has been supplemented by vast irrigation projects using the water from the melting snows. It is estimated that the population ruled over by the reigning Incas at the time of the coming of the Spaniards reached five millions.

Inca culture attained a highly perfected organization of society. The ruling Inca was a benevolent despot, and according to history unique in that he practiced most diligently all of the laws he promulgated for his people. There was no poverty, want or crime. Every man, woman and child was specifically provided with all necessities. The entire amount of tillable land was divided so that every man, woman and child had his assigned parcel. Everyone worked as assigned by the proper official.

While it is not appropriate here to go into details, it is important that we have a bird's eye view of this great culture for which I will quote a paragraph from Agnes Rothery's "South America, The West Coast and The East."

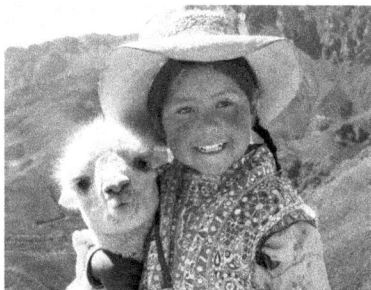

The people who erected this temple lived in order and health, under the most successful communism the world has ever seen. Their land was divided into three portions—one portion for the Inca, one for the Sun, and one for the people, with seventy square meters for every boy and thirty-five for every girl. The live stock and implements were similarly apportioned and the land was ploughed, planted, and the crops gathered in strict rotation.

First the fields of the Sun were cultivated, and then the land of the aged, the sick, widows, and orphans was tended; then the lands of the people, neighbors assisting one another; and last of all the lands of the Inca, with songs of praise and joy, because this was the service of their King.

To every living soul was given his tasks, according to his physical and mental capacities. He was prevented from overwork, prohibited from idleness, cared for in illness and old age. Children were taken by the Government when they were five and trained to the profession where they were most needed. There was no hunger, no crime in the whole empire.

The Inca held his kingly office over the docile, industrious, and contented mass not only through his royal blood, but through his wisdom and kindness in caring for and guiding his subjects, his bravery in war, and his statesmanship at home. Although he set an example to his subjects by following every law which he promulgated (astonishing idea to our modern lawmakers!), he lived, as became his rank, in luxury.

In his garden were rows of corn moulded from pure gold with leaves of pure silver, and a tassel of spun silver, as fine as silk, moving in the air. Llamas and alpacas, life-sized and cunningly fashioned from the same metal, stood upon his lawns, as they did in the courts of the Temple of the Sun.

The journey is made by train up through Arequipa and over the western Cordillera Range of the Andes into the plateau country and from there northward to Cuzco. So great is this natural barrier that the detour requires many days, and the crossing of several divides ranging from fourteen to sixteen thousand feet above the sea.

This was not necessary for the Incas who had built roads and suspension bridges through these mountains from Cuzco to all parts of the great empire. It is in this mountain vastness that the Inca rulers had constructed their most superb fortresses. While the early Spanish conquerors of the country knew that the nobility had great defenses to which they might retreat, the location of the fortresses was not known.

Their greatest fortress was discovered and excavated by Professor C. W. Bingham of Yale, under the auspices of Yale University and the American Museum of Natural History. This fortress and retreat is now world famous as Macchu Piccu, and probably represents the highest development of engineering, ancient and in some respects modern, on the American continent.

We are particularly concerned with the type of men that were capable of such great achievement, since they were required to carry forward their great undertakings without the use of iron or the wheel.

While the great Inca culture dominated the Sierras and the coast for several centuries prior to the coming of the Spanish, and while they had their seat of government and vast agricultural enterprises in the high Sierras, it is of special interest that many of the most magnificent monuments remaining today in stone were not constructed by the Inca culture, but by the Tauhuanocan culture which preceded the Inca.

The Incas were a part of the Quechu linguistic stock, while the Tauhuanocans were a part of the Aymara linguistic stock. The Incas had their capital in the high plateau country about the center of Peru. The earlier Tauhuanocan culture centered in southern Peru near Lake Titicaca where their most magnificent structures are to be found today.

One of the largest single stones to be moved and put into the building of a great temple in the history of the world is to be found near Lake Titicaca. According to engineers, there is no quarry known in an easily reached locality where such a stone could be quarried. It is conjectured that it was brought two hundred miles over mountainous country.

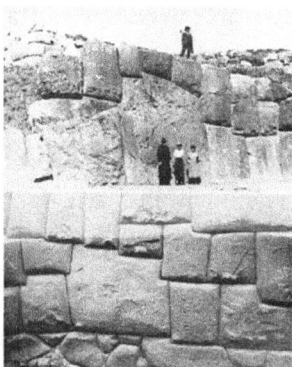

The primitive peoples of the Andean Sierra built wonderful fortresses and temples of cut stones which are assembled without mortar and cut to interlock. The central stone, above, is estimated to weigh one hundred and forty thousand pounds. Below the largest stone has twelve faces and twelve angles.

It is important to note that many magnificent structures, evidently belonging to this ancient Tauhaunocan culture, are found distributed through the Andean Plateau from Bolivia to Equador. Their masonry was characterized by the fitting together of large stones faced so perfectly that in many of the walls it was difficult to find a crevice which had enough space to allow the passage of the point of my pen knife, notwithstanding that these stones were many-sided with some of them fifteen to twenty feet in length.

While examining a section of wall of the great fortress Sacsahuaman, modern engineers seem unable to provide a satisfactory answer as to how these people were able to cut these stones with the limited facilities available, nor is it explained how they were able to transport and hoist some of their enormous monoliths.

The walls and fortress of Macchu Piccu, as well as the residences and temples, were built of white granite which apparently was taken from quarries in the bank of the river Urabamba, two thousand feet below the fortress. Without modern hoisting machinery, how did they raise those mammoth stones? One stone shown has twelve faces and twelve angles, all fitting accurately its boundary stones. It is as though the stones were plastic and pressed into a mould.

These wonderful fortresses and temples of cut stones were assembled without mortar and cut to interlock. The central stone is estimated to weigh one hundred and forty thousand pounds.

The country is rugged. Over it passes the highest standard-gage railroad in the world,—about 16,000 feet above sea level. The banks of this river are protected for long distances by ancient stone retaining walls.

The native Indians live and herd their flocks of llamas and alpacas up near the snow line, largely between 15,000 and 18,000 feet. The Incas and their descendants now occupying the high Sierras in the Andes have been thrifty agriculturists. They turn the soil with a very narrow, long, slender bladed spade which they force into the ground, and with which they pry the ground up in chunks. They then break up the chunks. These spades were originally made of copper which they mined themselves.

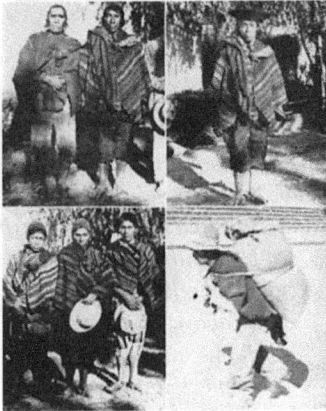

The Quichua Indians living in the high Andes are descendants of the Incas. They live at high elevations, up to 18,000 feet, where they raise herds of llamas and alpacas. They weave their own garments and have great physical endurance. They can carry over 200 pounds all day at high altitudes in the manner shown at the lower right.

Cuzco is the archeological capital of South America, but its glory is in the ancient fortresses and temples, rather than in the modern structures. As one passes through the streets, he will note that in many instances the foundations and parts of the walls of many of the modern Spanish cathedrals and public buildings are of old Inca construction, of fine stone work surmounted by cheap rubble work and mortar superstructure.

Whereas the original Cuzco had running water and an excellent sanitation system, modern Cuzco has deplorable sanitary conditions. The following is quoted from the West Coast Leader, published in Lima, dated July 20, 1937: "Of a total 3,600 houses in the city of Cuzco, 900 are without water or drainage; 2,400 are without light (windows) and 1,080 completely lack any sanitary systems. It is not surprising, therefore, that in some years the death rate exceeds the birth rate.

We are particularly concerned in studying these people to know the sources of their great capacity for developing art, engineering, government and social organization. Can such a magnificent culture be brought about unless founded on a superb physical development resulting from purely biologic forces?

It is important to note the roundness of the features of the Aymaras, the wide development of the nostrils for air intake and the breadth of the dental arches. Many of them had been transported several hundreds of miles to a coffee plantation because of their adeptness and skill in sorting imperfect coffee beans from the run.

As I watched them I found it difficult to move my eyes fast enough to follow their fingers and pick out from the moving run the undesired or imperfectly formed kernels. This revealed a superb development of coordination.

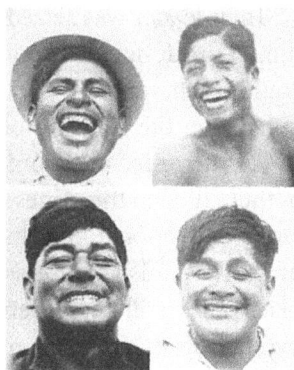

Some descendants of the ancient Chimu culture are still living in a few villages in the north of Peru. They live like their ancestors. Typical faces of this native stock are shown in this photograph. Note the breadth of the dental arches and full development of the facial bones.

The Quichua Indians living in the high Andes are descendants of the Incas. They live at high elevations, up to 18,000 feet, where they raise herds of llamas and alpacas. They weave their own garments and have great physical endurance.

The Indians of this region are able to carry all day two hundred to three hundred pounds at high altitudes, and they can do this day after day. At several of the ports, these mountain Indians have been brought down to the coast to load and unload coffee and freight from the ships. Their strength is phenomenal.

In approaching the study of the descendants of the Inca culture, it is important to keep in mind a little of their history and persecution under the Spanish rule. To this day they are bitter against the white man for the treachery that has been meted out to them on many occasions.

Their leader was seized under treachery. The agreement to free him, if the designated rooms were filled with gold as high as a man could reach, was broken and their chief killed after the gold was obtained.

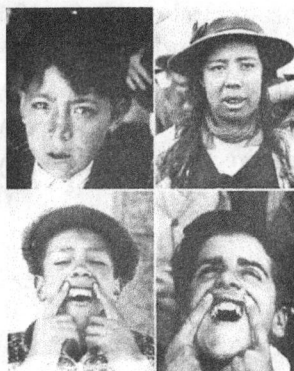

It is recorded that some six million of them died in the mines under forced labor and poor foods under the lash of their Spanish oppressors. In many places they still keep themselves aloof by staying in the high mountains of the Andes with their flocks of llamas and alpacas. They come down only for trading.

As in the past, they still weave their own garments. Indeed, they provide practically all of their necessities from the local environment. Their capacity for enduring cold is wonderful. They can sleep comfortably through the freezing nights with their ponchos wrapped about their heads and with their legs and feet bare. They wear two types of head cover, one inside the other. Many of them have faces that show strong character and personality.

The chest development, of necessity, must have large lung capacity for living

The modernization of the Sierra Indians through the introduction of foods of modern commerce has produced a sad wreckage in physique and often character. The boy at the upper left is a mouth breather because his nostrils are too small to carry sufficient air. The girl at the upper right has a badly underdeveloped chin and pinched nostrils. Both boys below have badly narrowed arches with crowding teeth.

in the rare atmosphere of the high Andes. They have a magnificent physique, including facial and dental arch development. Even in frosty weather they are bare below the knees.

Extensive wear of the teeth at the upper left was noted. Much of the food is eaten cold and dry as parched corn and beans. Such rough foods as these wear the teeth down.

One man we saw was said to be very old yet he climbs the mountains up into the snows herding the llamas and alpacas. The teeth have a very high state of perfection. Long and vigorous use has worn the teeth of the old people.

Market days which usually occur on Sunday present an interesting scene. The Indians travel long distances with their wares for exchange. They have no currency and exchanges are made by bargaining.

Where these Indians have become modernized, the new generation shows typical changes in facial and dental arch form as reported for the other groups. In some places, foods of the white man are displacing the native dietary.

The modernization of the Sierra Indians through the introduction of foods of modern commerce has produced a sad wreckage in physique and often character. Many children were found to be mouth breathers because their nostrils were too small to carry sufficient air. Some girls had badly underdeveloped chin and pinched nostrils while others had badly narrowed arches with crowding teeth. Tooth decay, needless to say was rampant.

51.

60000 Years And Still Going Strong

The Sentinelese - A Tale of Survival and A Lesson To The Civilized

The Sentinelese are one of the Andamanese indigenous peoples of the Andaman Islands, located in the Bay of Bengal. They exclusively inhabit North Sentinel Island which lies westwards off the southern tip of the Great Andaman archipelago. They are noted for vigorously maintaining their independence and sovereignty over the island, and resisting attempts of contact by outsiders.

By their long-standing separation from any other human society they are among the most isolated and unassimilated peoples on Earth, their social practices being almost entirely free of any recorded external influence.

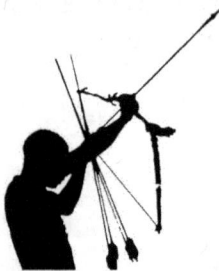

The Sentinelese maintain an essentially hunter-gatherer society, obtaining their subsistence through hunting, fishing, and collecting wild plants.

Their dwellings are either shelter-type huts with no side walls and a floor sometimes laid out with leaves, which provide enough space for a nuclear family of 3 or 4 and their belongings, or larger communal dwellings which may be some dozen square metres and are more elaborately constructed, with raised floors and partitioned family quarters.

Sentinelese wear no clothes, but utilize leaves, fibre strings or similar material as decorations, and they fashion belts which are apparently worn to provide some protection to the groin during potentially dangerous activity such as hunting or when encountering potentially hostile strangers.

Their weaponry consists of javelins, and an excellent flatbow with high accuracy against human-sized targets up to nearly 100 metres. At least 3 varieties of arrows, apparently for fishing and hunting, and untipped ones for shooting warning shots have been documented.

Perhaps no people on Earth remain more genuinely isolated than the Sentinelese and are believed to have lived on their island home for 60,000 years.

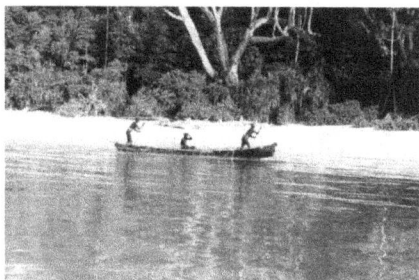

Like so many isolated tribal people with a fearsome reputation, the Sentinelese are often inaccurately described as 'savage' or 'backward'. Their hostility to outsiders, though, is easily understandable, for the outside world has brought them little but violence and contempt.

In 1879, for example, an elderly couple and some children were taken by force and brought to the islands' main town, Port Blair. The colonial officer in charge of the kidnapping wrote that the entire group, 'sickened rapidly, and the old man and his wife died, so the four children were sent back to their home with quantities of presents.'

Despite being responsible for the deaths of at least two people, and quite possibly starting an epidemic amongst the islanders, the same officer expressed no remorse, but merely remarked on the Sentinelese's 'peculiarly idiotic expression of countenance, and manner of behaving.'

The Sentinelese enjoy excellent health, unlike those Andamans tribes whose lands have been destroyed.

The islanders are clearly healthy, alert and thriving, in marked contrast to the two Andaman tribes who have 'benefited' from Western civilization, the Onge and the Great Andamanese. Their numbers have crashed and they are now largely dependent on state handouts just to survive.

Pressure from Survival and other organizations has led the Indian government to alter its policy towards the Sentinelese, from attempting to make contact, to recognising that similar policies have proved disastrous for other Andaman tribes, and accepting that they have the right to decide for themselves how they wish to live. Underpinning this shift is the simple acknowledgment that the people themselves are best placed to decide what is in their own interests.

Sentinelese Unaffected By Tsunami

In the days after the cataclysmic tsunami of 2004, as the full scale of the destruction and horror wreaked upon the islands of the Indian Ocean became apparent, the fate of the tribal peoples of the Andaman Islands remained a mystery.

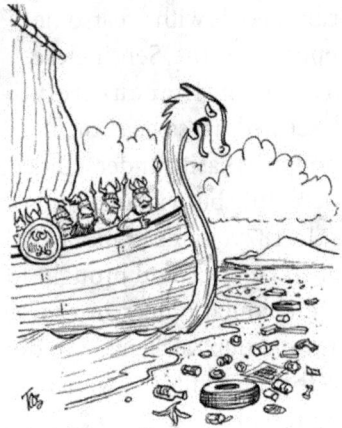

It seemed inconceivable, above all, that the Sentinelese islanders could have survived, living as they did on a remote island directly in the tsunami's path.

Yet when a helicopter flew low over the island, a Sentinelese man rushed out on to the beach, aiming his arrow at the pilot in a gesture that clearly said, 'We don't want

"Ok, we're raiding the next beach down."

you here'. Alone of the tens of millions of people affected by the disaster, the Sentinelese needed no help from anyone.

People in general do understand that civilization means a polished way of animal life. The animals eat what is fixed up by nature as its eatable but a civilized man eats not only what is fixed up by nature for him but also many other things which are outside the purview of his eatables. In other words a civilized person mishandles the problem of eating etc. and yet he calls himself something more than the animal.
~Srila Prabhupada (Back To Godhead, Who is a 'Sadhu'?)

52.

Diet of Mongolia

By Katherine Czapp

To 19th century Europeans, Central Asia represented vast tracts of unknown lands populated largely by the nomadic peoples of Mongolia, Turkestan and Tibet. Even as late as the mid-century, of the very few accounts available to Europeans of travels in this Terra Incognita, Marco Polo's 13th century adventures along the Silk Road and friendly visit with Genghis Khan's grandson, Kublai Khan, remained the most informative.

Isolated contemporary forays into the region by Christian missionaries produced largely inaccurate or incomplete information, although perhaps the most interesting of these was written by Evariste Huc, a French Lazarist missionary of the Roman Catholic Church who was sent with his brother missionary, Joseph Gabet, to evangelize the Mongols in 1844.

Abbé Huc wrote a lively, colorful and picaresque account of the two years of their travels which was translated into several languages and became immediately popular, although many of his readers assumed his nearly incredible adventures to be at least semi-fictional.

In 1870, the Russian Geographical Society (RGS) granted permission and funding for a small expedition of ten men led by Lieutenant-Colonel Nikolai Mikhailovich Przhevalsky to journey into Mongolia, on the western fringes of the Chinese empire.

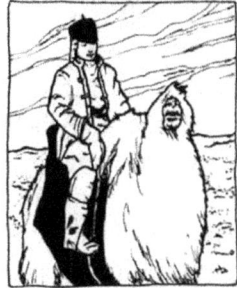

The impetus for this expedition was both political and scientific: recent uprisings among Muslim Tungans near the Chinese-Russian border exposed a weakness in Chinese authority, and the Russian government wanted Przhevalsky to reconnoiter these events. Przhevalsky would also be responsible for surveying and mapping the terrain and reporting on the flora and fauna of the regions he would travel through.

The Przhevalsky Journey

While a young officer in the Russian Army, Nikolai Przhevalsky had just two years earlier been sent by the RGS to survey new lands along the Amur and Ussuri Rivers in territory that had recently been ceded to Russia by China. Likely inspired by the immensely popular travel writings of David Livingstone and the colonizing of Africa and India by the British, Przhevalsky's aspirations for travel into Central Asia were fired by the race for influence and supremacy in Asia between Russia and Great Britain.

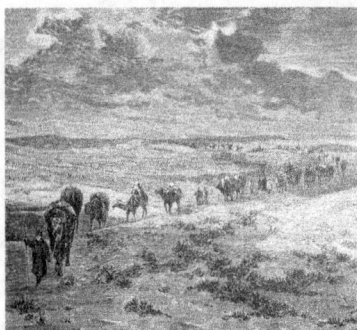

At the same time, Przhevalsky was a dedicated and talented naturalist, with great skills of observation. His original maps of exacting detail won him acclaim and medals of distinction from all the prominent geographical societies of Europe.

Traveling by horse and camel, and with a large herbarium in tow, Przhevalsky and his entourage first visited Beijing to secure passports for the rest of their journey through Chinese territory. Even with official permission from Beijing, Przhevalsky would meet with great difficulties as he traveled through regions ruled by local chieftains whose capricious chicanery and even cruelty would permanently sour his view of the Chinese, who were understandably suspicious of foreign presence.

Przhevalsky would learn to camp far from Chinese towns and closer to the Mongols, who were generally friendly and curious, and, once satisfied that the Russians were peaceful, would invite them inside their yurts for the ubiquitous cup of milk tea.

Ultimately, though, Przhevalsky's three-year sojourn in Western Mongolia was a great success. Along with his detailed maps and geographical notes, Przhevalsky brought back to St. Petersburg some 16,000 specimens of 1,700 botanical species, and introduced to Europe many species of yak, camel and other mammals. His most illustrious discovery was of the world's last extant wild horse which in his honor bears his name, Equus ferus przewalskii.

In 1875, the Imperial edition of Przhevalsky's Mongolia, the Tangut Country, and the Solitudes of Northern Tibet: Being a Narrative of Three Years' Travel in Eastern High Asia was published, and an English translation with notes appeared the very next year, published by the British Royal Geographical Society.

In his book, Przhevalsky dedicated an entire chapter to the ethnology of the Mongols, and in his descriptions of the details of their dress, habits and daily life, the reader finds both the keen eye of the observer as well as the chauvinistic sensibilities of the modern European much influenced by the then-popular notion of social Darwinism.

Przhevalsky views the Mongols, although not without sympathy, as a subjugated and weakened people, whose "glory days" of the empire-building great warriors Genghis Khan and Kublai Khan are sadly long past. His own certainty in the supremacy of the European "race" unfortunately clouds his understanding of aspects of Mongol culture that he nevertheless relates to the reader out of genuine interest and curiosity.

Mongol Diet

The food of the Mongols consists of milk prepared in various ways, either as butter, curds, whey or koumiss. The curds are made from the unskimmed milk, which is gently simmered over a slow fire, and then allowed to stand for some time, after which the thick cream is skimmed off and dried, and roasted millet often added to it. The whey is prepared from sour skimmed milk, and is made into small dry lumps of cheese.

Lastly, the koumiss is prepared from mares' or sheep's milk; all through the summer it is considered the greatest luxury, and Mongols are in the habit of constantly riding to visit their friends and taste the koumiss till they generally become intoxicated. They are all inclined to indulge too freely, although drunkenness is not so rife with them as it is in more civilized countries.

Tea and milk constitute the chief food of the Mongols all the year round, but they are equally fond of mutton. Sheep, like camels, are sacred; indeed all their domestic animals are emblems of some good qualities.

Mongolia has some of the harshest terrain in the world, as well as some of the highest altitudes. In the Russian version of Przhevalsky's descriptions of pastureland it is clear that "grass of poorest description" indicates that the alpine species growing in this arid range are only centimeters high, as opposed to the waving grasses of the steppes of Russia.

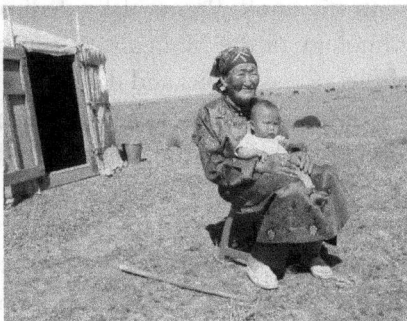

In fact, some 600 species of highly nutritious alpine grasses, herbs and flowers all comprise the high-altitude pastures where Mongols grazed their herds for barely four months during the year, yet during that brief time they fattened quickly.

Before eating, the lamas and the more religious among the laity, after filling their cups, throw a little onto the fire or the ground, as an offering; before drinking they dip the middle finger of the right hand into the cup and flick off the adhering drops.

The lamas will not touch meat, but have no objection to carrion. They do not habitually eat bread, but they will not refuse Chinese loaves, and sometimes bake wheaten cakes themselves.

Fowl or fish they consider unclean, and their dislike to them is so great that one of our guides nearly turned sick on seeing us eat boiled duck at lake Koko-nor; this shows how relative are the ideas of people even in matters which apparently concern the senses. The very Mongol, born and bred amid frightful squalor, who could relish carrion, shuddered when he saw us eat duck à l'Européenne.

Cattle - Their Life And Soul

Their only occupation and source of wealth is cattle-breeding, and their riches are counted by the number of their livestock, sheep, horses, camels, oxen, and a few goats—the proportion varying in different parts of Mongolia

As all the requirements of life: milk and meat for food, skins for clothing, wool for felt and ropes, are supplied by his cattle, which also earn him large sums by their sale, or by the transport of merchandise, so the nomad lives entirely for them. His personal wants, and those of his family, are a secondary consideration.

His movements from place to place depend on the wants of his animals. If they are well supplied with food and water, the Mongol is content. His skill and patience in managing them are admirable. The stubborn camel becomes his docile carrier; the half-tamed steppe-horse his obedient and faithful steed.

He loves and cherishes his animals; nothing will induce him to saddle a camel or a horse under a certain age; no money will buy his lambs or calves, which he considers it wrong to kill before they are full-grown.

Carefree Lifestyle

The most striking trait in their the Mongols' character is sloth. Their whole lives are passed in holiday making, which harmonizes with their pastoral pursuits. Their cattle are their only care, and even they do not cause them much trouble. The camels and horses graze on the steppe without any watch, only requiring to be watered once a day in summer at the neighboring well.

The women and children tend the flocks and herds. Milking the cows, churning butter, preparing their meals, and other domestic work, falls to the lot of the women. The men, as a rule, do nothing but gallop about all day long from yurta to yurta, drinking tea or koumiss, and gossiping with their neighbors.

An occasional pilgrimage to some temple, and horse-racing, are their favorite diversions.

The Mongol is an excellent father, and passionately fond of his children. Whenever we gave them anything they always divided it equally among all the members of their family, were it a lump of sugar, and the portion of each individual only a crumb.

The elders are always held in great respect, whose opinions and commands are implicitly followed. They are very hospitable. Any one who enters the yurta is regaled with tea and milk, and, for old acquaintance sake, a Mongol will open a bottle of koumiss.

On meeting an acquaintance, or even a stranger, the Mongol salutes him with, 'How are your cattle?' This is always one of the first questions, and they make no enquiry after your health until they have learned that your sheep, camels, and horses are fat and well to do.

We often had the most detailed questions asked us, such as: 'In whose care had we left our cattle before our departure on such a long journey?' 'What was the weight of the kurdiuk (fat tail) on each of our sheep?' 'How many good amblers did we possess and how many fat camels?'

"With the approach of autumn the Mongols throw off some of their laziness. The camels, which have been at pasture all the summer, are now collected together and driven to Kalgan or Kuku-Khoto to prepare for the transport of tea and merchandise to and from Kiakhta. Some are employed in carrying salt from the salt lakes of Mongolia to the nearest towns of China Proper.

In this way, during the autumn and winter, all the camels of Northern and Eastern Mongolia are earning large profits for their owners. With the return of April, the transport ceases, the wearied animals are turned loose on the steppe, and their masters repose in complete idleness for five or six months.

Extreme Hardiness

Endowed by nature with a strong constitution, and trained from early childhood to endure hardships, the Mongol enjoys excellent health, notwithstanding all the discomforts of life in the desert. In the depth of winter, for a month at a time, they accompany the tea caravans. Day by day the thermometer registers upwards of minus 20° F, with a constant wind from the northwest, intensifying the cold until it is almost unendurable.

But in spite of it they keep their seat on their camels for fifteen hours at a stretch, with a keen wind blowing in their teeth. A man must be made of iron to stand this; but a Mongol performs the journey backwards and forwards four times during the winter, making upwards of 3,000 miles."

Bartering

(Przhevalsky next describes the lengthy ritualized social etiquette of dickering for the price of a sheep, which the Mongols will never undersell.)

The difficulties in buying milk are also very considerable, and nothing will induce them to sell it in cloudy weather.

We were sometimes successful in overcoming the scruples of one of the fair sex by a present of needles or red beads, but in such case she begged us to cover the vessel over when removing it from the yurta, in order that the heavens should not witness the wicked deed.

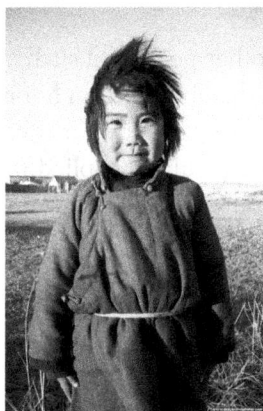

I may add that Mongols keep milk in the dirtiest way imaginable. It frequently happened that one of them would ride up to our tent with a jugful for sale, the lid and spout of the vessel having been smeared with fresh cow dung to prevent the liquid splashing out on the road. Cows' teats are never washed before milking, nor are the vessels into which the milk is poured."

The Magic of Dung

These last observations regarding issues of hygiene vis-à-vis milk present some challenging opportunities to stretch one's mind on the topic. First of all, the Mongolian high plains are a very arid region. Livestock do not find themselves in mud, nor do humid conditions exist. Cheese curds were commonly dried in the open air directly on the roofs of their gers.

Mountain peoples of other regions, such as Kyrgyzstan and Tajikistan, to name only two, traditionally soured milk in vessels (commonly wooden tubs) that were never washed, and in fact often stood outdoors. Morning and evening milk would be added to a continually fermenting mass. Tasty curd was scooped out when ready to eat, or was processed further by drying for long-term storage.

Likewise, traditional bakers worldwide never washed their wooden dough troughs in between bakings, and for the same reason: the stable cultures living in the crevices reliably produced the desired soured results, and the strength of the healthy culture deterred contamination by other microorganisms.

The use of fresh cow dung as an antiseptic, sanitary and healing agent has been practiced for centuries in India and Nepal. The first time I learned of the use of fresh cow dung as a housekeeping aid was in a modern Indian cookbook.

The author mentioned that her grandmother possessed such a fanatical obsession with cleanliness that she had her kitchen floor resurfaced with fresh cow dung not weekly, or even daily, but after every single meal. Fresh cow dung would be regularly applied to the floor of the kitchen, as well as to the floors of the sitting and sleeping areas of well-kept Indian homes.

Along with antiseptic qualities, the fresh dung repelled flies, mosquitoes and other insects. Farmers would reserve the dung for their customers.

Fresh cow dung has been used in Ayurvedic medicine and veterinary practice, applied to open wounds to speed healing, and in cases of psoriasis and eczema, to name but a few conditions for which it is prescribed. It is also used as a substrate for compound remedies, while urine has numerous medicinal uses as well.

Modern Indian practitioners today caution that the medicinal and antiseptic qualities of cow dung have been deteriorating in recent years due largely to unnatural foodstuffs fed to the animals. These include everything from invading leguminous weed species in pastures to fishmeal fed on farms. The resulting dung from these animals may not prevent infection.

These observations on alternative uses of cow dung are not an apology for careless hygiene, but they might suggest another, unconsidered dimension beyond our "fear of filth."

Harmonious ecosystems, in which humans are only one part, achieve balance through the cooperation and interdependence of many visible and invisible components. When the balance is upset, the wisdom of the entire system is deranged, and illness results.

(It is interesting to note that in Przhevalsky's account no one in his entourage falls ill from consuming any of the dairy products they purchase from the Mongols during their three years of travel. In fact, their primary complaint is that the butter and milk are always so expensive!)

Will The Traditional Mongolian Diet Reassert Itself?

The following are excerpts from an article by N. Oyunbayar, originally printed in Ger Magazine, which hints that Mongolians may be reconsidering the changes a free market economy is wreaking on their health and traditional diet:

When the Russians pulled the plug on Mongolia's aid in 1991, the economy went into a severe crisis. For many Mongolians it was their first experience of serious hunger. The staple traditional diet saw many people through this crisis. Mongolians traditionally have turned to foods that are high in protein and minerals, relying less on more seasonable foods like vegetables and fruits.

Out of necessity Mongolians have found creative and ingenious ways to use the milk of all five of the domestic animals in the country: sheep, cows, goats, camels and horses. Orom is the cream that forms on top of boiled milk; aaruul are dried curds and can be seen baking in the sun on top of gers in the summer; eetsgii is the dried cheese; airag is fermented milk of mares; nermel, is the home-brewed vodka that packs a punch; tarag is the sour yogurt; shar tos, melted butter from curds and orom, and tsagaan tos, boiled orom mixed sometimes with flour, natural fruits or eetsgii.

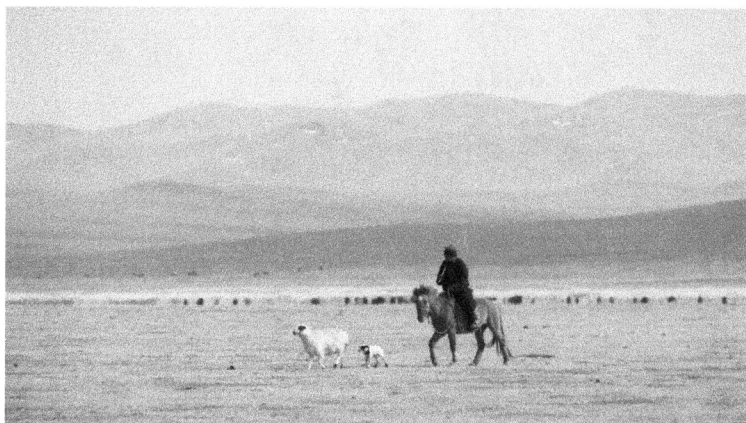

The method of drying the dairy products is common in preparing them. The Mongolians prepare enough dairy products for the long winter and spring. The traditions of using, producing and preparing these foods are stronger outside the main cities, where the population is more reliant on the vast herds for food. Dairy products, when sour in the summertime were thought to clean the stomach.

B. Baljmaa, a dietitian and nutritionist at the National Nutrition Research Centre, says there is a genetic compatibility for the food. "Before 1992 there wasn't much research in this area. But now we know from our research that Mongolians are better able to absorb foods with more acid. So, traditional food should be kept in the country..."

There is a big problem of importing poisonous foods and food which probably will cause the nutrition-related diseases common in more developed countries.... . For example, fast food made with more oil, salt and sugar are considered the biggest dangers for human health. On the plus side prices for these imported foods are higher and only the wealthiest people can afford them; the poor people can't buy and eat them no matter how much they desire them.

This means their poverty is protecting their health. We should boost our efforts to raise awareness on what foods protect your health.

53.

Characteristics Of Primitive And Modernized Dietaries

By Dr. Weston A. Price

If primitive races have been more efficient than modernized groups in the matter of preventing degenerative processes, physical, mental and moral, it is only because they have been more efficient in complying with Nature's laws.

We have two procedures that we can use for evaluating their programs: first, the interpretation of their data in terms of our modern knowledge; and second, the clinical application of their procedures to our modern social problems.

Specifically, since the greater success of the primitives in meeting Nature's laws has been based primarily on dietary procedures, it becomes desirable first, to evaluate their dietary programs on the basis of known biologic requirements for comparison with the foods of our modern civilization; and second, to test their primitive nutritional programs by applying their equivalents to our modern families.

The advancements in our knowledge of body-building and body-repairing materials from a biochemical standpoint makes it possible even with our limited knowledge of organic catalysts, to draw comparisons between the primitive and modernized dietaries.

If we use the generally accepted minimal and optimal quantities of the various minerals and vitamins required, as indicated by Sherman, (Chemistry of Foods and Nutrition. New York, Macmillan, 1933) we shall have at once a yardstick for evaluating the primitive dietaries.

Of the eighteen elements of which the human body is composed, all of which are presumably essential, several are needed in very small quantities. A few are required in liberal quantities. The normal adult needs to receive from the foods eaten one-half to one gram of calcium or lime per day. Few people receive more than one-half of the minerals present in the food. The requirements of phosphorus are approximately twice this amount.

Of iron we need from one-seventh to one-third of a gram per day. Smaller amounts than these are required of several other elements. In order to utilize these minerals, and to build and maintain the functions of various organs, definite quantities of various organic catalysts which act as activating substances are needed. These include the known and unknown vitamins.

Unlike some experimental animals human beings don't have the ability to create some special chemical substances (not elements) such as vitamins within their bodies. Several animals have this capacity. For example, scurvy, which is due to a lack of vitamin C, cannot be produced readily in rats because rats can manufacture vitamin C. Similarly, rickets cannot be produced easily in guinea pigs, because they can synthesize vitamin D. The absence of vitamin D and adequate minerals produces rickets in young human beings. Neither rickets nor scurvy can be produced readily in dogs because of the dogs' capacity to synthesize both vitamins C and D.

We are not so fortunate. Similarly, the absence of vitamin B (B1) produces in birds and man severe nervous system reactions, such as beri-beri. These symptoms are often less pronounced, or quite different, in other animals.

From our knowledge of the dietaries used by the various primitive racial stocks we can calculate the approximate amounts of the minerals and vitamins provided by those dietaries, for comparison with the amounts provided by modernized foods.

Our problem is simplified by the fact that the food of the white man in various parts of the world being built from a few fundamental food factors, has certain quite constant characteristics. Hence the displacing diets are similar for the several modernized groups herewith considered.

As a further approach to our problem, it is important to keep in mind that, in general, the wild animal life has largely escaped many of the degenerative processes which affect modern white peoples. We ascribe this to animal instinct in the matter of food selection. It is possible that man has lost through disuse some of the normal faculty for consciously recognizing body requirements.

In other words, the only hunger of which we now are conscious is a hunger for energy to keep us warm and to supply power. In general, we stop eating when an adequate amount of energy has been provided, whether or not the body building and repairing materials have been included in the food. The heat and energy factor in our foods is measured in calories. In planning an adequate diet, a proper ratio between body building and energy units must be maintained.

It is important to keep in mind that while the amount of body-building and repairing material required is similar for different individuals of the same age and weight, it is markedly different for two individuals, one of whom is leading a sedentary, and the other, an active life. Similarly, there is a great difference between the amount of body-building and repairing material required by a growing child or an expectant mother and an average adult.

There are certain characteristics of the various dietaries of the primitive races, which are universally present when that dietary program is associated with a high immunity to disease and freedom from deformities. In general, these are the foods that provide adequate sources of body-building and body-repairing material. The use by primitives, of foods relatively low in calories has resulted in forcing them to eat large quantities of these foods, in order to provide the heat and energy requirements of the body.

The primitives have obtained, often with great difficulty, foods that are scarce but rich in certain elements. In these rare foods were elements which the body requires in small quantities, including minerals such as iodine, copper, manganese and special vitamins. In connection with the vitamins it should be kept in mind that our knowledge of these unique organic catalysts is limited.

The medical profession and the public at large think of vitamin D as consisting of just one chemical factor, whereas, investigations are revealing continually new and additional factors. A recent review (C.E. Bills, New Forms and Sources of Vitamin D) describes in considerable detail eight distinct factors in vitamin D and refers to information indicating that there may be at least twelve.

Clearly, it is not possible to undertake to provide an adequate nutrition simply by reinforcing the diet with a few synthetic products which are known to represent certain of these nutritional factors. By the mass of the people at large, as well as by members of the medical profession, activated ergosterol is considered to include all that is necessary to supply the vitamin D group of activators to human nutrition.

I do not use the term vitamins exclusively because as yet little is known about the whole group of organic catalysts, although we have considerable knowledge of the limited number which are designated by the first half dozen letters of the alphabet. Most lay people and members of the medical and dental professions assume that the six or eight vitamins constitute practically all that are needed in an adequate nutrition.

These organic activators can be divided into two main groups, water-soluble and fat-soluble. An essential characteristic of the successful dietary programs of primitive races has been found to relate to a liberal source of the fat-soluble activator group.

When we discuss the successful dietary programs of the various groups from the standpoint of their ability to control tooth decay and prevent deformity we find that for the people in the high and isolated Alpine valleys their nutrition is dependent largely on entire rye bread and dairy products with meat only about once a week and various vegetables, fresh in the summer season and stored for the winter season.

An analysis in my laboratory of the dairy products obtained from the Loetschental Valley in Switzerland through a series of years has shown the vitamin content to be much higher than the average throughout the world for similar foods during the same seasons. The milk in these high valleys is produced from green pasturage and stored green hay of exceptionally high chlorophyll content. The milk and the rye bread provided minerals abundantly.

It is unfortunate that as the white man has come into contact with the primitives in various parts of the world he has failed to appreciate the accumulated wisdom of the primitive racial stocks.

Much valuable wisdom has been lost by this means. I have referred to the skill of the Indians in preventing scurvy and to the many drugs that we use which the white man has learned of from the primitives.

In this connection the Indians of British Columbia, who have been so efficient in preventing scurvy, have a plant product for the prevention and cure of diabetes. This has recently become known to the white man through the experience of a patient who was brought into the hospital at Prince Rupert, British Columbia, as reported in the Canadian Medical Journal, July 1938.

Prince Rupert is near the boundary between British Columbia and Alaska on the coast. The patient came to that hospital for an operation and suddenly showed signs of diabetes, which required treatment with large doses of insulin. Dr. Richard Geddes Large asked him regarding the history of his affection and what he had been taking. He was told that for several years he had been using an Indian preparation which was a hot water infusion of a root of devil's-club which is a spiny, prickly shrub.

This medicine was in common use by the British Columbia Indians. The material was obtained and used in this hospital for the treatment of diabetes and was found to be quite as efficient as insulin and had the great advantage that it would be taken by mouth whereas the insulin which is destroyed in the stomach by the process of digestion must be injected.

They could see very little difference in the efficiency of this preparation whether taken internally or used hypodermically. This promises to be a great boon to a large group of individuals suffering from diabetes. It is also probable that its use will prevent the development of diabetes and since the Indians used it for other affections it may also become a very important adjunct in modern preventive medicine.

It is also of interest that among the group in the Andes, among those in central Africa, and among the Aborigines of Australia, each knapsack contained a ball of clay, a little of which was dissolved in water. Into this they dipped their morsels of food while eating. Their explanation was to prevent "sick stomach." This is the medicine that is used by the native in these countries for combating dysentery and food infections.

It is the treatment that was given to me when I developed dysentery infection in central Africa while making studies there. The English doctor in Nairobi whom I called in said he would give me the native treatment of a suspension of clay. It proved very effective.

An illustration of the way in which modern science is slowly adopting practices that have been long in use among primitive races, is to be found in the recent extensive use that is made of clay (kaolin) in our modern medicine. This is illustrated in the following(Lawson, A., A Clay Adjunct To Potato Dietary):

In the course of an expedition to Lake Titicaca, South America, financed by the Percy Slade Trustees in which one of us took part, an interesting observation was made in regard to the diet of the Quetchus Indians on the Capachica Peninsula near Puno. These people are almost certainly descendants of the Incas and at the present time live very primitively. They exist largely on a vegetable diet of which potatoes form an important part. Immediately, before being eaten, the potatoes are dipped into an aqueous suspension of clay, a procedure which is said to prevent "souring of the stomach."

We have examined this clay and found it to consist of kaolin containing a trace of organic material, possibly coumarin, and presumably a decomposition product of the grass from underneath which the clay is dug. The local name for the clay is Chacco, and the Indians distinguish between good and bad qualities. This dietetic procedure is universal among the Indians of the Puno district, and is probably of very ancient origin.

Such a practice by a primitive people would appear rather remarkable in view of the comparatively recent introduction of kaolin into modern medicine as a protective agent for the gastric and intestinal mucosa and as a remedy for bacterial infections of the gut.

It is of interest that both the British and American Pharmacopeias have added kaolin to their list during the last two decades.

The Indians of the past buried, with their dead, foods to carry them on their journey. From an examination of these one learns that in many respects the Indians living in the high Sierras are living today very much as their ancestors did during past centuries.

Items of importance now and in the past are parched corn and parched beans which are nibbled as the people walk along carrying their heavy burdens. Today these are the only foods eaten on many long journeys. We found the parched beans pleasant to taste and very satisfying when we were hungry.

Few people will realize how reluctant members of the primitive races are, in general, to disclose secrets of their race. The need for this is comparable to the need for secrecy regarding modern war devices.

The Indians of the Yukon have long known the cure for scurvy and history makes an important contribution to their wisdom in treating this disease. It is of interest that W. N. Kemp (The sources of clinical importance of the vitamins) of Vancouver states:

> The earliest recorded successful treatment of scurvy occurred in Canada in 1535 when Jacques Cartier, on the advice of a friendly Indian, gave his scurvyprostrated men a decoction of young green succulent 'shoots' from the spruce trees with successful results. These happy effects apparently were not appreciated in Europe, for scurvy continued to be endemic.

Since that time untold thousands of mariners and white land dwellers have died with this dreaded disease.

Shortly before our arrival in Northern Canada a white prospector had died of scurvy. Beside him was his white man's packet of canned foods. Any Indian man or woman, boy or girl, could have told him how to save his life by eating the buds of trees.

The problem of estimating the mineral and activator contents, in other words the body-building and repairing qualities of the displacing foods used by the various primitive races, is similar in many respects to estimating these qualities in the foods used in our modern white civilizations, except that modern commerce has transported usually only the foods that will keep well. These include chiefly white flour, sugar, polished rice, vegetable fats and canned goods.

Even though calcium is present in spinach children cannot utilize it. Data have been published showing that children absorb very little of the calcium or phosphorus in spinach before six years of age. Adult individuals vary in the efficiency with which they absorb minerals and other chemicals essential for mineral utilization. It is possible to starve for minerals that are abundant in the foods eaten because they cannot be utilized without an adequate quantity of the fat-soluble activators.

A boy four and onehalf years of age suffered from convulsions due to malnutrition. His fracture occurred when he fell in a convulsion. There was no healing in sixty days. After reinforcing his nutrition with butter vitamins the healing at the right occurred in thirty days. Whole milk replaced skim milk and a whole wheat gruel made from freshly ground whole wheat replaced white bread.

Following are the details of this case. A minister in an industrial section of our city, during the period of severe depression, telephoned me stating that he had just been called to baptize a dying child. The child was not dead although almost constantly in convulsions. He thought the condition was probably nutritional and asked if he could bring the boy to the office immediately.

The boy was badly emaciated, had rampant tooth decay, one leg in a cast, a very bad bronchial cough and was in and out of convulsions in rapid succession. His convulsions had been getting worse progressively during the past eight months. His leg had been fractured two or three months previously while walking across the room when he fell in one of his convulsions. No healing had occurred.

His diet consisted of white bread and skimmed milk. For mending the fracture the boy needed minerals, calcium, phosphorus and magnesium. His convulsions were due to a low calcium content of the blood. All of these were in the skimmed milk for the butter-fat removed in the cream contains no calcium nor phosphorus, except traces.

The program provided was a change from the white flour bread to wheat gruel made from freshly ground wheat and the

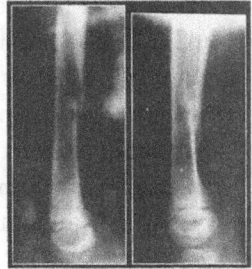

This figure shows the rapid healing of a fractured femur of a boy four and one half years of age suffering from convulsions due to malnutrition. His fracture occurred when he fell in a convulsion. There was no healing in sixty days. After reinforcing his nutrition with butter vitamins the healing at the right occurred in thirty days. Whole milk replaced skim milk and a whole wheat gruel made from freshly ground whole wheat replaced white bread.

substitution of whole milk for skimmed milk, with the addition of about a teaspoonful of a very high vitamin butter with each feeding. He was given this meal that evening when he returned to his home.

He slept all night without a convulsion. He was fed the same food five times the next day and did not have a convulsion. He proceeded rapidly to regain his health without recurrence of his convulsions. In a month the fracture was united.

Six weeks after this nutritional program was started the preacher called at the home to see how the boy was getting along. His mother stated that the boy was playing about the doorstep, but they could not see him. She called but received no answer.

Presently they spied him where he had climbed up the downspout of the house to the second story. On being scolded by his mother, he ran and jumped over the garden fence, thus demonstrating that he was pretty much of a normal boy. This boy's imperative need, that was not provided in white bread and skimmed milk, was the presence of the vitamins and other activators that are in whole milk but not in skimmed milk, and in whole wheat, freshly ground, but not in white flour. He was restored to health by the simple process of having Nature's natural foods restored to him.

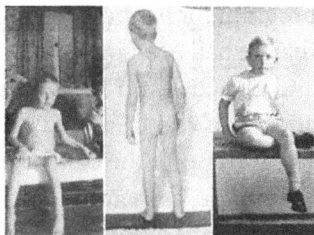

This boy, age 5, had suffered for two and one-half years from inflammatory rheumatism, arthritis and heart involvement. Upper left shows limit of movement of neck, left wrist, swollen knees and ankles. The middle upper view shows the change in six months after improvement of his nutrition, and at right his change in one year.

This problem of borrowing from the skeleton in times of stress may soften the bones so that they will be badly distorted. This is frequently seen as bow legs. An illustration of an extreme condition of bone softening by this process was seen in the skeleton of a monkey that was a house pet.

It became very fond of sweets and was fed on white bread, sweetened jams, etc., as it ate at the same table with its mistress. Note that the bones became so soft that the pull of the muscles distorted them into all sorts of curves. Naturally its body and legs were seriously distorted.

In this condition my patient, whom I was serving professionally, asked me for advice regarding her monkey's deformed legs and distorted body. I suggested an improved nutrition and provided fat-soluble vitamins consisting of a mixture of a high vitamin butter oil and high vitamin cod liver oil with the result that minerals were deposited on the borders of the vertebrae and joints and on the surfaces of the bones.

The necessity that the foods selected and used shall provide an adequate quantity of fat-soluble activators (including the known fatsoluble vitamins) is so imperative and is so important in preventing a part of our modern degeneration that I shall illustrate its need with another practical case.

A mother asked my assistance in planning the nutritional program for her boy. She reported that he was five years of age and that he had been in bed in hospitals with rheumatic fever, arthritis and an acute heart involvement most of the time for the past two and a half years. She had been told that her boy would not recover, so severe were the complications. As is so generally the case with rheumatic fever and endocarditis, this boy was suffering from severe tooth decay.

In this connection the American Heart Association has reported that 75 per cent of heart involvements begin before ten years of age. My studies have shown that in about 95 per cent of these cases

---

Agriculture is the noblest profession. Give him some land, he cuts the wood, makes cottages. The land is clear, now till it, keep cows and grow food grains.

Pusta Krishna: Doesn't put any local men out of work.

Prabhupada: Simple thing. And then live comfortably, eat comfortably, chant Hare Krishna. Comfortably means we require primary necessities, to eat something, to sleep somewhere and to defend, that's all. These are the primary necessities. That can be arranged anywhere. God has given all facilities. Grow your own food, eat, and live anywhere. Just this place was rough like that, now it is handled nicely, it is very attractive.

Any damn place, you cleanse it, it becomes home. And any nasty man, you decorate him, he becomes a bridegroom. (laughs)

~ Srila Prabhupada (New Vrindaban, June 24, 1976: Room Conversation)

there is active tooth decay. The important change that I made in this boy's dietary program was the removal of the white flour products and in their stead the use of freshly cracked or ground wheat and oats used with whole milk to which was added a small amount of specially high vitamin butter produced by cows pasturing on green wheat.

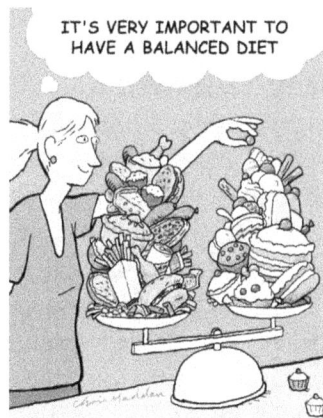

IT'S VERY IMPORTANT TO HAVE A BALANCED DIET

At this time the boy was so badly crippled with arthritis, in his swollen knees, wrists, and rigid spine, that he was bedfast and cried by the hour. His spine so rigid that he could not rotate his head.

With the improvement in his nutrition which was the only change made in his care, his acute pain rapidly subsided, his appetite greatly improved, he slept soundly and gained rapidly in weight.

On the same day, in the presence of his scientist-disciples, Srila Prabhupada met with an Indian scientist who was a specialist in nutrition. The man explained that his work benefited mankind by finding the cause of and treating protein deficiencies. Srila Prabhupada replied, "Suppose the birds and beasts have no research institute. Yet there is sufficient protein supplied by nature. An elephant has got a big body and so much strength, but they have not found that by your scientific research. The nature is supplying. Prakrteh kriyamanani gunaih karmani sarvasah. It is being done. Why you are wasting time in this way? You study what is nature and what is behind nature. That is real study. The protein supply is already being done. Just like a cow is eating grass. And she is supplying milk, full of protein. So do you think that the protein is coming from the grass? Can you eat grass?"

Scientist: "Something must be -- "

Prabhupada: "That is something, that is not perfect knowledge. Everyone knows the cow does not take any protein food. She takes on the grass."

Scientist: "Grass is quite rich in protein."

Prabhupada: "Then you take. Why are you searching after protein?"

This occurred six years ago. As I write this a letter has been received from the boy's mother. She reports that he is taller and heavier than the average, has a good appetite and sleeps well.

In the newer light regarding the cause of rheumatic fever, or inflammatory rheumatism, there appear to be three underlying causes: a general lowered defense against infection in which the fat-soluble vitamins play a very important part; minute hemorrhages in joint tissues as part of the expression of deficiency of vitamin C, a scurvy symptom, and a source of infecting bacteria such as streptococcus. This could be provided by his infected teeth.

These typical expressions of modern degeneration could not occur in most of the primitive races studied because of the high factor of safety in the minerals and vitamins of their nutrition. It is important to emphasize the changes that were made in our modern dietary program to make this boy's nutrition adequate for recovery.

Sugars and sweets and white flour products were eliminated as far as possible. Freshly ground cereals were used for breads and gruels. A liberal supply of whole milk, green vegetables and fruits were provided. In addition, he was provided with a butter that was very high in vitamins having been produced by cows fed on a rapidly growing green grass. The best source for this is a pasturage of wheat and rye grass. All green grass in a state of rapid growth is good, although wheat and rye grass are the best found. Unless hay is carefully dried so as to retain its chlorophyll, which is a precursor of vitamin A, the cow cannot synthesize the fat-soluble vitamins.

These two practical cases illustrate the fundamental necessity that there shall not only be an adequate quantity of body-building minerals present, but also that there shall be an adequate quantity

aho prajapati-patir
bhagavan harir avyayah
vanaspatin osadhis ca
sasarjorjam isam vibhuh

The Supreme Personality of Godhead, Sri Hari, is the master of all living entities, including all the prajapatis, such as Lord Brahma. Because He is the all-pervading and indestructible master, He has created all these trees and vegetables as eatables for other living entities.

(Srimad Bhagavatam 6.4.8)

of fat-soluble vitamins. Of course, water-soluble vitamins are also essential.

It is of interest that the diets of the primitive groups which have shown a very high immunity to dental caries and freedom from other degenerative processes have all provided a nutrition containing at least four times these minimum requirements; whereas the displacing nutrition of commerce, consisting largely of white-flour products, sugar, polished rice, jams, canned goods, and vegetable fats have invariably failed to provide even the minimum requirements.

The ratio in the Swiss native diets (rye bread, milk, cheese and butter) to that in the displacing diet was for calcium, 3.7 fold; for phosphorus, 2.2 fold; for magnesium, 2.5 fold; for iron, 3.1 fold; and for the fat-soluble activators, at least ten fold.

It is a pity that so much of their wisdom has been lost through lack of appreciation by the whites who made contact with them.

There are eight million four hundred thousand forms of living entities. Jalaja nava-laksani. In the water there are nine hundred thousand forms of living entity. Then, jalaja nava-laksani sthavara laksa-vimsati. Sthavarah means the living entities who cannot move, just like the trees, plants, grass, vegetables. They are standing in one place. They are also called "having no leg." Ahastani sahastanam apadani catus-padam. This is nature's law, that the living entities which have no hands, they are eatable for the living entities who have hands. Ahastani sahastanam apadani catus-padam. And the living entities which cannot move, they are the food for the living entities which has got four legs. Phalguni mahatam tatra jivo jivasya jivanam.

In this way the weak is the food for the strong. This is the law of nature, that one living entity is the food for another living entity. So when a person eats another living entity, it is not unnatural. This is nature's law. But when you come to the human form of living entity, you must use your discrimination. Just like one living entity is food for the another living entity. It does not mean... In the lower animals sometimes the father-mother eat the offspring, but in the history of human society it has not come into notice that the father and mother eating the offspring. But time has come when the mother is killing offspring. That has come already. This is due to Kali-yuga. ~Srila Prabhupada (Lecture, Bhagavad-gita 13.1-3, Durban, October 13, 1975)

54.

Nutrition And Healthy Reproduction

Traditional Wisdom For Continuation Of Human Race

By Dr. Weston A. Price

It is significant that while these important factors are just coming to light in our modernized civilization, the evidence clearly indicates that several so-called primitive races have been conscious of the need for safeguarding motherhood from reproductive overloads which would reduce the capacity for efficient reproduction. For example, G. T. Baden in his book "Among the Ibos of Nigeria" states:

It is not only a matter of disgrace but an actual abomination, for an Ibo woman to bear children at shorter intervals than about three years...The idea of a fixed minimum period between births is based on several sound principles. The belief prevails strongly that it is necessary for this interval to elapse in order to ensure the mother being able to recuperate her strength completely, and thus be in a thoroughly fit condition to bear another child. Should a second child be born within the prescribed period the theory is held that it must inevitably be weak and sickly, and its chances jeopardized.

Similarly, the Indians of Peru, Ecuador and Columbia have been familiar with the necessity of preventing pregnancy overloads of the mother. Whiffen in his book "North-West Amazons" states:

The numbers (of pregnant women) are remarkable in view of the fact that husbands abstain from any intercourse with their wives, not only during pregnancy but also throughout the period of lactation—far more prolonged with them than with Europeans. The result is that two

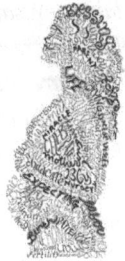

and a half years between each child is the minimum difference of age, and in the majority of cases it is even greater.

It may also be important to note that the Amazon Indians have been conscious of the fact that these matters are related to the nutrition of both parents. Whiffen states that:

> These Indians share the belief of many peoples of the lower cultures that the food eaten by the parents—to some degree of both parents—will have a definite influence upon the birth, appearance, or character of the child.

This problem of the consciousness among primitives of the need for spacing children has been emphasized by George Brown in his studies among Melanesians and Polynesians in which he reports relative to the natives on one of the Solomon Islands as follows:

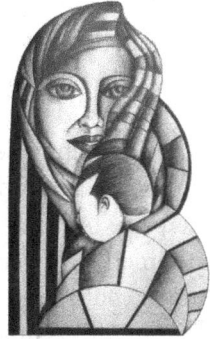

> After the birth of a child the husband was not supposed to cohabit with his wife until the child could walk. If a child was weak or sickly, the people would say, speaking of the parents, "Ah, well, they have only themselves to blame.

In approaching this problem as it applies to human beings, much can be learned from a study of domestic and wild animals.

Until recent years it has been common knowledge among the superintendents of large zoos of America and Europe that members of the cat family did not reproduce efficiently in captivity, unless the mothers had been born in the jungle.

Formerly, this made it necessary to replenish lions, tigers, leopards and other felines from wild stock as fast as the cages were emptied by death or as rapidly as new stock should be added by enlargement.

The story is told of a trip to Africa made by a wild animal specialist from the London zoo for the purpose of obtaining additional lions and studying this problem. While in the lion country, he observed the lion kill a zebra. The lion proceeded then to tear open the abdomen of the zebra and eat the entrails at the right flank. This took him directly to the liver. After spending some time selecting different internal organs, the lion backed away and turned and pawed dirt over the carcass which he abandoned to the jackals.

The scientist hurried to the carcass and drove away the jackals to study the dead zebra to note what tissues had been taken. This gave him the clue which when put into practice has entirely changed the history of the reproduction of the cat family in captivity.

The addition of the organs to the foods of the captive animals born in the jungle supplied them with foods needed to make reproduction possible. Their young, too, could reproduce efficiently.

As I studied this matter with the director of a large lion colony, he listed in detail the organs and tissues that were particularly selected by animals in the wilds and also those that were provided for animals reproducing in captivity. He explained that, whereas the price of lions used to be fifteen hundred dollars for a good specimen, they were now so plentiful that they would scarcely bring fifteen cents. If we observe the parts of an animal that a cat eats when it kills a small rodent or bird, we see that it does not select exclusively the muscle meat.

During my biological investigations using animals, I have had barn rats gnaw their way into the room where the rabbits were kept and kill several animals during a night. On two different occasions, only the eyes of the rabbits had been eaten, and the blood may have been sucked. On another occasion the brains had been eaten. It was evident that these rats had a conscious need for special food elements that were provided by these tissues.

One of the outstanding changes which I have found takes place in the primitive races at their point of contact with our modern civilization is a decrease in the ease and efficiency of the birth process.

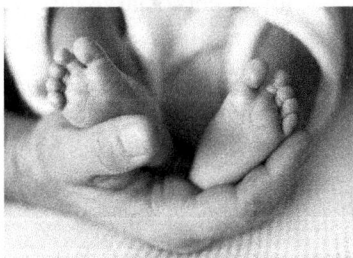

When I visited the Six Nation Reservation at Brantford, Ontario, I was told by the physician in charge that a change of this kind had occurred during the period of his administration, which had covered twenty-eight years and that the hospital was now used largely to care for young Indian women during abnormal childbirth.

A similar impressive comment was made to me by Dr. Romig, the superintendent of the government hospital for Eskimos and Indians at Anchorage, Alaska.

He stated that in his thirty-six years among the Eskimos, he had never been able to arrive in time to see a normal birth by a primitive Eskimo woman. But conditions have changed materially with the new generation of Eskimo girls, born after their parents began to use foods of modern civilization.

Many of them are carried to his hospital after they had been in labour for several days. One Eskimo woman who had married twice, her last husband being a white man, reported to Dr. Romig and myself that she had given birth to twenty six children and that several of them had been born during the night and that she had not bothered to waken her husband, but had introduced him to the new baby in the morning.

I have presumed in this discussion that the primitive races are able

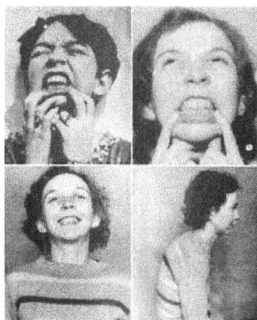

This girl suffered with a serious deformity of her face. She also had very contracted pelvic arch. The facial deformity was improved as shown. She nearly lost her life with the birth of her first baby which was removed by Caesarian operation. Note her badly deformed back from the overload of reproduction.

to provide us with valuable information. In the first place, the primitive peoples have carried out programs that will produce physically excellent babies. This they have achieved by a system of carefully planned nutritional programs for mothers-to-be.

It is important to note that they begin this process of special feeding long before conception takes place, not leaving it, as is so generally done until after the mother-to-be knows she is pregnant.

In some instances special foods are given the fathers-to-be, as well as the mothers-to-be. The cattle tribes of Africa, the Swiss in isolated high Alpine valleys, and the tribes living in the higher altitudes of Asia, including northern India, have depended upon a very high quality of dairy products.

Among the primitive Masai in certain districts of Africa, the girls were required to wait for marriage until the time of the year when the cows were on the rapidly growing young grass and to use the milk from these cows for a certain number of months before they could be married. In several agricultural tribes in Africa the girls were fed on special foods for six months before marriage.

Another important feature of the control of excellence of child life among the primitive races has been the systematic spacing of children by control of pregnancies. The interval between children ranged from two and a half to four years. For most of the tribes in Africa this was accomplished by the plural-wife system. The wife with the youngest child was protected.

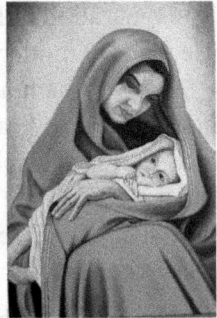

The original Maori culture of New Zealand accomplished the same end by birth control and definite planning. In one of the Fiji Island tribes the minimum spacing was four years.

These practices are in strong contrast with the haphazard, entirely unorganized programs of individuals in much of our modern civilization.

The question arises immediately: what can be done in the light of the data that I have presented in this volume to improve the condition of our modern civilization? A first requisite and perhaps by far the most important is that of providing information indicating why our present haphazard or over-crowded programs of pregnancies are entirely inadequate. This should include, particularly, the education of the highschool-age groups, both girls and boys.

In the matter of instruction of boys and girls it is of interest that several of the primitive races have very definite programs. In some, childbirth clinics supervised by the midwife are held for the growing girls. With several of these tribes, however, the ease with which childbirth is accomplished is so great that it is looked upon as quite an insignificant experience.

Among the ancient Peruvians, particularly the Chimu culture, definite programs were carried out for teaching the various procedures in industry, home-building and home management.

This was accomplished by reproducing in pottery form, as on practical water jugs, the various incidents to be demonstrated. The matter of childbirth was reproduced in detail in pottery form so that it was common knowledge for all young people from earliest observation to the time the practical problems arose. Many of the problems related directly were similarly illustrated in pottery forms.

It is not sufficient that information shall be available through maternal health clinics to young married couples. If pigs need several months of special feeding in order that the mothers-to-be may be prepared for adequate carrying forward of all of the inheritance factors in a high state of perfection, surely human mothers-to-be deserve as much consideration.

It is shown that it is not adequate that sufficient vitamin A be present to give the appearance of good health. If highly efficient reproduction is to be accomplished there must be a greater quantity than this.

There is no good reason why we, with our modern system of transportation, cannot provide an adequate quantity of the special foods for preparing women for pregnancy quite as efficiently as the primitive races who often had to go long distances on foot to procure special foods.

The primitive care of a newborn infant has been a matter of severe criticism by modernists especially those who have gone among them to enlighten them in modern ways of child rearing. It is common practice among many primitive tribes to wrap the newborn infant in an absorbent moss, which is changed daily. A newborn infant, however, does not begin having regular all over baths for a few weeks after birth.

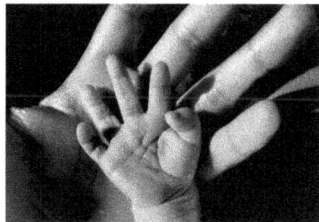

While this method is orthodox among the primitives it is greatly deplored as a grossly cruel and ignoble treatment by most moderns. Dr. William Forest Patrick of Portland, Oregon was deeply concerned over the regularly occurring rash that develops on newborn infants shortly after they are first washed and groomed. He had a suspicion that Nature had a way of taking care of this.

In 1931 he left the original oily varnish on several babies for two weeks without the ordinary washing and greasing. He found them completely free from the skin irritation and infection which accompanies modern treatment.

This method was adopted by the Multanomah County Hospital of Oregon which now reports that in 1,916 cases of unwashed, unanointed babies only two cases of pyodermia occurred. They record that each day the clothing was changed and buttocks washed with warm water. Beyond this the infants were not handled.

Dr. Patrick states that within twelve hours after birth by Nature's method the infant's skin is clear, and Nature's protective film has entirely disappeared.

In my observations of the infant's care among primitive races I have been continually impressed with the great infrequency with which we ever hear a primitive child cry or express any discomfort from the treatment it receives. Of course, when hungry they make their wants known. The primitive mother is usually very prompt, if possible, to feed her child.

I always found that primitive people went out of their way to gather special foods, sometimes walking for hours on end. These people understood the necessity for special foods:

1)before marriage, 2)during gestation, 3)during the nursing period and 4) for rebuilding before the next pregnancy.

As an illustration of the remarkable wisdom of these primitive tribes, I found them using for the nursing period two cereals with unusual properties. One, was a red millet which was not only high in carotin but had a calcium content of five to ten times that of most other cereals. They used also for nursing mothers in several tribes in Africa, a cereal called by them linga-linga. This proved to be the same cereal under the name of quinua that the Indians of Peru use liberally, particularly the nursing mothers. The botanical name is quinoa.

This cereal has the remarkable property of being not only rich in minerals, but a powerful stimulant to the flow of milk. I have found no record of the use of similar cereals among either the English or American peoples. As I have noted earlier, special nutrition was provided for the fathers by tribes in the Amazon jungle, as well as by the coastal tribes.

Professor Drummond, a British bio-chemist, in discussing the question of the modern decline in fertility, before the Royal Society of Medicine suggested that the decline in the birth rate in European countries, during the last fifty years, was due, largely, to the change in national diets which resulted from the removal of vitamins B and E from grains when the embryo or germ was removed in the milling process.

He called attention to the fact that the decline in the birth rate corresponded directly with the time when the change was made in the milling process so that refined flour was made available instead of the entire grain product.

Of the many problems on which the experience of the primitive races can throw light, probably none is more pressing than practical procedures for improving child life. Since this has been shown to be largely dependent upon the architectural design, as determined by the health of the parental germ cells and by the prenatal environment of the child, the program that is to be successful must begin early enough to obviate these various disturbing forces.

The normal determining factors that are of hereditary origin may be interrupted in a given generation but need not become fixed characteristics in the future generations. This question of parental nutrition, accordingly, constitutes a fundamental determining factor in the health and physical perfection of the offspring.

One of the frequent problems brought to my attention has to do with the responsibility of young men and women in the matter of the danger of transmitting their personal deformities to their offspring. Many, indeed, with great reluctance and sense of personal loss decline marriage because of this fear, a fear growing out of the current teaching that their children will be marked as they have been.

The problem of maternal responsibility with regard to the physical capacity of their offspring to reproduce a healthy new generation comprises one of the most serious problems confronting modern degenerating society.

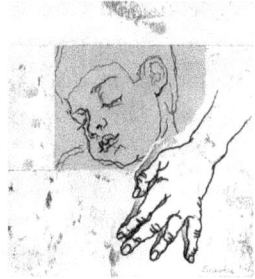

It is a matter of great importance that the most serious disturbances in reproduction and childbirth are occurring in the most civilized parts of the world.

Probably the most indelible impression that is left by my investigations among primitive races, is that which came from examining 1,276 skulls of the people who had been buried hundreds of years ago along the Pacific Coast of Peru and in the high Andean Plateau, without finding a single skull with the typical marked narrowing of the face and dental arches, that afflicts a considerable proportion not only of the residents in modernized districts in Peru, but in most of the United States and many communities of Europe today.

You'll find so many animals; they are eating differently. The hog is eating stool, the tiger is eating fresh blood, another animal is eating something, something. All facilities are there. Open hotel: you come on and take whatever you like. And the witness... God is so kind, this person has no discrimination of eating, so let him become dog, hog. The hog has no discrimination. Whatever you think: you give him halava, he will eat; you give him stool, it will eat. There are goats, so many animals, and no discrimination. The human being, there must be discrimination. Everything is eatable? So why don't you eat stool? No. Your eatable is different. It must be different from the animal eatables. Your teeth is different, your nature is different. A child, a child, you cannot give anything. She wants, he wants to drink milk only. Natural food. Artificially, the child is taught to eat something else. If you, if the child simply drinks mother's milk for six months, it becomes stout and strong for whole life. Because that is natural food. But there is no milk in the mother's breast. Artificial. So how the child will be healthy? This is modern civilization. Otherwise, if we get our natural food, there is no question of disease, there is no question of doctor's bill.

So that is science; that is human civilization. One who knows how to eat, how to sleep, how to have sex life, how to defend, that is human civilization. Without knowing, in the modes of ignorance -- simply animal life. They are simply like animals. They, that is not civilization.

~Srila Prabhupada (Lecture, Srimad-Bhagavatam 1.2.24 -- Los Angeles, August 27, 1972)

I know of no problem so important to our modern civilization as the finding of the reason for this, and the elimination of the cause of error. Perhaps few will recognize the significance of this important point. This may be the reason why the prospect is not encouraging.

One of the important lessons we should learn from the primitive races is that of the need for maintaining a balance between soil productivity, plant growth and human babies. Even in a country with so low a fertility as obtains in the greater part of Australia, the Aborigines for a very long period were able to maintain this balance. Their system of birth control was very efficient and exacting.

55.

Malnutrition, Personality Disorder And Crime

Dr. Weston A. Price

Malnutrition is a cause of not only physical injury, but also personality disturbances, the most common of which is a lower than normal mental efficiency and acuteness, chiefly observed as so-called mental backwardness which includes the group of children in the schools who are unable to keep up with their classmates.

Their I.Q.'s are generally lower than normal and they readily develop inferiority complexes growing out of their handicap. From this group or parallel with it a certain percentage develop personality disturbances which have their expression largely in unsocial traits.

A government survey has shown that 66 per cent of the delinquents who have been treated in the best institutions and released as cured, later have developed their unsocial or criminal tendencies, strongly emphasizes the urgent necessity that if preventive methods are to be applied these must precede and forestall the primary injuries themselves.

While it has been known that certain injuries were directly related to an inadequate nutrition of the mother during the formative period of the child, my investigations are revealing evidence that the problem goes back still further to defects in the germ plasms as contributed by the two parents. These injuries, therefore, are related directly to the physical condition of one or of both of these individuals prior to the time that conception took place.

A very important phase of my investigations has been the obtaining of information from these various primitive racial groups indicating that they were conscious that such injuries would occur if the parents were not in excellent physical condition and nourishment.

Indeed, in many groups I found that the girls were not allowed to be married until after they had had a period of special feeding. In some tribes a six months period of special nutrition was required before marriage. An examination of their foods has disclosed special nutritional factors which are utilized for this purpose.

The forces involved in heredity have in general been deemed to be so powerful as to be able to resist all impacts and changes in the environment. These data will indicate that much that we have interpreted as being due to heredity is really the result of intercepted heredity.

Incidents in the life of the individual such as disappointments, fright, etc., are largely responsible for disturbed behavior. Normal brain functioning has not been thought of as being as biologic as digestion. It can be safely said that associated with disturbances in the development of the bones of the head, disturbances may at the same time occur in the development of the brain.

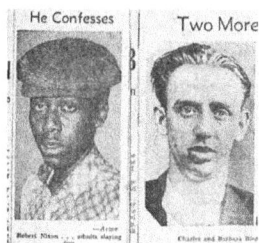

He Confesses   Two More

Such structural defects usually are not hereditary factors even though they appear in other members of the family or parents. They are products of the environment rather than hereditary units transmitted from the ancestry.

In the light of these data important new emphasis is placed on the quality of the germ cells of the two parents as well

Note the marked lack of normal facial development of these notorious young criminals. Nixon is only 18. These are typical samples seen frequently in the daily press.

as on the environment provided by the mother. The new evidence indicates that the paternal contribution may be an injured product and that the responsibility for defective germ cells may have to be about equally divided between the father and mother.

The blending of races has been blamed for much of the distortion and defects in body form in our modern generation. It will be seen that these face changes occur in all the pure blood races studied in even the first generation, after the nutrition of the parents has been changed.

There is an intimate relationship between delinquency and physical deficiency.

Most repeated offenders are far from robust; they are frail, sickly, and infirm. Indeed, so regularly is chronic moral disorder associated with chronic physical disorder that many have contended that crime is a disease, or at least a symptom of disease, needing the doctor more than the magistrate, physic rather than the whip.

The frequency among juvenile delinquents of bodily weakness and ill health has been remarked by almost every recent writer. In my own series of cases nearly 70 per cent were suffering from such defects; and nearly 50 per cent were in urgent need of medical treatment. . . . Of all the psychological causes of crime, the commonest and the gravest is usually alleged to be defective mind. The most eminent authorities, employing the most elaborate methods of scientific analysis, have been led to enunciate some such belief.

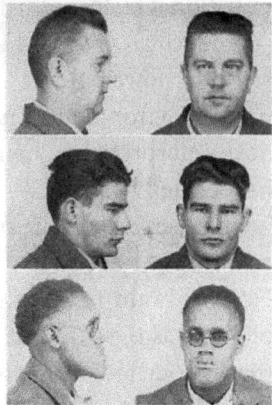

Criminals. Were their unsocial traits related directly to incomplete brain organization associated with prenatal injury?

In England, for example, Dr. Goring has affirmed that "the one vital mental constitutional factor in the etiology of crime is defective intelligence." In Chicago, Dr. Healy has likewise maintained that among the personal characteristics of the offender "mental deficiency forms the largest single cause of delinquency." And most American investigators would agree.

Thrasher, (The Gang, University of Chicago Press, 1936) in discussing the nature and origin of gangs, expresses this very clearly:

Gangs are gangs, wherever they are found. They represent a specific type or variety of society, and one thing that is particularly interesting about them is the fact that they are, in respect to their organization, so elementary, and in respect to their origin, so spontaneous.

Formal society is always more or less conscious of the end for which it exists, and the organization through which this end is achieved is always more or less a product of design. But gangs grow like weeds, without consciousness of their aims, and without administrative machinery to achieve them.

They are, in fact, so spontaneous in their origin, and so little conscious of the purposes for which they exist, that one is tempted to think of them as predetermined, foreordained, and "instinctive," and so, quite independent of the environment in which they ordinarily are found.

No doubt, many cities have been provided, as has Cleveland, with a special school for delinquent boys. The institution there has been given the appropriate title, the "Thomas A. Edison School." It usually has an enrollment of 800 to 900 boys. Dr. Watson, (Organization and administration of a public school for pre-delinquent boys in a large city) who has been of outstanding service in the organization of this work, makes an important comment on the origin of the student population there:

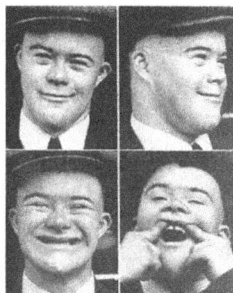

This is a typical mongoloid defective. Note the marked lack of development of the middle third of the face and nose with the upper arch too small for the lower. Individuals of this type look alike and act alike and all have typical speech and behavior defects. These are now associated with definite defects in the brain. Nearly all are either a first or last child. A large percentage are born to mothers over forty years of age.

The Thomas A. Edison student population consists of a group of truant and behavior boys, most of them in those earlier stages of mal-adjustment which we have termed predelinquency. .... In general, they are the products of unhappy experiences in school, home and community. They are sensitive recorders of the total complex of social forces which operate in and combine to constitute what we term their community environment.

It will be seen from these quotations that great emphasis has been placed upon the influence of the environment in determining factors of delinquency.

Very important contributions have been made to the forces that are at work in the development of delinquents through an examination of the families in which affected individuals have appeared. Sullenger, (Social Determinants in Juvenile Delinquency) in discussing this phase, states:

Abbott and Breckinridge found in their Chicago studies that a much higher percentage of delinquent boys than girls were from large families. However, Healy and Bronner found in their studies in Chicago and Boston that the large family is conducive to delinquency among children in that the larger the family the greater percentage of cases with more than one delinquent. They were unable to detect whether or not this fact was due to parental neglect, poverty, bad environmental conditions, or the influence of one child on another. In each of the series in both cities the number of delinquents in families of different sizes showed general similarity.

There is distinct possibility of children being born without sufficient spacing and being brought up with poor nutrition in large families. Hence this assertion by Abbott and Breckinridge.

The problems of modern degeneration can in general be divided into two main groups, those which relate to the perfection of the physical body and those which relate to its function. The latter

> *What is the distinction between the human form of life and the life of the hogs and dogs? What is the difference? The difference is that the hogs and dogs, whole day they are searching after eatables: "Where there is some food? Where there is some food?" That is hogs' and dogs' life, the condemned life. They cannot have any peaceful life. They cannot do any intelligent work. They cannot produce food from the earth. They have no intelligence. The same earth is there, the dogs and hogs are there, the human being is also there, but human being has developed a civilization, comfortable life; the hogs and dogs, they cannot do that. Although they have got the same opportunity, but they cannot do it. So human life is meant for living very comfortably, brain clear to understand what is Absolute Truth, what is our life, what is the goal of life, because the hogs and dogs, they will also die and we will also die, but we can understand what is the goal of life; the dogs and hogs, they do not know what is the goal of life.*
>
> *~Srila Prabhupada (Lecture, Srimad-Bhagavatam 1.2.6 -- Mauritius, October 5, 1975)*

include character as expressed in behavior of individuals and of groups of individuals which thus relate to national character and to an entire culture.

In an enumeration of the phases in which there is a progressive decline of modern civilization, it is essential that we keep in mind that in addition to an analysis of the forces responsible for individual degeneration, the ethical standards of the whole group cannot be higher than those of the individuals that compose it. That recent mass degeneration is in progress is attested by daily events throughout the world.

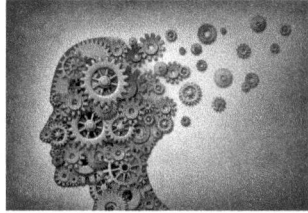

Sir Alfred Zimmern in his address on the decline of international standards said that "Recent events should convince the dullest mind of the extent to which international standards have deteriorated and the anarchy which threatens the repudiation of law and order in favour of brute force."

As we study the primitives we will find that they have had an entirely different conception of the nature and origin of the controlling forces which have molded individuals and races.

Buckle, in writing his epoch-making "History of Civilization" about the middle of the last century, summed up his years of historical studies with some very important conclusions, some of which are as follows:

- It is proved by history, and especially by statistics, that human actions are governed by laws as fixed and regular as those which rule in the physical world.

- Climate, soil, food, and the aspects of Nature are the principal causes of intellectual progress.

By the time the age of Kali ends, the bodies of all creatures will be greatly reduced in size,

Cows will be like goats, Most plants and herbs will be tiny, and all trees will appear like dwarf sami trees. and all human beings will have become like asses.

~ Srimad Bhagavatam - 12.2.12-16

- Religion, literature, and government are, at best, but the products, and not the cause of civilization.

Mayor Harold Burton of Cleveland, stressed very important phases. He stated that the American boys "are making irrevocable choices" between good and bad citizenship which "may make or wreck the nation. It may be on the battlefield of crime prevention that the life of democracy will be saved." He described great industrial cities as battlefields where "the tests of democracy are the newest and sharpest." "For centuries," he said, "we have fought crime primarily by seeking to catch the criminal after the crime has been committed and then through his punishment to lead or drive him and others to good citizenship. Today the greater range of operation and greater number of criminals argue that we must deal with the flood waters of crime. We must prevent the flood by study, control and diversion of the waters at their respective sources."

One such source of flood waters of crime is our ignorance on how to conceive, nurture and bring up good progeny.

56.

Idyllic Nauru

A Chubby Heaven

Imagine a Pacific Island that has all the elements of paradise, except fruits and vegetables. Tiny Nauru in the South Pacific is the last place a vegetarian would want to find him or herself. Since the American meat industry turned the island into a haven of canned meats like Spam and Corned Beef just a couple of decades back, the region has acquired the world's highest obesity rates, along with associated chronic diseases.

According to the latest data from the World Health Organisation (WHO), Pacific island nations occupy the top seven places in the global obesity rankings. Diet is the main reason: people who once subsisted on root vegetables, coconuts and fish, now eat imported processed foods that are high in sugar and fat.

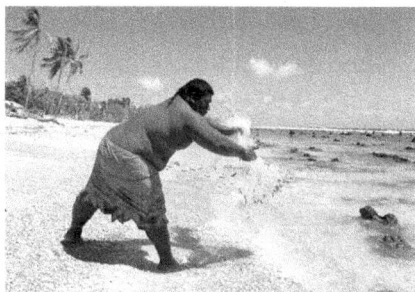

The statistics are alarming. In Nauru 97 per cent of men and 93 per cent of women are overweight or obese. Preventable conditions such as heart disease and cancer are responsible for three-quarters of deaths in this apparently carefree corner of the planet.

In the past, only chiefs achieved a large girth; nowadays, with higher incomes and Western diets, it has become far more common to be fat. At the Pacific Food Summit in Vanuatu this year, Temo Waqanivalu, a senior WHO official, bemoaned the decline of traditional foods. "They are unable to compete with the glamour and flashiness of imported food."

In Nauru, where 45 per cent of those aged 55-64 have diabetes, health authorities are trying to address the problem. Every Wednesday, locals are encouraged to walk around the three-mile airport perimeter. There are also regular exercise classes and sporting activities.

But it is proving difficult to wean people off processed foods such as tinned beef and mutton, which represent, to those who

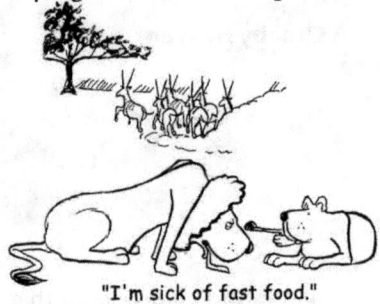

"I'm sick of fast food."

can afford them, a Western lifestyle. In Nauru, a popular snack is a whole fried chicken, washed down with a bucket-sized beaker of Coke.

The Pacific, of course, is not the only place where weight and preventable diseases are a big issue. Number eight in the WHO's league table is the United States, where more than 78 per cent of people are overweight or obese. In Britain, the figure is just over 61 per cent.

The island has the appearance of a health timebomb. Chen Ken, the WHO representative for the South Pacific, says: "We're now seeing extreme diabetes rates, and people ill and dying from diseases that were once uncommon in the Pacific."

(Source: The Independent, Sunday 26 December 2010)

They are now killing animal, but animal lives on this grass and grains. When there will be no grass, no grains, where they will get animal? They'll kill their own children and eat. That time is coming. Nature's law is that you grow your own food. But they are not interested in growing food. They are interested in manufacturing bolts and nuts.
-Srila Prabhupada (Morning Walk — June 22, 1974, Germany)

Section - V

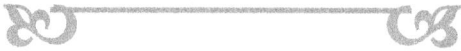

Killer Foods
of Modern Industrial Era

"Don't eat anything your great-grandmother wouldn't recognize as food."
~ Michael Pollan

57.

A New Era

Of Convenience And Calamity

Civilization has entered a new era, an era of convenience and expediency, in which virtually every aspect of our lives contains a seemingly unavoidable association with unhealthy foods of one kind or another.

For years, we have been subjected to every conceivable form of marketing and advertising, designed to convince us that the incredible array of manufactured, processed, tinned, packaged and bottled foods are superior to the fresh, natural foods of our forefathers. The processing removes most of the natural goodness and flavor of the food and it is turned into an almost indigestible form due to the complete absence of natural enzymes – destroyed through processing and cooking. Regular ingestion of these foods over a period of years, places an extreme load on the pancreas, liver and digestive system, as a whole, causing the body to wear out much sooner than it should.

As if this is not bad enough, further strain is placed on the body by the assortment of chemicals needed to preserve color, dry, flavor and tenderize processed food, in order to get people to eat it. By this stage,

---

"That eating should be foremost about bodily health is a relatively new and, I think, destructive idea-destructive not just the pleasure of eating, which would be bad enough, but paradoxically of our health as well. Indeed, no people on earth worry more about the health consequences of their food choices than we Americans-and no people suffer from as many diet-related problems. We are becoming a nation of orthorexics: people with an unhealthy obsession with healthy eating."

~Michael Pollan, In Defense of Food: An Eater's Manifesto

---

it is not really food but more a composition of reconstituted, chemical-laden organic matter. A recent study has shown that the average person now consumes about three kilograms of chemicals per year, in the form of food additives. The human body was never designed to be so constantly abused. It becomes overloaded and develops allergies to all the unnatural rubbish with which it has been constantly fed.

It is again a matter of degree. A little processed food, now and again, may not be a big problem for a healthy body. But, when it is eaten on a daily basis, year after year, as the main ingredients of the diet, the body will lose its capacity to cope, and an insidious form of ill health will result.

In this section, we will examine these killer 'foods' of the modern industrial era.

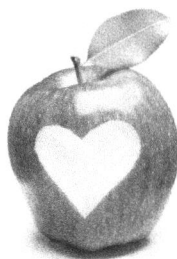

58.

The Whiter The Bread, The Quicker You're Dead!

The Scourge of Refined White Flour

The scourge of the 21 century is not war, famine, or plague. While most of the worlds population still struggles with these problems, there is even a bigger scourge that is taking its toll. Its called carbohydrate poisoning and it is caused by processed & refined foods, and an eating style promoted by corporate marketing and the medical community and it is now killing people more then ever before.

Here's an important rule to remember: the more a food is refined, the more you should stay away from it.

What are refined foods? Refined foods are highly processed foods that have been stripped of their original nutrient content and fibre. Refined white flour, white pasta, and white sugar are just some examples.

To get the conveniences of high-tech food processing, mass-production, mass-marketing, long shelf life, uniformity of final product, even coloration, and soft texture, we create nutritional deficiencies. The food processing industry deceptively markets its products as more convenient versions of what grandmother once did in her kitchen. That is far from the truth!

Most of today's mass-produced foods are seriously depleted of nutrients and are highly chemicalized with additives. Processed foods today are not just more sophisticated and more convenient versions of the foods eaten by our ancestors. The basic molecular structure of what remains is also degraded and nutritionally inferior.

Processed refined foods deliver a double whammy to your system. While overloading the body with glucose that raises insulin levels in the blood which shuts down fat burning, the chemicals used in processing to increase shelf life and promote taste, slowly damages the body's ability to properly use these foods as fuel by damaging the very cells this fuel is intended for.

Consider a loaf of sliced white bread. First, the wheat is stripped of bran and fibre, and then it's pulverised into the finest white flour. The baking process puffs it up into light, airy slices of bread. No wonder your stomach makes such quick work of it. A slice of white bread hits your bloodstream with the same jolt you'd get by eating a tablespoon of sugar right from the bowl!

Genuine 100-per cent whole-wheat or whole-grain bread, on the other hand – the coarse, chewy kind with a thick crust and visible pieces of grain – puts your stomach to work. It too is made of wheat, but the grains haven't been processed to 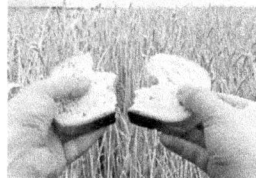 death. It contains starches, which are just chains of sugars, but they are bound up with the fibre, so digestion takes longer. As a result, the sugars are released gradually into the bloodstream. If there's no sudden surge in blood sugar, your pancreas won't produce as much insulin, and you won't get the exaggerated hunger and cravings for more sugary and starchy carbs.

Until recently, grains were ground between large stones to make flour. Everything in the original grain remained in the finished product, including the germ, the fiber, the starch, and a wide spectrum of vitamins and minerals. The final product contained all the naturally occurring vitamins, minerals and micronutrients.

In the absence of refrigeration, stone-ground flour spoils quickly. After wheat has been ground, natural wheat-germ oil becomes rancid at about the same rate that milk becomes sour.

Hippocrates, a physician in ancient Greece, once recommended stone-ground flour, complete with its vitamins, minerals, natural bran and dietary fiber, for beneficial effects on the digestive tract. Today, three-fourths of that dietary fiber is removed from commercial flour. Partially as a result, constipation is very common.

During the industrial revolution in the nineteenth century, assembly-line techniques for mass-producing flour and bread were developed. Grinding stones were not fast enough for mass-production. High-speed, steel roller mills were invented, to produce flour very rapidly. Grain mills thus earned higher profits.

High-speed mills do not grind the germ and the bran properly and it is ejected. Much of the original grain, including the most nutritious portion, is taken out and sold as "byproducts" for animals. Animals are often better nourished than people are. It's been cynically observed that more profit can be made from healthy animals and sick people.

High-speed mills run very hot, at 400 degrees Fahrenheit, just under the temperature that will burn and discolor the flour. That high heat destroys many vitamins. (While baking, the interior of bread does not get much hotter than 170 degrees, which is much less harmful to vitamins.) Since the late nineteenth century, white bread, biscuits and cakes made from white flour and sugar have become mainstays in the diets of industrialized nations.

Most bread is now manufactured in large factories capable of producing up to a quarter million loaves per day. This mass-produced bread is soft, gooey, devitalized, and nutritionally deficient--laced with chemical additives. Public taste is accustomed to such bread. People have forgotten how real bread tastes. Chemical

---

Flour Treatments - Bleaching Makes The Flour Whiter

The term "bleaching" is a traditional baking industry term that describes the process of whitening.

Through the years, various chemicals have entered the picture to "improve" white flour, including benzoyl peroxide, potassium bromate, ammonium persulfate, alloxan and chlorine dioxide for bleaching. Chlorine dioxide destroys the remaining vitamin E in flour, thus causing the starch to swell; something the baker actually appreciates not knowing how and why it happens.

As early as 1919, the US Public Health Service announced a definite connection between over-refined flour and the diseases beri-beri and pellagra (both of which are vitamin-deficiency diseases). But why is the public still given white flour and white bread as the predominant options today? Because we prefer to buy them.

preservatives allow bread to be shipped long distances and to remain on the shelf for many days without spoiling and without refrigeration. Again, resulting in higher profits.

To make bread a brighter white, at the expense of consumer health, flour is treated with chemical bleach, similar to Clorox. The bleaching process leaves residues of toxic chlorinated hydrocarbons and dioxins. Methionine, an essential amino acid, reacts with bleaching chemicals to form methionine sulfoxine. That toxic residue causes nervousness and seizures in animals.

The bleaching process destroys many vitamins (those not already destroyed by the high heat of milling). Bleaching agents have therefore been banned for breadmaking in Germany since 1958. In the United States, however, no such ban exists and the bleached bread continues to be the mainstay. Most white flour used in supermarket bread, rolls, cakes, pastries, spaghetti, noodles, pasta, and breakfast cereals, has been bleached.

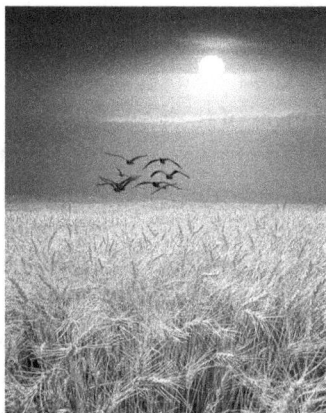

Grain millers in the nineteenth century soon discovered that highly refined flour would keep without spoiling for prolonged periods, even before the days of chemical preservatives and refrigeration. It's now clear refined flour is so depleted of essential vitamins and minerals that it will not support life. Even the insects and rodents cannot live on it! Can humans be expected to fare any better?

Dr Weston A. Price showed effect of different wheat products in an experiment on rats.

The experiment was conducted with three rats all of which received the same diet, except for the type of bread. The first rat (at the left) received whole-wheat products freshly ground, the center one received a white flour product and the third (at the right) a bran and middlings product. The amounts of each ash, of calcium as the oxide, and of phosphorus as the pentoxide; and the amounts of iron and copper present in the diet of each group are shown by the height of the columns beneath the rats.

Clinically it will be seen that there is a marked difference in the physical development of these rats. Several rats of the same age were in each cage. The feeding was started after weaning at about twenty-three days of age. The rat at the left was on the entire grain product. It was fully developed. The rats in this cage reproduced normally at three months of age. The rats in this first cage had very mild dispositions and could be picked up by the ear or tail without danger of their biting.

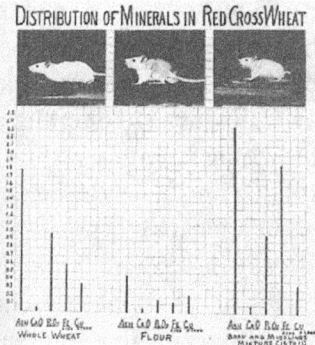

DISTRIBUTION OF MINERALS IN RED CROSS WHEAT

Effect of different wheat products on rats. Left: whole wheat. Center: white flour. Right: bran and middlings mixture. The graphs record actual amount of indicated minerals present, as milligrams per cent. Only the rats on the whole wheat developed normally without tooth decay. Those on white flour had tooth decay, were underweight, had skin infections and were irritable. They did not reproduce. The third group were undersize. The balance of the ration was the same for all.

The rats represented by the one in the center cage using white flour were markedly undersized. Their hair came out in large patches and they had very ugly dispositions, so ugly that they threatened to spring through the cage wall at us when we came to look at them. These rats had tooth decay and they were not able to reproduce.

The rats in the next cage (illustrated by the rat to the right) which were on the bran and middlings mixture did not show tooth decay, but were considerably undersized, and they lacked energy.

The flour and middlings for the rats in cages two and three were purchased from the miller and hence were not freshly ground. The wheat given to the first group was obtained whole and ground while fresh in a hand mill.

It is of interest that notwithstanding the great increase in ash, calcium, phosphorus, iron and copper present in the foods of the last group, the rats did not mature normally, as did those in the first group.

This may have been due in large part to the fact that the material was not freshly ground, and as a result they could not obtain a normal vitamin content from the embryo of the grain due to its oxidation.

This is further indicated by the fact that the rats in this group did not reproduce, probably due in considerable part to a lack of vitamins B and E which were lost by oxidation of the embryo or germ fat.

Enriched Flour

When grain is made into refined white flour, more than 30 essential nutrients are largely removed. Only four of those nutrients are added back in a process called "enrichment." Using this same logic, if a person were robbed of 30 dollars and the thief then returned 4 dollars to his victim for cab fare home, then that person should be considered "enriched" by 4 dollars, not robbed of 26 dollars.

How would you feel in that situation? You should feel the same about "enriched" white flour and bread? Only vitamins B1, B2, B3, and iron are added back. Nutrients which are removed and not

White flour contains diabetes-causing contaminant alloxan. You may want to think twice before eating your next sandwich on white bread. Studies show that alloxan, the chemical that makes white flour look "clean" and "beautiful," destroys the beta cells of the pancreas.

In June, 2005 Mr. Dani Veracity reported on Natural News issue, "The FDA and the white flour industry could counter-argue that, if alloxan were to cause diabetes, a higher proportion of Americans would be diabetic. After all, more consumers consume white flour on a regular basis than are actually diabetic."

In September 2008, three years after the report of Mr. Dani Veracity, the U.S. Department of Health and Human Services - Centers for Disease Control and Prevention issued the following report:

"New evidence shows that at least 57 million people in the United States have prediabetes. Coupled with the nearly 24 million who already have diabetes, this places more than 25% of our population at risk for further complications and suffering. Together, we can and must do more to prevent and control this growing epidemic."

returned include 44% of the vitamin E, 52% of the pantothenic acid, 65% of the folic acid, 76% of the biotin, 84% of the vitamin B6, and half or more of 20 minerals and trace elements, including magnesium, calcium, zinc, chromium, manganese, selenium, vanadium, and copper.

Removal of natural nutrients and substituting them with a few synthetic ones, is in itself a dangerous practice. Body can never handle the synthetic nutrients in the same way as it does the natural ones.

If consumers would just educate themselves in the principles of good nutrition and show an educated preference at the checkout counter, the food industry would be forced to respond with more nutritious products.

Iron, the single mineral added back to enriched white flour, is present in toxic amounts in the bodies of many older people. Iron as an additive contributes widely to premature atherosclerosis, heart attacks, strokes, arthritis, cancer and other age-related diseases.

It is quite possible that enrichment of flour with iron has been poisoning the public for decades. Avoidance of unneeded iron supplementation is reason enough in itself not to buy so-called "enriched" flour products.

Deceptive marketing practices are widespread. Much of the bread now marketed as "whole-wheat bread" is the same old refined white bread with a little brown coloring added. That coloring is usually burnt sugar, listed on the label as caramel.

One manufacturer even added sawdust to replace the lost bran, calling it cellulose on the label and advertising it as "high-fiber" bread. It is legal to describe inferior flour as "whole wheat" on the label, even when the bran and germ have been removed in high-speed roller mills.

It is slow and more expensive to mass-produce bread made with l00% stone-ground whole-wheat flour. Manufacturers go to great lengths to mislead the public by making inferior products appear of higher quality.

Without chemical preservatives bread spoils rapidly. It quickly becomes stale, hard and moldy. To market nutritious whole-grain, unrefined bread over long distances would require refrigerator trucks for delivery and refrigerator storage in super-markets. Even under refrigeration, spoilage would be faster than with chemicalized bread. That would add greatly to expense. Profits would be smaller. Production of truly nutritious bread therefore falls to small local bakeries, which sell direct or deliver daily to nearby stores.

Scientific evidence implicates a low-fiber diet of refined flour as one cause of bowel cancer. Without bran, transit time through the digestive tract is greatly lengthened. Constipation results, causing hemorrhoids, diverticulitis and increased risk of colon and rectal cancer.

Dr. Barrie (Nutritional anterior pituitary deficiency) reports that partial deficiency of vitamin E, as shown in the case of the female rat, results in the prolongation of gestation which may be continued as long as ten days beyond the normal period. The offspring under these conditions are abnormal. Further, animals deficient in vitamin E, occasionally give birth to a litter, but fail to lactate.

When we realize that one of the best sources of vitamin E is wheat germ, most of which is removed from white flour, usually along with four-fifths of the mineral, we see one cause of the tragedy that is overwhelming so many individuals in our modern civilization.

I am 94 years old and in good health for my age. I walk 2-3 km daily.

In my youth, due to various reasons, we were not allowed to eat anything not made in our house. As a child, I never saw biscuits, buns, breads or other white flour items in Tiruvaiyaru, (South India), at least not in the shops near our house. We ate two meals of rice, vegetables, sambar, rasam and pickles, at 11am and 7 pm. In between we drank coffee or mostly buttermilk. We walked everywhere. The lucky ones rode bicycles.

I find my grandchildren and great grandchildren eating and drinking all the time. Most of it is impulsive eating or absent-minded eating. Often they don't realize that they ate! There is a lot of refined and highly processed food, mostly of white flour and sugary, fizzy drinks.

All my grandchildren--in their 30s and early 40s--have health problems. My great-grandchildren are all overweight. The culprit: refined food, no vigorous exercise. They say my childhood eating pattern is primitive. I'm the one laughing at them!

~N.Mahalingam, Mar 17, 2012

Investigations indicate that Nature has put just the right amount of embryo in each grain of wheat to accompany that quantity of food. If the whole wheat is prepared and eaten promptly after grinding and exposing the embryo to oxidation, the effect desired by Nature is adequately provided.

Make Your Own Whole Grain Flour, Fresh At Home

Many companies are selling Home Grain Mills. These are also called mini or domestic flour mills. With one such mill, you can make your own healthy wholesome flour, right in your kitchen. They don't occupy much space either. These mills can grind any type of grain. Freshly ground flours have all their nutrients intact and the taste is also very different. It doesn't take much time or effort to grind the flour for a small family. Some of the brands can be ordered online. One such popular brand is WonderMill Grain Mill. You can create super fine flour or coarse flour at temperatures that preserve nutrients. The WonderMill can grind over 100 pounds of flour in an hour. It not only grinds wheat, rice and other small grains, but also legumes and beans as large as garbanzos.

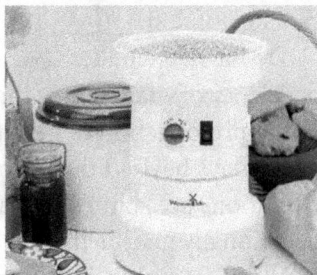

> So I see in your this Mauritius land, you have got enough land to produce food grains. You produce food grain. I understand that instead of growing food grains, you are growing sugar cane for exporting. Why? And you are dependent on food grains, on rice, wheat, dahl. Why? Why this attempt? You first of all grow your own eatables. And if there is time and if your population has got sufficient food grains, then you can try to grow other fruits and vegetables for exporting. The first necessity is that you should be self-sufficient. That is God's arrangement. Everywhere there is sufficient land to produce food grains, not only in your country. I have traveled all over the world -- Africa, Australia, and other, in America also. There are so much land vacant that if we produce food grains, then we can feed ten times as much population as at the present moment. There is no question of scarcity. The whole creation is so made by Krishna that everything is purnam, complete.
>
> ~ Srila Prabhupada (Lecture, Srimad-Bhagavatam 7.5.30, Mauritius, October 2, 1975)

59.

White Sugar

The Sweet Assassin

Almost everyone on planet loves "sweet foods" or "dessert". The sweet taste in these foods comes from sugar. Sugar, or table sugar as we know it, is the white crystalline substance produced by industrial processes (mostly from sugar cane or sugar beets) by refining it down to pure sucrose, after taking away all the vitamins, minerals, proteins, enzymes and other beneficial nutrients.

It has 12 carbon atoms, 22 hydrogen atoms, 11 oxygen atoms, and absolutely nothing else to offer. Simply put, sugar is a concentrated unnatural substance, which the human body is not able to handle, at least not in quantities that is ingested in today's lifestyle.

Most of the products we consume daily are loaded with sugar! The average healthy digestive system can digest and eliminate from half to one teaspoons of sugar daily, usually without noticeable problems (if damage is not already present).

World consumption of sugar varies significantly from country to country. In India the per capita consumption of white sugar is 54.3 pounds where as an average North American consumes a whopping 149 pounds of sugar every year.

To get a feel of what it means, stack 149 one-pound bags up in your kitchen and you'll know just how much that is. You will barely have room for anything else.

"Not me," you may quip, or "I couldn't possibly eat that much sugar, someone else is making up for me." While that may be possible, it is not very likely. Even if you rarely consume desserts, you may be surprised to learn some of the ways that sugar sneaks into your diet. Of course there are all the obvious places, such as soft drinks (the average North American drinks 486 ten-ounce cans of soda pop every year; each one contains about eight teaspoons of sugar), ice cream, cake, and cookies.

Nancy Appleton, author of the best-selling book Lick the Sugar Habit, identified some of the following lesser-known sources of sugar.

What about that hamburger you ate last weekend? Shockingly, the meat was most likely injected with a sugar solution to prevent it from shrinking. Many meat packers feed sugar to animals prior to slaughter. This "improves" the flavour and colour of cured meat, at least according to the food industry.

The average bottle or package of "juice" may not even contain a single drop of juice from any fruit. More likely, it is loaded with sugar, colours, and artificial flavours to give it that "natural" fruit juice flavour. Dry-roasted nuts, peanut butter, flavored yogurt, salad dressings, and many dry cereals (even many of your so-called healthy favourites) contain sugar. This one may shock you: some salts contain sugar! Almost half the calories found in most condiments, such as ketchup, come from sugar.

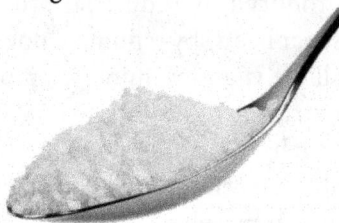

Blocking The Body's Immune Response

Refined sugar, in the large doses we consume, may be one of the worst poisons we put into our bodies. Sugar blocks your body's immune response for between four and six hours. That means your body is more likely to fall prey to the thousands of viruses, bacteria, and other infectious diseases present in our environment and in our bodies during that time.

Although we are quick to blame those pesky pathogens, we rarely look to that decadent triple chocolate cake or that delicious sundae. How could anyone fault something that looks and tastes so sweet?

The proper functioning of white blood cells is integral to a healthy immune system. Research shows that both sugar and alcohol consumption inhibit white blood cell activity. The amount of sugar in one soft drink will stop white blood cell activity within thirty minutes and normal activity will not resume for four to five hours. You are more vulnerable to bacterial and viral infections after consuming sweets because your white blood cells are unable to function properly to fight these foreign invaders.

Plenty of studies link sugar consumption to cancer, hormonal disruptions, arthritis, osteoporosis, cataracts, and many other degenerative diseases, the list of which is massive.

In one study hamsters were fed diets high in sucrose (refined white sugar). Some were also fed calcium supplements in their food. The calcium made no difference—the hamsters developed osteoporosis, regardless of how much calcium was in their food. Researchers credited high sugar consumption as the primary cause of osteoporosis in this study.

Sugar makes the pH in your body very acidic. Countless studies link acidic body chemistry with disease. The same diseases that thrive in an acidic body rarely exist if the body is returned to a more neutral pH. In the case of osteoporosis, your body recognizes that acidic blood can cause damage to your arteries, organs, and central nervous system.

In its wisdom, your body recognizes that drawing calcium from the bones neutralizes the body's pH. This mechanism is fine for short-term amounts of acidity but it is a contributing factor to osteoporosis over the long term.

Sugar also contains over sixty synthetic chemicals left over from the many processes it endures to transform a thick, fibrous, brownish stalk of sugar cane into the white crystalline substance we call sugar.

Although you will not find bleach, deodorizers, and all kinds of other garbage listed on the label, you would find it present in small amounts if you took some sugar to a laboratory for analysis. Not to mention that government regulations insist that white sugar must have all the vitamins and minerals removed so that it can be labelled "sucrose." These nutrients and fibre "waste" products are the substances that help your body digest sugar without massive blood sugar fluctuations.

High sugar products give instant energy and a feeling of "high" which is why they are now being consumed to the level of addiction by the younger generation.

You could say that sugar tends to throw off the homeostatic balance of the whole body by increasing the production of adrenaline by many times. In essence, sugar stimulates the nervous system by inducing a flight or fight response.

Sugar also adversely affect body weight and hormones; it also causes fatigue, increased hyperactivity and tooth decay.

Refined sugar provides empty calories and if a lot of your food contains sugar, there's no room for the nutrients you need to stay healthy. When sugar isn't needed, it's stored as fat, and by eating sugar, you're also raising levels of the hormone insulin in your blood. Insulin stores fat, a risk factor of diabetes, and can damage artery walls, making it easier for cholesterol and fat to build up and cause heart disease.

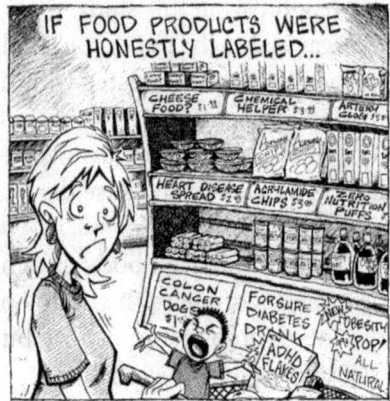

Refined sugar, because it is devoid of all nutrients, robs the body of its stores of various vitamins, minerals and enzymes. If the body is lacking the nutrients used to metabolize sugar, it will not be able to properly handle and rid itself of the poisonous residues. These wastes accumulate through the brain and nervous system, which speeds up cellular death. The bloodstream becomes over-loaded with waste products and symptoms of carbonic poisoning result.

Research has also shown that refined sugar may be one of the major dietary risk factors in gallstone disease. Gallstones are composed of fats and calcium. Sugar can disturb the natural mineral balance in the body, and one of the minerals, calcium, can become toxic or nonfunctioning, depositing itself anywhere in the body, including the gallbladder.

The escalating aggressive behavioural pattern in adolescents perturbs everyone today. While many believe that the violence shown on television and cinemas is to be blamed, there is one hidden cause for this. Refined sugar are now being linked to various mental problems. Our brains are very sensitive and react to quick chemical changes within the body. As sugar is consumed, our cells are robbed of their B vitamin, which destroys them, and insulin production is inhibited. Low insulin production means a high sugar (glucose) level in the bloodstream, which can lead to a confused mental state or unsound mind, and has also been linked with juvenile criminal behavior.

Many nutritionists believe that sugar can be addictive and it is difficult to break the habit of excess sugar intake. In fact, sugar does more damage than any other poison, drug or narcotic because :

-It is considered a "food" and ingested in such massive quantities.

-The damaging effects begin early, from the day a baby is born and is fed sugar in its formula. Even mothers milk is contaminated with it if the mother eats sugar.

-Practically 95% of people are addicted to it to some degree or other

You don't have to be a physician or a scientist to notice the expanding waistline. All you have to do is stroll through a shopping mall or a schoolyard, or perhaps glance in the mirror.

Sugar - Role In Shaping The World History

The consumption of sugar and its history gives a great insight into various inter-related issues, such as economics, human rights, slavery, environmental issues, health, consumerism issues and so on. We also see a hint at the "hidden costs" and impacts to society.

Historically, around 1000 years ago, sugar was used in a variety of ways, such as:

- For medicinal purposes (because unrefined sugar is beneficial in limited quantities)

- As a preservative

- As a spice

- As a sweetener, of course.

Records show that in India it was extensively used. In Europe, up to the seventeenth century, it was an expensive luxury item.

To be consumed by the masses, this luxury had to be turned into a necessity and be available in abundance to drive prices down.

Colonialism, Slavery And Sugar Plantations

Sugar was a lucrative trade in the fifteenth and sixteenth centuries. The growing of Spain and Portugal's sugarcane was expanded into the Caribbean and parts of South America. From there, it would be shipped to places like Lisbon for refining.

While this led to an industry growing from this, it also came with some costs. One such cost was slavery.

The slave trade was a major factor in the expansion of the sugar industries. The growing demand for and production of sugar created the plantation economy in the New World and was largely responsible for the expansion of the Atlantic slave trade in the sixteenth, seventeenth and eighteenth centuries. From 1701 to 1810 almost one million slaves were brought to Barbados and Jamaica to work the sugar plantations.

Sugar became the focus of an industry, a sugar complex that combined the sugar plantations, the slave trade, long-distance shipping, wholesale and retail trade, and investment finance. Slave children were also used on sugar plantations. (Richard Robbins, Global Problems and the Culture of Capitalism, pp. 215-216)

With the rise in consumerism, there has been a rise in sugar use and with the increasing work demands, partly a result of rising consumerism, there has been a rise in convenience and fast foods. This implies more sugar!

Just take a look at the sugar consumption trends of the past 300 years in the developed countries:

- In 1700, the average person consumed about 4 pounds of sugar per year.

- In 1800, the average person consumed about 18 pounds of sugar per year.

- In 1900, individual consumption had risen to 90 pounds of sugar per year.

- In 2009, the average person consumed a whopping 149 pounds of sugar per year!

Children – The Ultimate "Market"

The increasing consumption of sugar and related products has of course also been directed towards children and Eric Schlosser, author of New York Times bestseller, Fast Food Nation, is worth quoting:

"Liquid Candy," a 1999 study by the Center for Science in the Public Interest, describes who is not benefiting from the beverage industry's latest marketing efforts: the children.

- In 1978, the typical teenage boy in the United States drank about seven ounces of soda every day; today he drinks nearly three times that amount, deriving 9 percent of his daily caloric intake from soft drinks.

- Soda consumption among teenage girls has doubled within the same period, reaching an average of twelve ounces a day.

- A significant number of teenage boys are now drinking five or more cans of soda every day.

Each can contains the equivalent of about ten teaspoons of sugar. Coke, Pepsi, Mountain Dew, and Dr Pepper also contain caffeine. These sodas provide empty calories and have replaced far more nutritious beverages in the American diet.

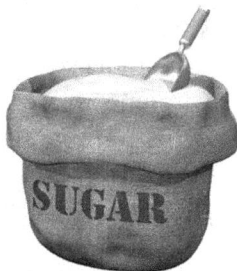

- Excessive soda consumption in childhood can lead to calcium deficiencies and a greater likelihood of bone fractures.

- About twenty years ago, teenage boys in the United States drank twice as much milk as soda; now they drink twice as much soda as milk.

Soft-drink consumption has also become commonplace among American toddlers.

- About one-fifth of the nation's one—and two-year olds now drink soda.

- "In one of the most despicable marketing gambits," Michael Jacobson, the author of "Liquid Candy" reports, "Pepsi, Dr Pepper and Seven-Up encourage feeding soft drinks to babies by licensing their logos to a major maker of baby bottles, Munchkin Bottling, Inc."

- A 1997 study published in the Journal of Dentistry for Children found that many infants were indeed being fed soda in those bottles.

An Enormous Employer Of Labor, Capital And Resources. But Is It Productive?

Sugar production and consumption has increased. Given the rise in consumption of other sweet foods, such as chocolates, jams, sugar in bread, and later, in soda drinks and other confectioneries, candies, sweets and fast foods etc, the amount of land to produce sugar, refine it, and support the industry has also increased. That is, even more resources have been expended.

Centralized mass production of refined sugar affects the environment in numerous ways:

-Forests must be cleared to plant sugar.
-Wood or fossil fuel is needed in processing steps.
-Waste products from processing affect the environment.
-Parallel consumption of other items related to sugar, including coffee, tea, chocolate, etc all collectively put additional resource requirements on the environment.
-Then there are 'numerous' "hidden" or "external" costs.

Furthermore, some of the industries involved in sugar (or sugar related products) have caused some problems that other segments of society have to deal with. Cultural, health and economic problems arising out of Coke's colonization of Latin America, can be cited as an example. (Kari Lydersen, Sugar and Blood: Coke in Latin America, Lip Magazine, 28 May 2002)

Note here how a luxury-turned-necessity product consumed en masse has produced so many negative side effects. It can even be suggested that almost the entire sugar industry of the present day (and all the things dependent on it) wastes many resources and that the true costs (economic, political, social, health, environmental etc) are not accounted for by the industry. After all, the way economic progress is measured today, through things like growth rates, GDP, GNP etc, all these industries contribute to those measures.

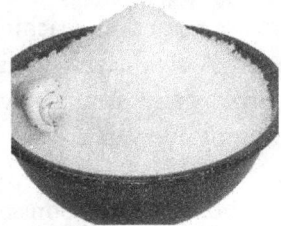

Modern sugar industry has emerged from a dark era of colonial oppression. But the exploitation continues, from slavery it has moved to consumers and children (albeit in another form), while the environment continues to suffer.

Fat or Sugars : Which Is Worse?

According to Andrew Weil, M.D., the saturated fat lauded in this menu won't kill you. It may even be the safest element of the meal.

Saturated fat is made of fatty acid chains that cannot incorporate additional hydrogen atoms. It is often of animal origin, and is typically solid at room temperature. Its relative safety has been a theme in nutrition science for at least the last decade, but a significant exoneration took place recently. An analysis that combined the results of 21 studies, published in The

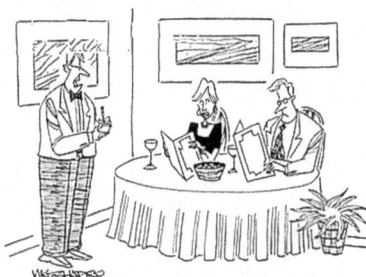

"Our menu is divided into three sections: Cancer causing foods, artery clogging foods, and foods that are being boycotted for political or environmental reasons."

American Journal of Clinical Nutrition found that "saturated fat was not associated with an increased risk" of coronary heart disease, stroke or coronary vascular disease.

Although this was not a true study, it was a big analysis. It aggregated information from nearly 348,000 participants, most of whom were healthy at the start of the studies. They were surveyed about their dietary habits and followed for five to 23 years. In that time, 11,000 developed heart disease or had a stroke. Researcher Ronald M. Krauss of the Oakland Research Center in California found that there was no difference in the risk of heart disease or stroke between people with the lowest and highest intakes of saturated fat.

This contradicts nutritional dogma we've heard repeated since 1970, when a physiologist named Ancel Keys published his "Seven Countries" study that showed animal fat consumption strongly predicted heart attack risk. His conclusions influenced dietary guidelines for decades to come, but other researchers pointed out that if 21 other countries had been included in that study, the association that Keys observed would have been seen as extremely weak.

Meanwhile, in the years since, there has been increasing evidence that added sweeteners in foods may contribute to heart disease. Sweeteners appear to lower levels of HDL cholesterol (the higher your HDL, the better) and raise triglycerides (the lower the better). That's according to a study of more than 6,000 adults by Emory University and the Centers for Disease Control and Prevention, and published in The Journal of the American Medical Association.

People who received at least 25 percent of their daily calories from any type of sweetener had more than triple the normal risk of having low HDL levels than those who consumed less than five percent of their calories from sweeteners. Beyond that, those whose sugar intake made up 17.5 percent or more of daily calories were 20 to 30 percent more likely to have high triglycerides.

Science writer Gary Taubes has done more than anyone else to deconstruct the Keys mythos and replace it with a more sensible view. In his revolutionary book, Good Calories, Bad Calories: Challenging the Conventional Wisdom on Diet, he presents more than 600 pages of evidence that lead to these conclusions:

1. Dietary fat, whether saturated or not, is not a cause of obesity, heart disease or any other chronic disease of civilization.

I have been on a journey for the last ten years to find the best "diet" for my family. My son has already fought cancer, he was 5, and two of my boys are autistic. All three were diagnosed with ADHD. We had nutritionists and oncologists recommend diets for our kids and ourselves, but we never got healthy or better. So I started researching, and came across such conflicting reports, studies, opinions. I was overwhelmed. Being pushed by all large "forces" in our country into this food pyramid, we tried hard to do it the right way. To no avail. Then I happened to read about white sugar.

My kids are all off their ADHD meds, they are cured! The funny thing is, the doctors can't believe it, and just seem to shrug off that removing white sugar cured them. Why can't they see the obvious? I am sure glad I have.

~ Carolyn, Alberta, March 22, 2012

2. The problem is the carbohydrates in the diet, their effect on insulin secretion, and thus the hormonal regulation of homeostasis - the entire harmonic ensemble of the human body. The more easily digestible and refined the carbohydrates, the greater the effect on our health, weight and well-being.

3. Sugars - sucrose and high-fructose corn syrup specifically — are particularly harmful, probably because the combination of fructose and glucose simultaneously elevates insulin levels while overloading the liver with carbohydrates.

4. Through their direct effects on insulin and blood sugar, refined carbohydrates, starches and sugars are the dietary cause of coronary heart disease and diabetes. They are the most likely dietary causes of cancer, Alzheimer's disease and other chronic diseases of modern civilization.

Looks like we would be much better off if we stopped worrying so much about fats, and instead made a concerted effort to avoid processed, quick-digesting carbohydrates — especially added sugars. Our obscene amount of sugar intake is the principal driver of the "diabesity" epidemic, sharply increases coronary risks and promises to put this generation of children at risk of dying sooner than their parents.

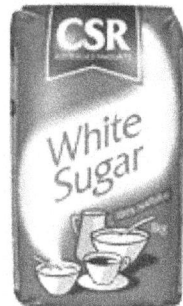

Whole or minimally processed foods - especially vegetables and fruits - have low glycemic loads. That means consuming these foods keeps blood sugar levels relatively stable, which in turn lowers both fat deposition and heart-disease risk. If you make a concerted effort to eat such foods and avoid sugar, you'll soon lose your taste for it. The natural sugars in fruits and vegetables will provide all the sweetness you desire.

Finally Andrew Weil has an advice; while saturated fat appears to have no effect on heart health, eating too much can crowd out vitamins, minerals and fiber needed for optimal health. So he suggests sticking to a "saturated fat budget" which can be "spent" on some butter, or high quality, natural cheese a few times a week.

76 Additional Ways Sugar Can Ruin Your Health

In addition to throwing off your body's homeostasis and wreaking havoc on your metabolic processes, excess sugar has a number of other significant consequences.

Nancy Appleton, PhD, author of the book Lick the Sugar Habit, contributed an extensive list of the many ways sugar can ruin your health from a vast number of medical journals and other scientific publications.

1. Sugar can suppress your immune system and impair your defenses against infectious disease. [1] [2] [3]

2. Sugar upsets the mineral relationships in your body: causes chromium and copper deficiencies and interferes with absorption of calcium and magnesium. [4] [5][6] [7] [8]

3. Sugar can cause a rapid rise of adrenaline, hyperactivity, anxiety, difficulty concentrating, and crankiness in children. [9] [10] [11]

4. Sugar can produce a significant rise in total cholesterol, triglycerides and bad cholesterol and a decrease in good cholesterol. [12] [13] [14] [15]

5. Sugar causes a loss of tissue elasticity and function. [16] [17] [18]

6. Sugar feeds cancer cells and has been connected with the development of cancer of the breast, ovaries, prostate, rectum, pancreas, biliary tract, lung, gallbladder and stomach.[19] [20] [21] [22] [23] [24] [25]

7. Sugar can increase fasting levels of glucose and can cause reactive hypoglycemia.[26] [27]

8. Sugar can weaken eyesight.[28]

9. Sugar can cause many problems with the gastrointestinal tract including: an acidic digestive tract, indigestion, malabsorption in patients with functional bowel disease, increased risk of Crohn's disease, and ulcerative colitis.[29] [30] [31] [32] [33]

10. Sugar can cause premature aging.[34] In fact, the single most important factor that accelerates aging is insulin, which is triggered by sugar.

11. Sugar can lead to alcoholism.[35]

12. Sugar can cause your saliva to become acidic, tooth decay, and periodontal disease.[36] [37] [38]

13. Sugar contributes to obesity. [39]

14. Sugar can cause autoimmune diseases such as: arthritis, asthma, and multiple sclerosis.[40] [41] [42]

15. Sugar greatly assists the uncontrolled growth of Candida Albicans (yeast infections) [43]

16. Sugar can cause gallstones.[44]

17. Sugar can cause appendicitis.[45]

18. Sugar can cause hemorrhoids.[46]

19. Sugar can cause varicose veins.[47]

20. Sugar can elevate glucose and insulin responses in oral contraceptive users.[48]

21. Sugar can contribute to osteoporosis.[49]

22. Sugar can cause a decrease in your insulin sensitivity thereby causing an abnormally high insulin levels and eventually diabetes.[50] [51] [52]

23. Sugar can lower your Vitamin E levels.[53]

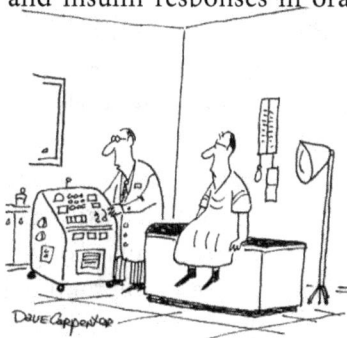

"First we're going to run some tests to help pay off the machine."

24. Sugar can increase your systolic blood pressure.[54]

25. Sugar can cause drowsiness and decreased activity in children.[55]

26. High sugar intake increases advanced glycation end products (AGEs),which are sugar molecules that attach to and damage proteins in your body. AGEs speed up the aging of cells, which may contribute to a variety of chronic and fatal diseases. [56]

27. Sugar can interfere with your absorption of protein.[57]

28. Sugar causes food allergies.[58]

29. Sugar can cause toxemia during pregnancy.[59]

30. Sugar can contribute to eczema in children.[60]

31. Sugar can cause atherosclerosis and cardiovascular disease. [61] [62]

32. Sugar can impair the structure of your DNA.[63]

33. Sugar can change the structure of protein and cause a permanent alteration of the way the proteins act in your body[64] [65]

34. Sugar can make your skin age by changing the structure of collagen.[66]

35. Sugar can cause cataracts and nearsightedness.[67] [68]

36. Sugar can cause emphysema.[69]

37. High sugar intake can impair the physiological homeostasis of many systems in your body.[70]

38. Sugar lowers the ability of enzymes to function.[71]

39. Sugar intake is higher in people with Parkinson's disease.[72]

40. Sugar can increase the size of your liver by making your liver cells divide, and it can increase the amount of fat in your liver, leading to fatty liver disease.[73] [74]

41. Sugar can increase kidney size and produce pathological changes in the kidney such as the formation of kidney stones.[75] [76] Fructose is helping to drive up rates of kidney disease.

42. Sugar can damage your pancreas.[77]

43. Sugar can increase your body's fluid retention.[78]

44. Sugar is enemy #1 of your bowel movement.[79]

45. Sugar can compromise the lining of your capillaries.[80]

46. Sugar can make your tendons more brittle.[81]

47. Sugar can cause headaches, including migraines.[82]

48. Sugar can reduce the learning capacity, adversely affect your children's grades and cause learning disorders.[83] [84]

49. Sugar can cause an increase in delta, alpha, and theta brain waves, which can alter your ability to think clearly.[85]

50. Sugar can cause depression.[86]

51. Sugar can increase your risk of gout.[87]

52. Sugar can increase your risk of Alzheimer's disease.[88] MRI studies show that adults 60 and older who have high uric acid are four to five times more likely to have vascular dementia, the second most common form of dementia after Alzheimer's.

53. Sugar can cause hormonal imbalances such as: increasing estrogen in men, exacerbating PMS, and decreasing growth hormone.[89] [90] [91] [92]

54. Sugar can lead to dizziness.[93]

55. Diets high in sugar will increase free radicals and oxidative stress.[94]

56. A high sucrose diet of subjects with peripheral vascular disease significantly increases platelet adhesion.[95]

57. High sugar consumption by pregnant adolescents can lead to a substantial decrease in gestation duration and is associated with a twofold-increased risk for delivering a small-for-gestational-age (SGA) infant.[96] [97]

58. Sugar is an addictive substance.[98]

59. Sugar can be intoxicating, similar to alcohol.[99]

60. Sugar given to premature babies can affect the amount of carbon dioxide they produce.[100]

61. Decrease in sugar intake can increase emotional stability.[101]

62. Your body changes sugar into 2 to 5 times more fat in the bloodstream than it does starch.[102]

63. The rapid absorption of sugar promotes excessive food intake in obese subjects.[103]

64. Sugar can worsen the symptoms of children with attention deficit hyperactivity disorder (ADHD).[104]

65. Sugar adversely affects urinary electrolyte composition.[105]

66. Sugar can impair the function of your adrenal glands.[106]

67. Sugar has the potential of inducing abnormal metabolic processes in normal, healthy individuals, thereby promoting chronic degenerative diseases.[107]

68. Intravenous feedings (IVs) of sugar water can cut off oxygen to your brain.[108]

69. Sugar increases your risk of polio.[109]

70. High sugar intake can cause epileptic seizures.[110]

71. Sugar causes high blood pressure in obese people.[111]

72. In intensive care units, limiting sugar saves lives.[112]

73. Sugar may induce cell death.[113]

74. In juvenile rehabilitation centers, when children were put on low sugar diets, there was a 44 percent drop in antisocial behavior. [114]

75. Sugar dehydrates newborns.[115]

76. Sugar can cause gum disease.[116]

It should now be crystal clear just how damaging sugar is. You simply cannot achieve your highest degree of health and vitality if you are consuming a significant amount of it.

Fortunately, your body has an amazing ability to heal itself when given the basic nutrition it needs, and your liver has an incredible ability to regenerate. If you start making changes today, your health will begin to improve, returning you to the state of vitality that nature intended.

References:

[1] Johnson RJ and Gower T. (2009) The Sugar Fix: The High-Fructose Fallout That is Making You Sick and Fat, Pocket, 416 pp

[2] "What sweetener should you choose? Sugar? Honey? Agave nectar?" Fitnessspotlight

[3] Stanhope KL, Schwarz JM, Keim NL, Griffen SC, Bremer AA, Graham JL, Hatcher B, Cox CL, Dyachenko A, Zhang W, McGahan JP, Seibert A, Krauss RM, Chiu S, Schaefer EJ, Ai M, Otokozawa S, Nakajima K, Nakano T, Beysen C, Hellerstein MK, Berglund L and Havel PJ. "Consuming fructose-sweetened, not glucose-sweetened, beverages increases visceral adiposity and lipids and decreases insulin sensitivity in overweight/obese humans," J Clin Invest. 2009; 119(5):1322-1334

[4] Park A. "All sugars aren't the same: Glucose is better, study says," Time Magazine, April 21, 2009

[5] Appleton N. Lick the Sugar Habit (1996) Avery, 2nd Ed. 272 pp.

[6] Sanchez, A., et al. Role of Sugars in Human Neutrophilic Phagocytosis, American Journal of Clinical Nutrition. Nov 1973;261:1180_1184. Bernstein, J., al. Depression of Lymphocyte Transformation Following Oral Glucose Ingestion. American Journal of Clinical Nutrition.1997;30:613

[7] Ringsdorf, W., Cheraskin, E. and Ramsay R. Sucrose, Neutrophilic Phagocytosis and Resistance to Disease, Dental Survey. 1976;52(12):46_48

[8] Couzy, F., et al. "Nutritional Implications of the Interaction Minerals," Progressive Food and Nutrition Science 17;1933:65-87

[9] Kozlovsky, A., et al. Effects of Diets High in Simple Sugars on Urinary Chromium Losses. Metabolism. June 1986;35:515_518

[10] Fields, M.., et al. Effect of Copper Deficiency on Metabolism and Mortality in Rats Fed Sucrose or Starch Diets, Journal of Clinical Nutrition. 1983;113:1335_1345

[11] Lemann, J. Evidence that Glucose Ingestion Inhibits Net Renal Tubular Reabsorption of Calcium and Magnesium. Journal of Clinical Nutrition. 1976 ;70:236_245

[12] Goldman, J., et al. Behavioral Effects of Sucrose on Preschool Children. Journal of Abnormal Child Psychology.1986;14(4):565_577

[13] Jones, T. W., et al. Enhanced Adrenomedullary Response and Increased Susceptibility to Neuroglygopenia: Mechanisms Underlying the Adverse Effect of Sugar Ingestion in Children. Journal of Pediatrics. Feb 1995;126:171-7

[14] Scanto, S. and Yudkin, J. The Effect of Dietary Sucrose on Blood Lipids, Serum Insulin, Platelet Adhesiveness and Body Weight in Human Volunteers, Postgraduate Medicine Journal. 1969;45:602_607

[15] Albrink, M. and Ullrich I. H. Interaction of Dietary Sucrose and Fiber on Serum Lipids in Healthy Young Men Fed High Carbohydrate Diets. American Journal of Clinical Nutrition. 1986;43:419-

[16] Reiser, S. Effects of Dietary Sugars on Metabolic Risk Factors Associated with Heart Disease. Nutritional Health. 1985;203_216

[17] Lewis, G. F. and Steiner, G. Acute Effects of Insulin in the Control of Vldl Production in Humans. Implications for The insulin-resistant State. Diabetes Care. 1996 Apr;19(4):390-3 R. Pamplona, M. .J., et al. Mechanisms of Glycation in Atherogenesis. Medical Hypotheses. 1990;40:174-181

[18] Cerami, A., Vlassara, H., and Brownlee, M. "Glucose and Aging." Scientific American. May 1987:90. Lee, A. T. and Cerami, A. The Role of Glycation in Aging. Annals of the New York Academy of Science; 663:63-67

[19] Takahashi, E., Tohoku University School of Medicine, Wholistic Health Digest. October 1982:41:00

[20] Quillin, Patrick, Cancer's Sweet Tooth, Nutrition Science News. Ap 2000 Rothkopf, M.. Nutrition. July/Aug 1990;6(4)

[21] Michaud, D. Dietary Sugar, Glycemic Load, and Pancreatic Cancer Risk in a Prospective Study. J Natl Cancer Inst. Sep 4, 2002 ;94(17):1293-300

[22] Moerman, C. J., et al. Dietary Sugar Intake in the Etiology of Biliary Tract Cancer. International Journal of Epidemiology. Ap 1993.2(2):207-214.

[23] The Edell Health Letter. Sept 1991;7:1

[24] De Stefani, E."Dietary Sugar and Lung Cancer: a Case control Study in Uruguay." Nutrition and Cancer. 1998;31(2):132_7

[25] Cornee, J., et al. A Case-control Study of Gastric Cancer and Nutritional Factors in Marseille, France. European Journal of Epidemiology 11 (1995):55-65

[26] Kelsay, J., et al. Diets High in Glucose or Sucrose and Young Women. American Journal of Clinical Nutrition. 1974;27:926_936. Thomas, B. J., et al. Relation of Habitual Diet to Fasting Plasma Insulin Concentration and the Insulin Response to Oral Glucose, Human Nutrition Clinical Nutrition. 1983; 36C(1):49_51

[27] Dufty, William. Sugar Blues. (New York:Warner Books, 1975)

[28] Acta Ophthalmologica Scandinavica. Mar 2002;48;25. Taub, H. Ed. Sugar Weakens Eyesight, VM NEWSLETTER;May 1986:06:00

[29] Dufty.

[30] Yudkin, J. Sweet and Dangerous.(New York:Bantam Books,1974) 129

[31] Cornee, J., et al. A Case-control Study of Gastric Cancer and Nutritional Factors in Marseille, France, European Journal of Epidemiology. 1995;11

[32] Persson P. G., Ahlbom, A., and Hellers, G. Epidemiology. 1992;3:47-52

[33] Jones, T. W., et al. Enhanced Adrenomedullary Response and Increased Susceptibility to Neuroglygopenia: Mechanisms Underlying the Adverse Effect of Sugar Ingestion in Children. Journal of Pediatrics. Feb 1995;126:171-7

[34] Lee, A. T.and Cerami A. The Role of Glycation in Aging. Annals of the New York Academy of Science.1992;663:63-70

[35] Abrahamson, E. and Peget, A. Body, Mind and Sugar. (New York: Avon, 1977)

[36] Glinsmann, W., Irausquin, H., and Youngmee, K. Evaluation of Health Aspects of Sugar Contained in Carbohydrate Sweeteners. F. D. A. Report of Sugars Task Force. 1986:39:00 Makinen K.K.,et al. A Descriptive Report of the Effects of a 16_month Xylitol Chewing_gum Programme Subsequent to a 40_month Sucrose Gum Programme. Caries Research. 1998; 32(2)107_12

[37] Glinsmann, W., Irausquin, H., and K. Youngmee. Evaluation of Health Aspects of Sugar Contained in Carbohydrate Sweeteners. F. D. A. Report of Sugars Task Force.1986;39:36_38

[38] Appleton, N. New York: Healthy Bones. Avery Penguin Putnam:1989

[39] Keen, H., et al. Nutrient Intake, Adiposity, and Diabetes. British Medical Journal. 1989; 1:00 655_658

[40] Darlington, L., Ramsey, N. W. and Mansfield, J. R. Placebo Controlled, Blind Study of Dietary Manipulation Therapy in Rheumatoid Arthritis, Lancet. Feb 1986;8475(1):236_238

[41] Powers, L. Sensitivity: You React to What You Eat. Los Angeles Times. (Feb. 12, 1985). Cheng, J., et al. Preliminary Clinical Study on the Correlation Between Allergic Rhinitis and Food Factors. Lin Chuang Er Bi Yan Hou Ke Za Zhi Aug 2002;16(8):393-396

[42] Erlander, S. The Cause and Cure of Multiple Sclerosis, The Disease to End Disease." Mar 3, 1979;1(3):59_63

[43] Crook, W. J. The Yeast Connection. (TN:Professional Books, 1984)

[44] Heaton, K. The Sweet Road to Gallstones. British Medical Journal. Apr 14, 1984; 288:00:00 1103_1104. Misciagna, G., et al. American Journal of Clinical Nutrition. 1999;69:120-126

[45] Cleave, T. The Saccharine Disease. (New Canaan, CT: Keats Publishing, 1974)

[46] Ibid

[47] Cleave, T. and Campbell, G. (Bristol, England:Diabetes, Coronary Thrombosis and the Saccharine Disease: John Wright and Sons, 1960)

[48] Behall, K. Influ ence of Estrogen Content of Oral Contraceptives and Consumption of Sucrose on Blood Parameters. Disease Abstracts International. 1982;431437

[49] Tjäderhane, L. and Larmas, M. A High Sucrose Diet Decreases the Mechanical Strength of Bones in Growing Rats. Journal of Nutrition. 1998:128:1807_1810

[50] Beck, Nielsen H., Pedersen O., and Schwartz S. Effects of Diet on the Cellular Insulin Binding and the Insulin Sensitivity in Young Healthy Subjects. Diabetes. 1978;15:289_296

[51] Sucrose Induces Diabetes in Cat. Federal Protocol. 1974;6(97). diabetes

[52] Reiser, S., et al. Effects of Sugars on Indices on Glucose Tolerance in Humans. American Journal of Clinical Nutrition. 1986;43:151-159

[53] Journal of Clinical Endocrinology and Metabolism. Aug 2000

[54] Hodges, R., and Rebello, T. Carbohydrates and Blood Pressure. Annals of Internal Medicine. 1983:98:838_841

[55] Behar, D., et al. Sugar Challenge Testing with Children Considered Behaviorly Sugar Reactive. Nutritional Behavior. 1984;1:277_288

[56] Furth, A. and Harding, J. Why Sugar Is Bad For You. New Scientist. Sep 23, 1989;44

[57] Simmons, J. Is The Sand of Time Sugar? LONGEVITY. June 1990:00:00 49_53

[58] Appleton, N. New York: LICK THE SUGAR HABIT. Avery Penguin Putnam:1988. allergies

[59] Cleave, T. The Saccharine Disease: (New Canaan Ct: Keats Publishing, Inc., 1974).131

[60] Ibid. 132

[61] Pamplona, R., et al. Mechanisms of Glycation in Atherogenesis. Medical Hypotheses . 1990:00:00 174_181

[62] Vaccaro O., Ruth, K. J. and Stamler J. Relationship of Postload Plasma Glucose to Mortality with 19 yr Follow up. Diabetes Care. Oct 15,1992;10:328_334. Tominaga, M., et al, Impaired Glucose Tolerance Is a Risk Factor for Cardiovascular Disease, but Not Fasting Glucose. Diabetes Care. 1999:2(6):920-924

[63] Lee, A. T. and Cerami, A. Modifications of Proteins and Nucleic Acids by Reducing Sugars: Possible Role in Aging. Handbook of the Biology of Aging. (New York: Academic Press, 1990)

[64] Monnier, V. M. Nonenzymatic Glycosylation, the Maillard Reaction and the Aging Process. Journal of Gerontology 1990:45(4):105_110

[65] Cerami, A., Vlassara, H., and Brownlee, M. Glucose and Aging. Scientific American. May 1987:00:00 90

[66] Dyer, D. G., et al. Accumulation of Maillard Reaction Products in Skin Collagen in Diabetes and Aging. Journal of Clinical Investigation. 1993:93(6):421_22

[67] Veromann, S.et al."Dietary Sugar and Salt Represent Real Risk Factors for Cataract Development." Ophthalmologica. 2003 Jul-Aug;217(4):302-307

[68] Goulart, F. S. Are You Sugar Smart? American Fitness. March_April 1991:00:00 34_38. Milwakuee, WI

[69] Monnier, V. M. Nonenzymatic Glycosylation, the Maillard Reaction and the Aging Process. Journal of Gerontology. 1990:45(4):105_110

[70] Ceriello, A. Oxidative Stress and Glycemic Regulation. Metabolism. Feb 2000;49(2 Suppl 1):27-29

[71] Appleton, Nancy. New York; Lick the Sugar Habit. Avery Penguin Putnam, 1988 enzymes

[72] Hellenbrand, W. Diet and Parkinson's Disease. A Possible Role for the Past Intake of Specific Nutrients. Results from a Self-administered Food-frequency Questionnaire in a Case-control Study. Neurology. Sep 1996;47(3):644-650

[73] Goulart, F. S. Are You Sugar Smart? American Fitness. March_April 1991:00:00 34_38

[74] Ibid.

[75] Yudkin, J., Kang, S. and Bruckdorfer, K. Effects of High Dietary Sugar. British Journal of Medicine. Nov 22, 1980;1396

[76] Blacklock, N. J., Sucrose and Idiopathic Renal Stone. Nutrition and Health. 1987;5(1-2):9-Curhan, G., et al. Beverage Use and Risk for Kidney Stones in Women. Annals of Internal Medicine. 1998:28:534-340

[77] Goulart, F. S. Are You Sugar Smart? American Fitness. March_April 1991:00:00 34_38. Milwakuee, WI

[78] Ibid. fluid retention

[79] Ibid. bowel movement

[80] Ibid. compromise the lining of the capillaries

[81] Nash, J. Health Contenders. Essence. Jan 1992; 23:00 79_81

[82] Grand, E. Food Allergies and Migraine.Lancet. 1979:1:955_959

[83] Schauss, A. Diet, Crime and Delinquency. (Berkley Ca; Parker House, 1981)

[84] Molteni, R, et al. A High-fat, Refined Sugar Diet Reduces Hippocampal Brain-derived Neurotrophic Factor, Neuronal Plasticity, and Learning. NeuroScience. 2002;112(4):803-814

[85] Christensen, L. The Role of Caffeine and Sugar in Depression. Nutrition Report. Mar 1991;9(3):17-24

[86] Ibid,44

[87] Yudkin, J. Sweet and Dangerous.(New York:Bantam Books,1974) 129

[88] Frey, J. Is There Sugar in the Alzheimer's Disease? Annales De Biologie Clinique. 2001; 59 (3):253-257

[89] Yudkin, J. Metabolic Changes Induced by Sugar in Relation to Coronary Heart Disease and Diabetes. Nutrition and Health. 1987;5(1-2):5-8

[90] Yudkin, J and Eisa, O. Dietary Sucrose and Oestradiol Concentration in Young Men. Annals of Nutrition and Metabolism. 1988:32(2):53-55

[91] The Edell Health Letter. Sept 1991;7:1

[92] Gardner, L. and Reiser, S. Effects of Dietary Carbohydrate on Fasting Levels of Human Growth Hormone and Cortisol. Proceedings of the Society for Experimental Biology and Medicine. 1982;169:36_40

[93] Journal of Advanced Medicine. 1994;7(1):51-58

[94] Ceriello, A. Oxidative Stress and Glycemic Regulation. Metabolism. Feb 2000;49(2 Suppl 1):27-29

[95] Postgraduate Medicine.Sept 1969:45:602-07

[96] Lenders, C. M. Gestational Age and Infant Size at Birth Are Associated with Dietary Intake among Pregnant Adolescents. Journal of Nutrition. Jun 1997;1113-1117

[97] Ibid.

[98] Sugar, White Flour Withdrawal Produces Chemical Response. The Addiction Letter. Jul 1992:04:00 Colantuoni, C., et al. Evidence That Intermittent, Excessive Sugar Intake Causes Endogenous Opioid Dependence. Obes Res. Jun 2002 ;10(6):478-488. Annual Meeting of the American Psychological Society, Toronto, June 17, 2001 www.mercola.com/2001/jun/30/sugar.htm

[99] Ibid.

[100] Sunehag, A. L., et al. Gluconeogenesis in Very Low Birth Weight Infants Receiving Total Parenteral Nutrition Diabetes. 1999 ;48 7991_800

[101] Christensen L., et al. Impact of A Dietary Change on Emotional Distress. Journal of Abnormal Psychology.1985;94(4):565_79

[102] Nutrition Health Review. Fall 85 changes sugar into fat faster than fat

[103] Ludwig, D. S., et al. High Glycemic Index Foods, Overeating and Obesity. Pediatrics. March 1999;103(3):26-32

[104] Pediatrics Research. 1995;38(4):539-542. Berdonces, J. L. Attention Deficit and Infantile Hyperactivity. Rev Enferm. Jan 2001;4(1)11-4

[105] Blacklock, N. J. Sucrose and Idiopathic Renal Stone. Nutrition Health. 1987;5(1 & 2):9-

[106] Lechin, F., et al. Effects of an Oral Glucose Load on Plasma Neurotransmitters in Humans. Neurophychobiology. 1992;26(1-2):4-11

[107] Fields, M. Journal of the American College of Nutrition. Aug 1998;17(4):317_321

[108] Arieff, A. I. Veterans Administration Medical Center in San Francisco. San Jose Mercury; June 12/86. IVs of sugar water can cut off oxygen to the brain

[109] Sandler, Benjamin P. Diet Prevents Polio. Milwakuee, WI,:The Lee Foundation for for Nutritional Research, 1951

[110] Murphy, Patricia. The Role of Sugar in Epileptic Seizures. Townsend Letter for Doctors and Patients. May, 2001 Murphy Is Editor of Epilepsy Wellness Newsletter, 1462 West 5th Ave., Eugene, Oregon 97402

[111] Stern, N. & Tuck, M. Pathogenesis of Hypertension in Diabetes Mellitus. Diabetes Mellitus, a Fundamental and Clinical Test. 2nd Edition, (PhiladelphiA; A:Lippincott Williams & Wilkins, 2000)943-957

[112] Christansen, D. Critical Care: Sugar Limit Saves Lives. Science News. June 30, 2001; 159:404

[113] Donnini, D. et al. Glucose May Induce Cell Death through a Free Radical-mediated Mechanism.Biochem Biohhys Res Commun. Feb 15, 1996:219(2):412-417

[114] Schoenthaler, S. The Los Angeles Probation Department Diet-Behavior Program: Am Empirical Analysis of Six Institutional Settings. Int J Biosocial Res 5(2):88-89

[115] Gluconeogenesis in Very Low Birth Weight Infants Receiving Total Parenteral Nutrition. Diabetes. 1999 Apr;48(4):791-800

[116] Glinsmann, W., et al. Evaluation of Health Aspects of Sugar Contained in Carbohydrate Sweeteners." FDA Report of Sugars Task Force -1986 39 123 Yudkin, J. and Eisa, O. Dietary Sucrose and Oestradiol Concentration in Young Men. Annals of Nutrition and Metabolism. 1988;32(2):53-5

60.

Artificial Sweeteners

Dangerous Neurotoxins - Taking A Devastating Toll

Forget aspartame and saccharin and the myriad other artificial sweeteners— they are worse than refined sugar. Countless studies show that they are powerful health destroyers. Of course, the research that is conducted by the manufacturers of these chemicals never indicates any link to health concerns.

Research done by independent organizations that do not have a vested financial interest in these synthetic sweeteners links these products to many serious health problems, including birth defects, brain tumours, menstrual irregularities and premenstrual syndrome, migraines and headaches, epilepsy and seizures, psychiatric disorders, blindness, and even death. Which studies would you believe?

According to author Michelle Schoffro Cook, artificial sweeteners are synthetic chemicals your body has to break down, chemicals your body may find it impossible to break down, chemicals your body was never designed to digest. The manufacturers of these products know this information and twist it with slick marketing campaigns to make you think that something that travels through your body undigested (and therefore has no calories) is good for you. According to them, foods sweetened with these chemicals are just a fabulous way to eat sweets without paying the price. Wrong. Wrong. Wrong.

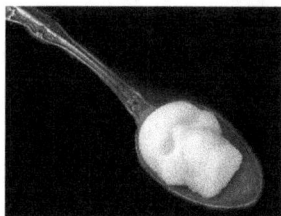

No matter what the slick advertisements or product packaging might suggest, there really is no such thing as a free lunch. Nature in its infinite wisdom designed your body to perform many functions on the food you ingest as part of the overall digestion process and there are many organs that interact with every morsel of food you ingest. Each one is designed to break that food down to extract any goodness it offers and eliminate the leftovers.

If something cannot be broken down, your body wastes energy in a futile effort to do its job. These chemical substances clog your body's natural detoxification mechanisms and make them less effective.

And there are a whole bunch of sugar substitutes, increasingly in use around the world.

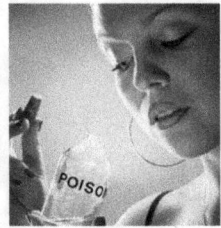

Non-nutritive Sweeteners

The use of non-nutritive sweeteners began with the need for cost reduction and continued on with the need for calorie reduction. It is interesting that artificial sweeteners were actually chemicals being developed for another purpose when the researcher tasted it, often accidently and found that it was sweet.

Since the 1950s, non-nutritive sweeteners have become a weight-loss wonder that allowed us to have our sweets without the calories and cavities. Between 1999 and 2004 more than 6,000 new products containing artificial sweeteners were launched. They are found in so many products now that people can be consuming them without even knowing it.

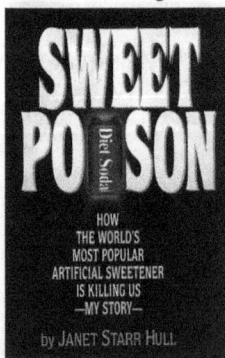

The National Household Nutritional Survey estimated that as of 2004, 15% of the population was regularly using artificial sweeteners. These non-nutritive sweeteners are also referred to as intense sweeteners, sugar substitutes, alternative sweeteners, very low-calorie sweeteners, and artificial sweeteners.

The names of the five FDA-approved non-nutritive sweeteners are saccharin, aspartame, acesulfame potassium, sucralose, and neotame. Each of these is regulated as a food additive.

High-Fructose Corn Syrup (HFCS)

Study after study are taking their place in a growing lineup of scientific research demonstrating that consuming high-fructose corn syrup is the fastest way to trash your health. It is now known without a doubt that sugar in your food, in all it's myriad of forms, is taking a devastating toll.

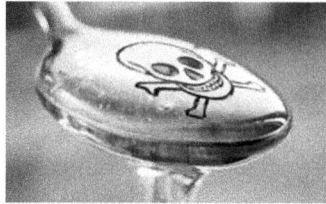

And fructose in any form — including high-fructose corn syrup (HFCS) and crystalline fructose — is the worst of the worst.

Fructose is a major contributor to:

- Insulin resistance and obesity
- Elevated blood pressure
- Elevated triglycerides and elevated LDL
- Depletion of vitamins and minerals.
- Cardiovascular disease, liver disease, cancer, arthritis and even gout.

If you received your fructose only from vegetables and fruits (where it originates) as most people did a century ago, you'd consume about 15 grams per day — a far cry from the 73 grams per day the typical adolescent gets from sweetened drinks. In vegetables and fruits, it's mixed in with fiber, vitamins, minerals, enzymes, and beneficial phytonutrients, all which moderate any negative metabolic effects. It isn't that fructose itself is bad — it is the massive doses of an artificial substance you're exposed to that make it dangerous.

There are two reasons fructose is so damaging:

1. Your body metabolizes fructose in a much different way than glucose. The entire burden of metabolizing fructose falls on your liver.

> "There is every reason to believe that corn has succeeded in domesticating us."
> ~Michael Pollan

2. People are consuming fructose in enormous quantities, which has made the negative effects much more profound.

Today, 55 percent of sweeteners used in food and beverage manufacturing are made from corn, and the number one source of calories is soda, in the form of HFCS.

Food and beverage manufacturers began switching their sweeteners from sucrose (table sugar) to corn syrup in the 1970s when they discovered that HFCS was not only far cheaper to make, it's about 20 percent sweeter than table sugar.

As we saw in the last chapter, the average American consumes a staggering 149 pounds a year of sugar! And the very products most people rely on to lose weight — the low-fat diet foods — are often the ones highest in fructose.

Fructose Metabolism Basics

Dr. Robert Lustig, Professor of Pediatrics in the Division of Endocrinology at the University of California, San Francisco, has been a pioneer in decoding sugar metabolism. His work has highlighted some major differences in how different sugars are broken down and used:

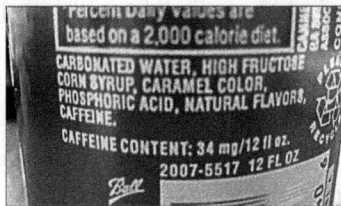

- After eating fructose, 100 percent of the metabolic burden rests on your liver. But with glucose, your liver has to break down only 20 percent.

- Every cell in your body, including your brain, utilizes glucose. Therefore, much of it is "burned up" immediately after you consume it. By contrast, fructose is turned into free fatty acids (FFAs), VLDL (the damaging form of cholesterol), and triglycerides, which get stored as fat.

- The fatty acids created during fructose metabolism accumulate as fat droplets in your liver and skeletal muscle tissues, causing insulin resistance and non-alcoholic fatty liver disease (NAFLD). Insulin resistance progresses to metabolic syndrome and type II diabetes.

- When you eat 120 calories of glucose, less than one calorie is stored as fat. 120 calories of fructose results in 40 calories being stored as fat. Consuming fructose is essentially consuming fat!

- The metabolism of fructose by your liver creates a long list of waste products and toxins, including a large amount of uric acid, which drives up blood pressure and causes gout.

If anyone tries to tell you "sugar is sugar," they are way behind the times. As you can see, there are major differences in how your body processes each one.

The bottom line is: fructose leads to increased belly fat, insulin resistance and metabolic syndrome — not to mention the long list of chronic diseases that directly result.

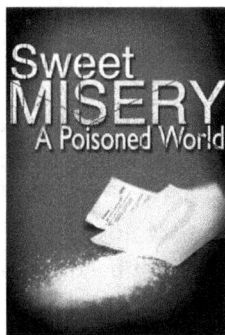

Panic in the Corn Fields

As the truth comes out about HFCS, the Corn Refiners Association is scrambling to convince you that their product is equal to table sugar, that it is "natural" and safe.

Of course, many things are "natural" — cocaine is natural, but you wouldn't want to use hundreds of pounds of it each year.

Fructose is the number one contributing factor to the current obesity epidemic.

By now you are probably aware of the childhood obesity epidemic in America—but did you know about childhood hypertension?

Until recently, children were rarely diagnosed with high blood pressure, and when they were, it was usually due to a tumor or a vascular kidney disease.

In 2004, a study showed hypertension among children is four times higher than predicted: 4.5 percent of American children have high blood pressure. Among overweight children, the rate is 10 percent. It is thought that obesity is to blame for about 50 percent of hypertension cases in adolescents today.

—Johnson RJ and Gower T. (2009) The Sugar Fix: The High-Fructose Fallout That is Making You Sick and Fat,

The food and beverage industry doesn't want you to realize how truly pervasive HFCS is in your diet — not just from soft drinks and juices, but also in salad dressings and condiments and virtually every processed food. The introduction of HFCS into the Western diet in 1975 has been a multi-billion dollar boon for the corn industry.

The FDA classifies fructose as GRAS: Generally Regarded As Safe, which pretty much means nothing and is based on nothing.

According to Dr. Joseph Mercola, there is plenty of data showing that fructose is not safe — but the effects on the people's health have not been immediate. That is why we are just now realizing the effects of the last three decades of nutritional misinformation.

As if the negative metabolic effects are not enough, there are other issues with fructose that disprove its safety:

- More than one study has detected unsafe mercury levels in HFCS.

In the past 30 years, qualitative features of refined sugar consumption have changed concurrently with the quantitative changes. With the advent of chromatographic fructose enrichment technology in the late 1970s, it became economically feasible to manufacture high-fructose corn syrup (HFCS) in mass quantity. A rapid and striking increase in HFCS use has occurred in the US food supply since its introduction in the 1970s.

HFCS is available in 2 main forms, HFCS 42 and HFCS 55, both of which are liquid mixtures of fructose and glucose (42% fructose and 53% glucose and 55% fructose and 42% glucose, respectively). Increases in HFCS occurred simultaneously, whereas sucrose consumption declined. On digestion, sucrose is hydrolyzed in the gut into its 2 equal molecular moieties of glucose and fructose. Consequently, the total per capita fructose consumption (fructose from HFCS and fructose from the digestion of sucrose) increased from 23.1 kg in 1970 to 28.9 kg in 2000. As was the case with sucrose, current Western dietary intakes of fructose could not have occurred on a population-wide basis before industrialization and the introduction of the food-processing industry.

~Hanover LM, White JS. (Manufacturing, composition, and applications of fructose)

- Crystalline fructose (a super-potent form of fructose the food and beverage industry is now using) may contain arsenic, lead, chloride and heavy metals.

- Nearly all corn syrup is made from genetically modified corn, which comes with its own set of risks.

Aspartame - The Deadly Neurotoxin Nearly Everyone Uses Daily

Aspartame was discovered in 1965 by James M. Schlatter and it was later purchased by Monsanto. He was working on an anti-ulcer drug and accidentally spilled some aspartame on his hand. When he licked his finger, he noticed that it had a sweet taste. It is about 200 times as sweet as sugar. Aspartame is one of the most common artificial sweeteners in use today. It is sold under the brand names NutraSweet® and Equal®.

According to statistics published by Forbes Magazine, based on Tate & Lyle estimates, aspartame had conquered 55 percent of the artificial sweetener market in 2003. One of the driving factors behind aspartame's market success is the fact that since it is now off patent protection, it's far less expensive than other artificial sweeteners like sucralose (Splenda).

Today, the statistics on the aspartame market are being kept so close to the vest, it has proven to be virtually impossible to find

In the Anbarra Aborigines of northern Australia, average honey consumption over four 1 month periods, chosen to be representative of the various seasons, was 2 kg per person per year. In the Ache Indians of Paraguay, honey represented 3.0% of the average total daily energy intake over 1580 consumer days. Consequently, current population-wide intakes of refined sugars in Westernized societies represent quantities with no precedent in human history.

~ Hawkes K, Hill K, (Why hunters gather: optimal foraging and the Ache of eastern Paraguay)

current data on usage. By 1984, three years after its initial approval for use in tabletop sweeteners and dry food, U.S. consumption of aspartame had already reached 6.9 million pounds per year. This number doubled the following year, and continued to climb well into the 90's. However, a 2009 Food Navigator article cites the current global market for aspartame as being roughly 37.5 million pounds and worth $637 million.

According to aspartame.org, diet soda accounts for 70 percent of the aspartame consumed. A 12 ounce can of diet soda contains 180 mg of aspartame, and aspartame users ingest an average of 200 mg per day.

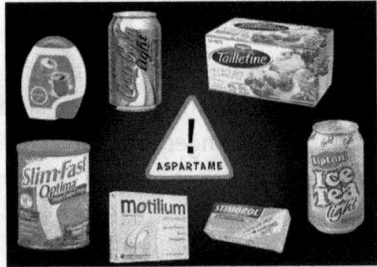

However, it can be quite difficult to calculate just how much you're really ingesting, especially if you consume several types of aspartame-containing foods and beverages. Dosing can vary wildly from product to product. For example, the amount of aspartame will vary from brand to brand, and from flavour to flavour. Some can contain close to twice the amount of aspartame as others, and some contain a combination of aspartame and other artificial sweeteners.

Ajinomoto, one of the leading aspartame manufacturers in the world next to NutraSweet, actually rebranded aspartame to AminoSweet last year, in order to dissociate itself from the negative associations of aspartame.

It also wanted to "remind the industry that aspartame tastes just like sugar, and that it's made from amino acids - the building blocks of protein that are abundant in our diet," - as opposed to a concoction of chemicals never before consumed by man, some ingredients of which are more toxic than others. They will probably deceive some consumers with this newer, more sweetly innocent name that does not bear the same controversial past as the word "aspartame."

Aspartame can already be found in some 6,000 food products and beverages, and the list is about to get even longer. Recently

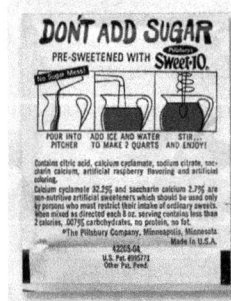

Ajinomoto announced a global R&D alliance agreement with Kellogg Company.

Your Brain And Aspartame

In a video entitled Sweet Misery, Dr. Russell Blaylock, a recently retired neurosurgeon and author of the book Excitotoxins - The Taste That Kills, says, because aspartame is "a poison that affects protein synthesis; affects how the synapses operate in the brain, and affects DNA, it can affect numerous organs. So you can get many different symptoms that seem unconnected."

> Ingredient List 成分
> Sugar, gum base, gluco** **orn syrup, humectant (422), sweeteners (95** 961), **lazing agent (903)
> 糖 · 膠基 栗米葡萄糖漿 · 水分保持劑(422) · 甜味劑 (955, 961) · 上光劑(903)

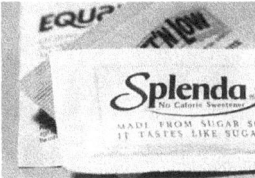

He's referring to a Department of Health and Human Services report that categorizes 10,000 adverse reaction reports logged by the FDA. (Department of Health and Human Services Quarterly Report on

---

I found out about the side effects of artificial sweeteners about 24 years ago. When diet pop first came out, I started drinking large amounts of it. I was 13. By the time I was fifteen I was having Grand Mal seizures. On new years eve at age 16, I had a really big seizure (body arched for fifteen minutes followed by convulsions and remained unconscious until the next day). It was absolutely terrible. Shortly following this incident my Aunt called me saying she had read an article in a health magazine all about the dangers of Aspartame. She informed me one of the things it could cause was seizures. I stopped ingesting anything with aspartame in it and have not had a seizure since. I have had a couple of times where I have ingested it by accident and felt like I was going to faint and have a seizure, so now I am extremely careful to check every label. As other artificial sweeteners have come out I have avoided them as well and do not allow my children to ingest anything with artificial sweeteners.

The effects of these poisons has been known for a very long time! Sadly our government seem to care more about the big corporations than they do for the health of the common people.

~ Lizz, Edmonton, Alberta, 01/21/2010

Adverse Reactions Associated with Aspartame Ingestion, DHHS, Washington, DC, October 1, 1986).

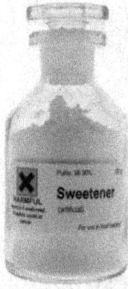

Two years prior to that, a CDC report dated November 2, 1984, discusses several hundred adverse reaction reports received, and at that time, the majority - 67 percent - of complainants also reported neurological/behavioral symptoms.

Some of the most commonly reported neurological symptoms include:
- Headaches
- Changes in behavior or mood
- 'Fuzzy' thinking
- Seizures
- Depression

A 1987 study published in the journal Environmental Health Perspectives states:

"If only 1% of the 100,000,000 Americans thought to consume aspartame ever exceed the sweetener's ADI (acceptable daily intake), and if only 1% of this group happen coincidentally to have an underlying disease that makes their brains vulnerable to the effects of an aspartame-induced rise in brain phenylalanine levels, then the number of people who might manifest adverse brain reactions attributable to aspartame would still be about 10,000, a number on the same order as the number of neutrally related consumer complaints already registered with the FDA and other federal agencies."

Published in the European Journal of Clinical Nutrition in 2008, a South African study offers the same conclusions about the potential workings of aspartame on human brain and concludes that excessive aspartame ingestion might be involved in the pathogenesis of certain mental disorders and also in compromised learning and emotional functioning.

H.J. Roberts, MD, coined the term "aspartame disease" in a book filled with over 1,000 pages of information about the negative health consequences of

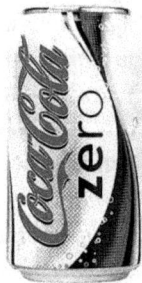

ingesting aspartame. Dr. Roberts reports that by 1998, aspartame products were the cause of 80% of complaints to the FDA about food additives. Aspartame users have reported side-effects like fibromyalgia symptoms, spasms, shooting pains, numbness in legs, cramps, vertigo, dizziness, headaches, tinnitus, joint pain, depression, anxiety attacks, slurred speech, blurred vision, or memory loss.

Don't Drink *Killer Coke* zero

zero Ethics!
zero Justice!
zero Health!

www.KillerCoke.org • StopKillerCoke@aol.com

This monster sweetner is a creation of another monster, Monsanto, who knows how deadly it is. Monsanto funds the American Diabetes Association, American Dietetic Association, Congress, and the Conference of the American College of Physicians. The New York Times, on November 15, 1996, ran an article on how the American Dietetic Association takes money from the food industry to endorse their products. Therefore, they can not criticize any additives or tell about their link to Monsanto.

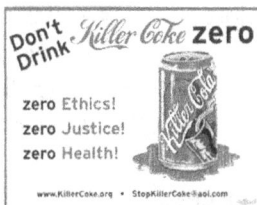

Saccharin

Saccharin was the first artificial sweetener and was originally synthesized in 1879 by Remsen and Fahlberg. Its sweet taste was

DANGER

☠ **POISON**

also discovered by accident. It is 300 to 500 times as sweet as sugar (sucrose) and is often used to improve the taste of toothpastes, dietary foods, and dietary beverages. The bitter aftertaste of saccharin is often minimized by blending it with other sweeteners.

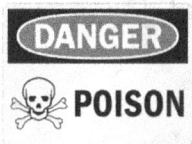

Fear about saccharin increased when a 1960 study showed that high levels of saccharin may cause bladder cancer in laboratory rats. In 1977, Canada banned saccharin due to the animal research. In the United States, the FDA considered banning saccharin in 1977, but Congress stepped in and placed a moratorium on such a ban. The moratorium required a warning label and also mandated further study of saccharin safety.

According to the International Agency for Research on Cancer, part of the World Health Organization, "Saccharin and its salts were

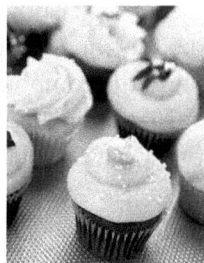

downgraded from Group 2B, possibly carcinogenic to humans, to Group 3, not classifiable as to carcinogenicity to humans.

In 2001 the United States repealed the warning label requirement, while the threat of an FDA ban had already been lifted in 1991. Most other countries also permit saccharin, but restrict the levels of use, while other countries have outright banned it.

The EPA has officially removed saccharin and its salts from their list of hazardous constituents and commercial chemical products. In a December 14, 2010 release the EPA stated that saccharin is no longer considered a potential hazard to human health.

Sucralose

Sucralose is a chlorinated compound that is about 600 times as sweet as sugar, twice as sweet as saccharin, and 3.3 times as sweet as aspartame. It is used in beverages, frozen desserts, chewing gum, baked goods, and other foods. Unlike other artificial sweeteners, it is stable when heated and can therefore be used in baked and fried goods. It belongs to a class of chemicals called organochlorides, some types of which are toxic or carcinogenic. It is nothing like sugar even though the marketing implies that it is.

Common brand names of sucralose-based sweeteners are Splenda, Sukrana, SucraPlus, Candys, Cukren and Nevella. Sucralose can be found in more than 4,500 food and beverage products.

Sucralose was discovered in 1976 by scientists from Tate & Lyle, at Queen Elizabeth College, London. While researching ways to use sucrose as a chemical intermediate in non-traditional areas, Phadnis, a scientist was told to 'test' a chlorinated sugar compound. Phadnis thought that he has been asked to 'taste' it, so he did. He found the compound to be exceptionally sweet.

These scientists were in fact trying to create a new insecticide. It may have started out as sugar, but the final product is anything but sugar. According to the book Sweet Deception, sucralose is made when sugar is treated with trityl chloride, acetic anhydride, hydrogen chlorine, thionyl chloride, and methanol in the presence

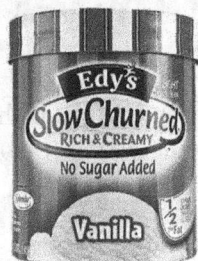

of dimethylformamide, 4-methylmorpholine, toluene, methyl isobutyl ketone, acetic acid, benzyltriethlyammonium chloride, and sodium methoxide, making it unlike anything found in nature. If you read the fine print on the Splenda web site, it states that "although sucralose has a structure like sugar and a sugar-like taste, it is not natural."

The name sucralose is misleading. The suffix -ose is used to name sugars, not additives. Sucralose sounds very close to sucrose, table sugar, and can be confusing for consumers. A more accurate name for the structure of sucralose was purposed. The name would have been trichlorogalactosucrose, but the FDA did not believe that it was necessary to use this so sucralose was allowed.

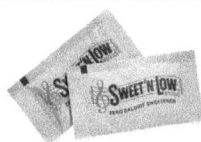

The presence of chlorine is thought to be the most dangerous component of sucralose. Chlorine is considered a carcinogen and has been used in poisonous gas, disinfectants, pesticides, and plastics. The digestion and absorption of sucralose is not clear due to a lack of long-term studies on humans. The majority of studies were done on animals for short lengths of time. The alleged symptoms associated with sucralose are gastrointestinal problems (bloating, gas, diarrhea, nausea), skin irritations (rash, hives, redness, itching, swelling), wheezing, cough, runny nose, chest pains, palpitations, anxiety, anger, moods swings, depression, and itchy eyes. The only way to be sure of the safety of sucralose is to have long-term studies on humans done.

This blend is increasingly found in restaurants, including McDonald's, Tim Hortons and Starbucks, in yellow packets, in contrast to the blue packets commonly used by aspartame and the pink packets used by those containing saccharin sweeteners.

Sucralose was first approved for use in Canada in 1991. Subsequent approvals came in Australia in 1993, in New Zealand in 1996, in the United States in 1998, and in the European Union in 2004. By 2008, it had been approved in over 80 countries, including Mexico, Brazil, China, India and Japan.

The disease tsunami sweeping the world has a definite correlation with the introduction of these synthetic food additives in the public diet.

Cyclamate

Cyclamate, an artificial sweetener, is 30–50 times sweeter than sugar, making it the least potent of the commercially used artificial sweeteners.

Cyclamate was discovered in 1937 at the University of Illinois by graduate student Michael Sveda. Sveda was working in the lab on the synthesis of anti-fever medication. He put his cigarette down on the lab bench, and, when he put it back in his mouth, he discovered the sweet taste of cyclamate.

On October 18, 1969, the Food and Drug Administration banned its sale in the United States with citation of the Delaney Amendment after reports that large quantities of cyclamates could cause liver damage, bladder cancer, birth mutations and defects, reduce testosterone or shrivel the testes. In the same month, cyclamate was approved for use in the United Kingdom and is still used in low-calorie drinks; it is still available without restriction in the UK and Europe. As cyclamate is stable in heat, it was and is marketed as suitable for use in cooking and baking. Commercially, it is available as Sucaryl™.

Cyclamate is approved as a sweetener in over 55 countries, including those in Europe.

In Taipei, Taiwan, a city health survey in 2010 found nearly 30% of tested dried fruit products failed a health standards test, most having excessive amounts of cyclamate, some at levels 20 times higher than the legal limit.

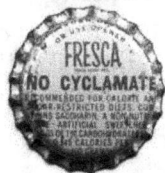

In the Philippines, Magic Sugar, a brand of cyclamate, has been banned. It was placed in coconut juices by local street-side vendors.

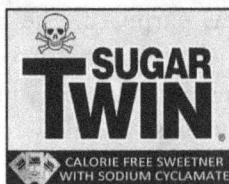

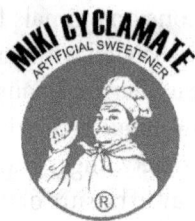

Acesulfame K

Acesulfame K has been an approved sweetener since 1988, and yet most people are not even aware that this is an artificial sweetener being used in their food and beverages. It is listed in the ingredients on the food label as acesulfame K, acesulfame potassium, Ace-K, or Sunett. It is 200 times sweeter than sucrose (table sugar) and is often used as a flavor-enhancer or to preserve the sweetness of sweet foods. The FDA has set an acceptable daily intake (ADI) of up to 15 mg/kg of body weight/day.

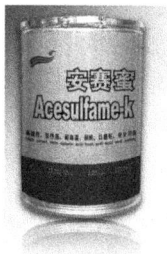

The problems surrounding acesulfame K are based on the improper testing and lack of long-term studies. Acesulfame K contains the carcinogen methylene chloride. Long-term exposure to methylene chloride can cause headaches, depression, nausea, mental confusion, liver effects, kidney effects, visual disturbances, and cancer in humans. There has been a great deal of opposition to the use of acesulfame K without further testing, but at this time, the FDA has not required that these tests be done.

Neotame

In 2002, the FDA approved a new version of aspartame called Neotame. It is much sweeter than aspartame with a potency of approximately 7,000 to 13,000 times sweeter than sugar.

Neotame is also being promoted for use as a flavor enhancer that "accentuates and lifts the flavors in food." The neotame web site states that it's safe for use by people of all ages, including pregnant or breastfeeding women, teens and children, and can be used in cooking. The FDA has set an acceptable daily intake (ADI) at 18 mg/kg of body weight/day.

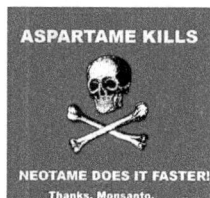

Neotame entered the market much more discreetly than the other artificial sweeteners. While the web site for neotame claims that there are over 100 scientific studies to support its safety, they are not readily available to the public. Opponents of neotame claim that the studies that have been done do not address the long-term health implications of using this sweetener. The chemical similarity that it has to aspartame may mean that it can cause the same problems that are associated with that. Without scientifically sound studies done by independent labs, there is no way to know if this is safe and for whom it is safe.

Sugar Alcohols

If you spend any time looking at nutrition labels, you've probably noticed some intriguing ingredients in sweet foods that are touted as diet-friendly, sugar-free, low-carb, or even formulated for people with diabetes. One ingredient, known as sugar alcohol, is a special type of sugar replacement that is frequently found in soft drinks, gums, cookies, and sugar-free candy. Ever wonder what sugar alcohol is doing in these supposedly healthy foods?

The term "sugar alcohol" is very misleading. Sugar alcohols get their name from their unique chemical structure, which resembles both sugar and alcohol. But they're neither sugars nor alcohols. In fact, sugar alcohols are a type of carbohydrate that sweetens foods, but with half the calories of sugar. There are several specific types of sugar alcohols (usually ending with the letters "-ol"). When reading a food label, the following ingredients are actually sugar alcohols:

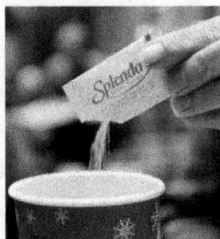

- Erythritol
- Hydrogenated starch hydrolysates
- Isomalt
- Lactitol
- Maltitol
- Mannitol
- Sorbitol
- Xylitol

You'll find sugar alcohols in a wide variety of foods (gums, pancake syrups, candies, ice creams, baked goods, and fruit spreads), health and beauty products (toothpastes, mouthwashes and breath mints), and even medicines (cough syrups, cough drops and throat lozenges). Also they are found in pie fillings, cake frostings, canned fruit, beverages, yogurt and tabletop sweeteners.

Stevia

Stevia is a type of leaf from the Sunflower family. Stevia has been used as a natural sweetener in countries like Japan for decades and in South America for centuries without any side effects. It is interesting to note that the powerful food industry has made it illegal to sell natural stevia as a sweetener in USA.

On December 17, 2008, the FDA did grant GRAS (Generally Recognized as Safe) status to rebaudioside which is one component of the whole stevia plant, and this specific purified component of stevia may be used as a food additive and sold as an alternative sweetener. Examples include Truvia and Purevia. The jury is still out, however, on whether consuming this one component of stevia is as safe as consuming extract from the whole plant, as all the synergistic, protective factors have been removed in these refined products.

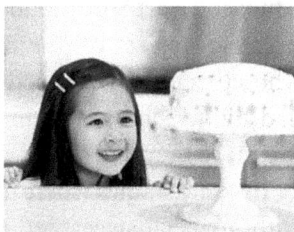

Agave Syrup

Agave syrup is 1.4 to 1.6 times sweeter than sugar. Agave nectar is often substituted for sugar or honey in recipes. Because it dissolves quickly, it can be used as a sweetener for cold beverages such as iced tea. It is added to some breakfast cereals as a binding agent.

Avoid agave syrup since it is a highly processed sap that is almost all fructose. Your blood sugar will spike just as it would if you were consuming regular sugar or HFCS. Agave's meteoric rise in popularity is due to a great marketing campaign, but any health benefits present in the original agave plant are processed out.

Agave nectar syrup is a triumph of marketing over science. True, it may have a low-glycemic index, but so does gasoline -- that doesn't mean it's good for you.

Artificial Sweeteners - The Myth of Weight Loss

The majority of the people who use these products often do so in order to save calories to lose or maintain weight. We are told that this is why we need to consume them and it would be upsetting to find out that they have actually been a part of the problem and not the solution.

The research that shows weight gain with artificial-sweetener consumption has been around since the 1970s. The Nurses' Health Study in 1970 found weight gain over eight years in 31,940 women using saccharin. In the early '80s, the American Cancer Society's study of 78,694 women found that after one year 2.7% to 7.1% more regular artificial-sweetener users gained weight compared to nonusers. The San Antonio Heart Study followed 3,682 adults over eight years on the early '80s. Those who consumed more artificial sweeteners had higher body mass index (BMIs), and the more they consumed, the higher the BMI.

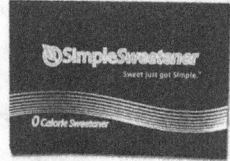

In some studies where they replaced sugar-sweetened beverages with artificial sweetened ones, no difference in weight loss was shown. The possible cause of this could be that artificial sugar actually increases sugar cravings. The theory is that our bodies sense the sweetness of the food and expect the calories. When you consume the artificial sweetener without the calories, your body continues to crave the calories so you end up eating more calories later on.

In rat studies, rats fed diets with artificial sweeteners ate more calories all day then those fed meals with sugar. There may also be a connection with a complex food reward pathway that drives our desire to eat. The sweetness without the calories interferes with the normal process of this pathway causing an increased craving for sweets.

Take a two-week sugar sabbatical and see how different you feel.

61.

Wholesome Goodness Of
Natural Sweeteners

After examining an impressive array of dangerous sweeteners, let us look at the options we are left with. After all, some sweetness is something no one can live without.

Commercial Brown Sugar - A Word of Caution

It is often said that brown sugar is a healthier option than white sugar. But you can chalk that up to clever marketing or plain and simple illusion. In reality, brown sugar is most often ordinary table sugar that is turned brown by the reintroduction of molasses. Normally, molasses is separated and removed when sugar is created from sugarcane plants.

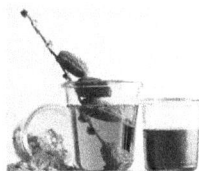

In some cases, brown sugar — particularly when it is referred to as "raw sugar" - is merely sugar that has not been fully refined. But more often than not, manufacturers prefer to reintroduce molasses to fine white sugar - creating a mixture with about 5 percent to 10 percent molasses - because it allows them to better control the color and size of the crystals in the final product.

So the two varieties of sugar are almost similar nutritionally. Because of its molasses content, brown sugar does contain certain minerals, most notably calcium, potassium, iron and magnesium (white sugar contains none of these). But since these minerals are present in only minuscule amounts, there is no real health benefit by using brown sugar.

A 1-teaspoon serving of brown sugar supplies just 0.02 milligrams of iron, for example -- a miniscule amount of the daily 8 milligram requirement for men and 18 milligrams for women of childbearing age.

Raw Sugar

Raw sugar is cane sugar which has been minimally processed. The precise definition varies, depending on who you talk to. Adherents to a raw food diet, for example, may have very specific definitions which involve temperature and handling, while others may view any sort of lightly refined sugar as raw sugar. In all cases, raw sugar is the product of the first stage of the cane sugar refining process, and as a result it has some very distinctive characteristics.

Because raw sugar is not heavily refined, it has a higher molasses content than table sugar, which lends the raw sugar a rich, complex flavor. The large granules are also delightfully crunchy. On nutrition scale, it scores little higher than commercial brown sugar and white sugar.

When Europeans started to explore Asia, one of the first products they were introduced to was raw sugar, and it proved to be a big hit; it was also one of the first crops established in the Caribbean colonies, demonstrating how readily people took to it.

There's nothing wrong with a little raw or brown sugar, consumed in moderation. And if you eat a lot of it, nothing is going to make it any healthier for you.

Unrefined Jaggery

It is advised to use healthy sugar alternative that is unrefined Jaggery. Unrefined jaggery has a mineral content of approximately 60 times that of refined white sugar. One teaspoon of jaggery contains approximately 4-5 mg calcium, 2-3 mg phosphorus, 8 mg magnesium, 48 mg potassium, 0.5 mg iron, as well as trace amounts of zinc, copper, thiamin, riboflavin, and niacin. The corresponding values for refined white sugar are all essentially zero.

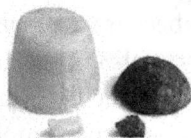

Rapadura

Rapadura is the Portuguese name for unrefined dried sugarcane juice. Probably the least refined of all sugarcane products, rapadura is made simply by cooking juice that has been pressed from sugarcane until it is very concentrated, and then drying and granulating it or, traditionally, pouring it into a mold to dry in brick form, which is then shaved. Because the only thing that has been removed from the original sugarcane juice is the water, rapadura contains all of the vitamins and minerals that are normally found in sugarcane juice, namely iron. A German company called Rapunzel markets pure, organic rapadura.

Raw Honey

Raw honey is a natural sweetener that is easily available. Honey has been used as a sugar substitute for centuries. You can mix it in milk or spread it on bread for a great breakfast. Since it has a low glycemic index, it's ideal for those who want to lose weight. If you're trying to lose weight, you should take some honey every morning. Honey is rich in antioxidants, which can protect your body from a variety of illnesses. It can also treat insomnia, beautify the skin, help wounds heal and promote digestion.

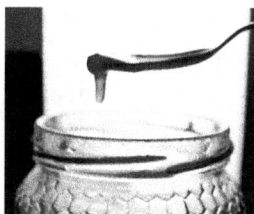

Not all honey is created equal – in fact far from it. The liquid honey that is normally sold in stores is a type of honey that has been processed. Most of this processing involves a high heat treatment, which actually eliminates most, if not all of the health benefits of honey and leaves you mainly with plain sugar.

Therefore, for maximum benefits, especially for one's health, honey should be raw, and preferably from organic sources.

Honey is a truly natural sweetener that was a part of the human diet since time immemorial. We know also that this substance was never eaten in large amounts. Honey has also been used regularly as a substance with healing properties in many ancient traditions, including Ayurveda. Honey should never be heated to maintain its benefits.

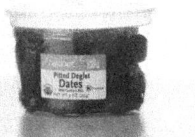

Date Sugar

Though it's called "date sugar," this sweetener is not a form of sugar. It's actually an extract taken from dehydrated dates. Date sugar is widely used as a substitute for regular sugar, because it is a healthier alternative. It contains essential minerals such as iron, calcium, phosphorus, magnesium, zinc and selenium, and it's effective in improving cognitive functions, maintaining healthy blood pressure, enhancing immune system and relieving migraine, asthma and sore muscles.

Blackstrap Molasses

Unlike other sugarcane sweeteners, it contains significant amounts of vitamins and minerals. "First" molasses is left over when sugarcane juice is boiled, cooled, and removed of its crystals. If this product is boiled again, the result is called second molasses. Blackstrap molasses is made from the third boiling of the sugar syrup and is the most nutritious molasses, containing substantial amounts of calcium, magnesium, potassium, and iron. When buying, consider choosing organic blackstrap molasses, as pesticides are more likely to be concentrated due to the production of molasses.

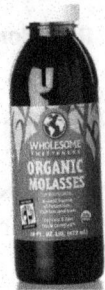

A tablespoon of viscous molasses packs about 15 percent of the daily iron requirement for a normal adult, as well as vitamin B6, magnesium, calcium, and more antioxidants than any other natural sweetener.

Maple Syrup

Maple syrup comes from the sap of maple trees, which is collected, filtered, and boiled down to an extremely sweet syrup with a distinctive flavor. It contains fewer calories and a higher concentration of minerals (like manganese and zinc) than honey. You can find it in bulk in some natural foods stores, but don't be fooled by fake maple syrups, which are cheaper and more readily available at the grocery store. "Maple-flavored syrups" are imitations of real maple syrup. To easily tell the difference, read the ingredients list on the nutrition label. True maple syrup contains nothing but "maple syrup." Imitation syrups are primarily made of high fructose corn syrup, sugar, and/or artificial sweeteners, and contain 3 percent maple syrup (or less).

Brown Rice Syrup

Brown rice syrup is made when cooked rice is cultured with enzymes, which break down the starch in the rice. The resulting liquid is cooked down to a thick syrup, which is about half as sweet as white sugar and has a mild butterscotch flavor. It is composed of about 50% complex carbohydrates, which break down more slowly in the bloodstream than simple carbohydrates, resulting in a less dramatic spike in blood glucose levels. It's worth noting that the name "brown rice syrup" describes the color of the syrup, not the rice it's made from, which is white.

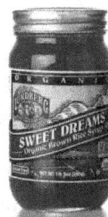

Grape and Orange Juice

You can juice your own grapes and get a very potent sweetener. If you buy grape juice, make sure it's not already supplemented with sugar or fructose. Orange juice is slightly less sweet and has a bit more of a specific taste, but does well in many bread and soup recipes.

Agave Nectar

Agave nectar is produced from the juice of the core of the agave, a succulent plant native to Mexico. Far from a whole food, agave juice is extracted, filtered, heated and hydrolyzed into agave syrup. Vegans often use agave as a honey substitute, although it's even sweeter and a little thinner than honey. It contains trace amounts of iron, calcium, potassium and magnesium. Agave nectar syrup is available in the baking aisle at most natural foods stores. The fructose content of agave syrup is much higher than that of high fructose corn syrup, which is of concern since some research has linked high fructose intake to weight gain (especially around the abdominal area), high triglycerides, heart disease and insulin resistance. High fructose corn syrup contains 55% fructose while agave nectar syrup contains 90%. Despite this, it has a low glycemic index because of its low glucose content.

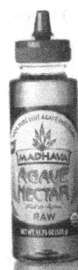

Sucanat

Sucanat stands for sugar-cane-natural, and is very similar to rapadura. It is made by mechanically extracting sugarcane juice, which is then heated and cooled until tiny brown (thanks to the molasses content) crystals form. It contains less sucrose than table sugar (88 percent and 99 percent, respectively).

Turbinado sugar

Turbinado sugar is often confused with sucanat, but the two are different. After the sugarcane is pressed to extract the juice, the juice is then boiled, cooled, and allowed to crystallize into granules (like sucanat, above). Next, these granules are refined to a light tan color by washing them in a centrifuge to remove impurities and surface molasses. Turbinado is lighter in color and contains less molasses than both rapadura and sucanat.

Evaporated Cane Juice

Evaporated cane juice is essentially a finer, lighter-colored version of turbinado sugar. Still less refined than table sugar, it also contains some trace nutrients (that regular sugar does not), including vitamin B2. In Europe, it's known as "unrefined sugar."

Coconut Sugar

Coconut sugar is made from coconut sap, resembles cane sugar, but is very low on the glycemic index. Very healthy, coconut sugar contains sulfur, healthy micronutrients, potassium and magnesium. It is easiest to find in Asian countries.

Mesquite

The mesquite tree, common to the American southwest, produces a beanlike pod that can be dried and pulverized for use as a sweetener or flour. It's gluten-free, with a low glycemic index, and high in fiber and protein. Sprinkle mesquite powder onto oatmeal, add it to smoothies, or replace a percentage of regular flour in baking recipes. Mesquite adds a warm, mellow caramel flavor to almost any food that needs a touch of sweetness.

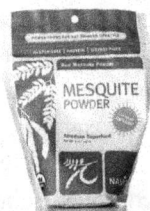

62.

White Rice

The Dead Food

Rice feeds the world! Three billion people worldwide depend on rice for over half of their daily calorie intake. Most of them eat white rice.

It is the predominant dietary energy source for 17 countries in Asia and the pacific, 9 countries in North and South America and 8 countries in Africa. Rice provides 20 percent of the world's dietary energy supply, while wheat supplies 19 percent and maize 5 percent.

As with all natural foods, the precise nutritional composition of rice varies slightly depending on the variety, soil conditions, environmental conditions and types of fertilizers.

When rice is made, it goes through a variety of processes, including going through a husker to remove the grain husks. Once that process is done, brown rice is made.

At various times, starting in the 19th century, brown rice and wild rice have been advocated as healthier alternatives. The bran in brown rice contains significant dietary fiber and the germ contains many vitamins and minerals.

White rice is the name given to milled rice that has had its husk, bran, and germ removed. This alters the flavour, texture and appearance of the rice and helps prevent spoilage and extend its storage life. After milling, the rice is polished using glucose, resulting in a seed with a bright, white, shiny appearance.

This may not seem like much of a difference, but it removes several important nutrients. To get those nutrients back, many companies then reintroduce some of these nutrients from synthetic sources. Enrichment of white rice with B1, B3, and iron is required by law in the United States. But nature can not be imitated and no one knows how good these synthetic additives are. A diet based on polished white rice leaves people vulnerable to many diseases that are prevalent today.

Even 'enriched' white rice is deficient in Vitamin E, Thiamin, Riboflavin, Niacin, Vitamin B6, Folacin, Potassium, Magnesium and Iron when compared to the brown rice. The dietary fiber of white rice is a quarter of what is in brown rice.

Rice bran is the brown coating between the rice kernel and the protective hull. Brown rice still has a thin layer of rice bran around the seed. White rice has none. That's why white rice is a nutritionally dead food.

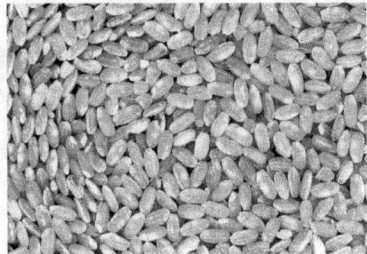

Rice bran is a storehouse of healing nutrients. Paul Pitchford in his book, Healing With Whole Foods, write about many health benefits of rice bran. Some of these health benefits are:

1) Aside from cancer protection, rice bran also contains over 70 anti-oxidants that can protect against cellular damage.

2) Rice bran has been shown to bolster the vitality of the internal organs, especially the adrenals, thymus, spleen, and thyroid, which increase in size and exhibit additional anti-stress effects.

3) Rice bran has rather remarkable effects on lowering high blood-sugar levels. It also produces a calming effect; a food which can foster serenity.

4) Rice bran contains healthy amounts of Alpha lipoic acid, SOD, and Coenzyme Q10. The first is used to restore the liver, the second, SOD, is used to treat cataracts, rheumatism, and osteo-arthritis, and the third, CO Q10, is a widely- respected supplement for all kinds of heart disease.

5) Rice bran contains Gamma-Oryzanol, a powerful anti-oxidant, that helps convert fat to muscle. Rice bran is the only food which contains this nutrient in meaningful amounts.

6) Rice bran contains GPx, an enzyme, anti-oxidant, that reduces mucus, boosts respiratory function, and helps detoxify the body.

7) Rice bran is a valuable source of lecithin, a substance that our brains need to function properly. Lecithin makes up 30 percent of the dry-weight of the brain.

To conclude, brown rice has:

Twice the manganese and phosphorus as white.

2 ½ times the iron.

3 times vitamin B3.

4 times the vitamin B1.

10 times the vitamin B6.

It contains manganese which is essential for energy production, antioxidant activity, and sex hormone production.

Brown rice has high fibre and selenium content which reduces colon cancer. Selenium has been shown to substantially reduce the risk of colon cancer.

Brown rice reduces metabolic problems and lowers cholesterol.

I am a macrobiotic professional with more than forty years of experience guiding many thousands of my clients on diet and lifestyle to recover and maintain their health. I have observed the power and benefits of the regular consumption of brown rice on the young and old over these forty years. My own children and their children follow these same dietary and lifestyle practices. You can easily observe that each generation following these practices is stronger, brighter, and more vibrant than the one before. This response is based on my personal experience along with my long-time observation and experience with people practicing macrobiotics, and not as a medical professional.

The benefits of proper macrobiotic practice are varied and all-embracing. They include recovery from cancer, allergies, diabetes, high cholesterol, arthritis and weight issues. Many of my clients have also followed my recommendations to successfully overcome infertility, to have healthy pregnancies, and to raise healthy children. Macrobiotic practice can also lead to a more positive attitude towards life in general, better moods, and a renewed or enhanced satisfaction and enjoyment from food.

One of the most common points of macrobiotic practice is the regular or daily consumption of brown rice along with a variety of other grains, grain products, beans and vegetables. ~ Denny Waxman

A study at Louisiana State University showed that rice bran and rice bran oil reduced LDL (bad) cholesterol. Also, brown Rice is gluten Free.

We could go on, but switching over from white rice to brown rice can make a great difference to your health. It might just help you to stay hale and hearty well into the autumn and winter years of your life.

Shelf Life

Like all dead foods, white rice has a long shelf life. And that is the only factor that most food-producing companies care about: not your life or my life, but shelf life!

Brown rice, because of the oil content in the attached bran, aleurone and germ, is susceptible to oxidation. As a result, brown rice has a shelf life of only 6-8 months. Keeping brown rice in a refrigerator or cooler will extend the shelf life. White rice, if stored properly, has an almost indefinite shelf life.

White Rice - A History

Rice was originally hulled/polished manually, which meant that it was only done roughly, leaving a lot of the bran still attached.

However just before the start of industrial revolution, technology advanced to the point of using water power for this purpose and the resulting rice became more refined (and thus more appealing to the palate).

In the beginning, this higher-quality rice was at first limited to mostly the urban upper-class due to its high price, but as polishing technique improved, especially in late 19th century, eating white rice became more commonplace.

An unfortunate result of this refined rice was the spread of vitamin B1 deficiency, known as Beriberi disease. As a result, people started mixing in other things (e.g. barley) with their rice to make up for the lost vitamins and try to fend off the disease.

> *We shifted to brown food 2 years ago–brown rice, brown bread and brown sugar. Since then, my bowel problems are long gone. And also, with just half a cup of brown rice I feel full already. I think this maybe the reason why I was able to maintain my weight. ~Diana Herrington*

But if brown rice is so nutritionally rich, why didn't we grow up eating it? Well, that's culture and social class snobbery for you. Because brown rice was cheaper, it was associated with being poor. In short, you only ate brown rice if you weren't rich enough to afford white rice. Polished white rice was a symbol of affluence.

In most of the Asian cultures, brown rice was for the poor rural folk. The irony, of course, is how the snobbery has worked against us. If it weren't for the fact that brown rice has now become fashionable, many would still probably stay away from it.

The even bigger irony is that now that brown rice has become all the rage especially for the health-conscious, it is no longer as inexpensive as it once was. Some brands of brown rice are even more expensive than white rice.

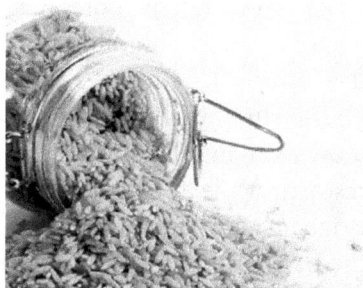

White Rice - An Accused In Diabetes And Obesity Epidemic

Like a runaway train, type 2 diabetes is speeding through many rapidly developing countries. Could a seemingly simple change in diet - from white rice to brown rice - slow the spread of this disease?

In a new study, researchers from the Harvard School of Public Health (HSPH) have found that eating five or more servings of white rice per week was associated with an increased risk of type 2

I would like to rather discuss my experience with brown rice. I have been raised eating white rice and have only begun incorporating brown rice into my meals a few months ago. I am so glad that I did! Brown rice, in my opinion, has a better taste and texture than white rice and I get all these health benefits to go along with it. The only advantage that white rice seems to have is that it has a shelf life of years while brown rice generally has one of 6-8 months; this is no problem for me because brown rice will not last long around me!

In conclusion, brown rice is an amazing grain to incorporate into your meals. It is so darn good-in both the healthy and tasty ways! It is possible to eat your cake and have it too, in the case of brown rice.

~ Laura Hernandez, Memphis, Tennessee

diabetes. In contrast, eating two or more servings of brown rice per week was associated with a lower risk of the disease. The researchers estimated that replacing 50 grams of white rice (just one third of a typical daily serving) with the same amount of brown rice would lower risk of type 2 diabetes by 16%. The same replacement with other whole grains, such as whole wheat and barley, was associated with a 36% reduced risk.

As brown rice is more of a whole grain than white rice, this makes sense; whole grains, across the board, seem to be correlated to a lower risk of diabetes.

The study is the first to specifically examine white rice and brown rice in relation to diabetes risk, says Qi Sun, who did the research while at HSPH and is now an instructor of medicine at Brigham and Women's Hospital in Boston. "Rice consumption in the U.S. has dramatically increased in recent decades. We believe

---

Brown rice has a number of qualities that I find endlessly fascinating. From my personal experience brown rice is the only whole grain that we can eat on a regular or daily basis and never get tired of it. In my early days I tried eating a number of other grains exclusively without any brown rice and found that I grew tired of them quickly and could not wait to get back to my brown rice. When I cook any of these other grains with brown rice I never get tired of them. The other grains I tried eating exclusively included barley, millet, bulgur and oats.

Anything that you cook with brown rice cooks in about the same time as the rice, even if that food takes a much longer time to cook on its own. For example chickpeas can take up to three hours to cook on their own and cook in about an hour with brown rice. It seems that most other foods align with brown rice. It is not the same with other grains.

More importantly, brown rice enhances the taste of all other foods. This is completely unique. Any other food cooked with brown rice tastes good. Brown rice combines well with all other grains, beans, vegetables, seeds, nuts, fresh or dried fruits, sugar, rice syrup, maple syrup and other sweeteners, cheese and other dairy products, herbs, spices and seasonings. In all of my years in practice, I have not been able to find an exception, though some are likely to exist. Brown rice has the ability to complement, embrace and harmonize with all foods and seasonings. I find this truly amazing! ~ Denny Waxman

---

replacing white rice and other refined grains with whole grains, including brown rice, would help lower the risk of type 2 diabetes," says Qi Sun.

The study appeared online on June 14, 2010, on the website of the journal Archives of Internal Medicine.

Brown rice does not generate as large an increase in blood sugar levels after a meal. Its fiber content helps deter diabetes by slowing the rush of sugar (glucose) into the bloodstream.

The researchers, led by Qi Sun, and senior author Frank Hu, professor of nutrition and epidemiology at HSPH, examined white and brown rice consumption in relation to type 2 diabetes risk in 157,463 women and 39,765 men participating in the Brigham and Women's Hospital-based Nurses' Health Study I and II and the Health Professionals Follow-up Study.

The researchers analyzed responses to questionnaires about diet, lifestyle, and health conditions which participants completed every four years. They documented 5,500 cases of type 2 diabetes during 22 years of follow-up in NHS 1 participants, 2,359 cases over 14 years in NHS II participants, and 2,648 cases over 20 years in HPFS participants.

Sun and his colleagues found that the biggest consumers of white rice were more likely to have a family history of diabetes.

I am 73. I am diabetic from last 2 years taking tablets. I strongly believe, after going through lot of health literature on the subject, the white rice is the culprit. In 1950's in my village we used to grow our own paddy. My uncle who was in medical profession, always used to tell me any number of times, while I take 2 bags of paddy to the Huller rice mill in the village, that I should insist with the operator and make sure that the paddy undergoes only the first process which removes the husk portion of the paddy leaving bran portion intact. I also used to notice that many of the other customers insist two and sometimes even three-step processing leaving the rice very very white. As I could recall none of my family members were affected by diabetes in those days. The fact of the matter is, white and overly polished rice consumption is the major cause for virulent spread of diabetes at least in South India...

~Kowtha, West Godavari, Mar 17, 2012

Eating brown rice was not associated with ethnicity but with a more health-conscious diet and lifestyle. In the analysis, researchers adjusted for a variety of factors that could influence the results, including age, body mass index, smoking status, alcohol intake, family history of diabetes, and other dietary habits, and found that the trend of increased risk associated with high white rice consumption remained.

Because ethnicity was associated with both white rice consumption and diabetes risk, the researchers conducted a secondary analysis of white participants only and found similar results.

"From a public health point of view, whole grains, rather than refined carbohydrates, such as white rice, should be recommended as the primary source of carbohydrates," says Hu, "These findings could have even greater implications for Asian and other populations in which rice is a staple food."

This study was supported by the National Institutes of Health. Qi Sun was supported by a postdoctoral fellowship from Unilever Corporate Research.

Another study by the Harvard School of Public Health correlated higher brown rice consumption to lower body weight. This 12-year study followed 74,000 nurses and concluded those that ate more whole grains, such as brown rice, had an easier time with weight loss. Furthermore, the study concluded that the consumption of such whole grains led to a 49% decreased risk of significant weight gain!

One big reason for this is probably brown rice's high fiber content, which means that the digestive system must use up more energy (easy calorie loss) in order to break it down and that the brown rice requires more time to be digested, thus making you feel

---

From my experience, a good way to introduce children or even adults to brown rice is to mix equal parts of cooked white rice and cooked brown rice. After a few times of this, then you serve just the brown rice and it won't be noticed. Brown rice taste different from white rice, to me brown rice has a nutty taste to it which I like.
~ Betty Moore, June 21, 2012

more full for longer periods of time. Therefore, brown rice should be incorporated into your diet if you seek any weight loss.

The Dreaded Pipeline

The biggest danger in the way we eat now lies in the pipeline effect. Obesity can lead to type 2 diabetes in just 5 to 10 years. In turn, diabetes can cause heart, eye, and kidney disease within 5 to 25 years. Dementia can also set in as diabetes takes a toll on the brain's vascular network.

One consequence of diabetes worldwide is that "It's going to generate huge social disparities and ethical issues," Walter Willett, chair of the HSPH Department of Nutrition, predicts. "Those who can afford it will push for dialysis and transplant services, but it's just not conceivable that we could ever build enough dialysis and transplant facilities. Who will live and who will die? The world faces harsh choices."

"Obesity and diabetes will be the public health challenge of the century around the globe," Willett says. "Latinos have at least as high a risk as Asians. The risk is rising in the Middle East and Africa, too."

If the numbers are staggering, consider the costs. According to the World Health Organization, China ranks second to India in total diabetes cases. (The United States is third.) WHO estimates that, between 2006 and 2015, China, one of the biggest white rice consumer, will lose $558 billion in income due to diabetes, heart disease, and stroke. Warns Willett: "No health system can afford it."

Parboiled Rice

In India, where millions depend on rice, the process of parboiling rice was discovered. Uncle Ben's later copied this process and termed it "converted rice." This process involves steaming the rice before the final stages of processing. This drives some of the

My husband thinks brown rice curbs down his appetite which encouraged him to eat more brown rice than white. And I notice too that since its high in fiber, it keeps you fuller longer. I love brown rice for its nutty taste esp. Jasmine brown rice.

~ Patricia, June 21, 2012

vitamins and minerals into the inner layers before the outer layers are removed. The result is 'white rice or semi-brown rice,' but with more nutrients.

Sprouted or Germinated Brown Rice

Germinated brown rice is easier to digest and the sprouting process adds certain nutrients.

Germinated rice contains much more fibre than conventional brown rice, say the researchers, three times the amount of the essential amino acid lysine, and ten times the amount of gamma-aminobutyric acid (GABA), another amino acid known to improve kidney function.

The researchers also found that brown rice sprouts – tiny buds less than a millimetre tall – contain a potent inhibitor of an enzyme called protylendopetidase, which is implicated in Alzheimer's disease.

To make the rice sprout, the researchers soaked it in water at 32 degrees C for 22 hours. The outer bran layer softened and absorbed water easily, making the rice easier to cook. Cooked sprouted rice has a sweet flavor, the researchers report, because the liberated enzymes break down some of the sugar and protein in the grain.

GABA promotes fat loss by stimulating the production of Human Growth Hormone (HGH). HGH increases the sleep cycle, giving deeper rest, boosts the immune system, lowers blood pressure, inhibits development of cancer cells, and assists the treatment of anxiety disorders.

Unique Phytonutrients

All whole grains have bound phytonutrients which are released by the action of intestinal bacteria.

I use brown rice for health reasons. I have type 2 diabetes.

According to my body's response with white rice, it causes spikes in blood sugar as much as 60 - 80 mg/dl when my body converts carbohydrates in white rice into sugar.

I find that brown rice to have a controlled spike in my blood sugar levels after a meal.

~ Julius S, June 21, 2012

These unique substances have the same health-promoting activity attributed to the free form phytonutrients found in vegetables and fruits. One example is a lignin called enterolactone thought to protect against breast cancer and heart disease.

White rice is regarded as an essential item in an Indian's diet. Growing up in a south Indian family, I consumed 3 portions of white rice with every meal. Having realized the nutritional value of brown rice and millets over white rice, I made a choice to consume more of the former than the latter. It wasn't easy when I started and it didn't feel right but slowly I got accustomed to short grain brown rice and started feeling healthier. The high fibre content helped in better digestion. I find that I eat considerably less but feel more full which has helped in weight loss. I don't think there is enough highlighting of the benefits of brown rice by the healthcare professionals. By making a few minor changes to our everyday diet and with some exercise, we can save ourselves the thousands of nasty pills and medicine we may end up taking. I strongly recommend that people at least give it a try. You will only be rewarded.

~Vijay, Nellore, March 19, 2012

63.

Refined Vegetable Oils And Fats

Leave Them on the Shelf

Oil and fat have always been an essential part of the human diet because of the energy they provide. Obtaining oil and fat from plants is a characteristic of many ancient cultures. Oil presses dating back as far as 3500 B.C. have been found and Indian Ayurvedic texts refer to a number of oils which are good for health. Chinese sources from 2800 B.C. show that soy and hemp plants were used to produce oils. In the late 1800s, archaeologists discovered a substance that they concluded was originally palm oil in a tomb at Abydos dating back to 3,000 BCE.

As vegetable oils and fats were goods in short supply, they gained an almost mythical reputation and were of immense commercial importance. Edible oils along with salt were among the first goods to be traded over long distances. A large part of the prosperity of the ancient cultures of the Mediterranean was based on the production of olive oil, the first widely used vegetable oil in Europe.

The basis of the industrial revolution was actually an agricultural revolution. Historically, edible vegetable oil is one of the dietary pillars, along with grains and sugar, on which any civilization stands.

> *"What was garbage in 1860 was fertilizer in 1870, cattle feed in 1880, and table food and many things else in 1890." -- Popular Science, on cottonseed.*

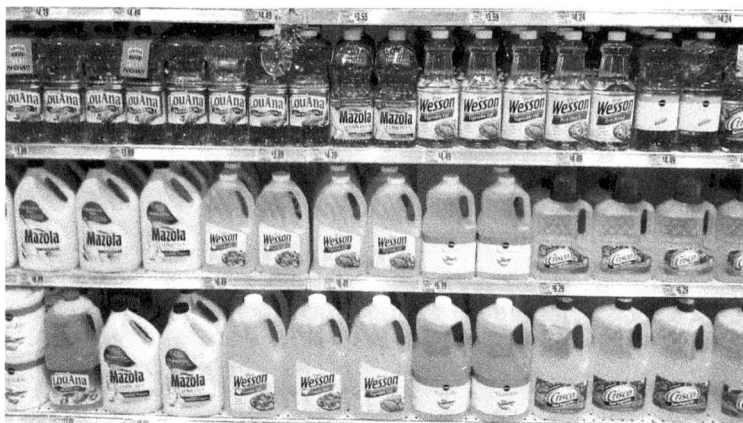

Essential Foods

High-quality fats and oils are one of the most essential foods to consume every day. They are needed for your brain and nervous system, for energy production and for making most of the body's vital hormones. Children, in particular, absolutely require plenty of quality fats which are needed for development of the brain and nervous system. Quality fats are also essential for transporting all vitamins, minerals and hormones in and out of every one of the body cells.

The right amount and types of high-quality fats and oils do not drive up one's insulin level, create insulin resistance and make one fat, as do sugar and carbohydrates. They also do not rob the body of minerals, as does eating sugars and many starches.

The idea of avoiding all high-quality fats because they may make you fat, or that quality fats clog your arteries, is one of the worst nutritional errors of our time.

Industrialization Of Edible Oils

A horrible dietary change has been the substitution of cheap soy, corn and other vegetable oils for the traditional fats used for

The process of refining oils is exactly analogous to the refining of whole wheat and whole sugar into white ones. In all cases, one takes a product full of natural vitamins, minerals, enzymes and other food factors and reduces the original natural food into a relative "nonfood" -- devitalized, stripped.

cooking and frying. These oils are very harmful because they are highly processed.

While butter, olive oil and other pressed oils have been around for millennia, Procter and Gamble researchers were innovators when they started selling cottonseed oil as a creamed shortening, in 1911 in USA. Ginning mills were happy to have someone haul away the cotton seeds.

In their book, The Happiness Diet, authors Drew Ramsey and Tyler Graham narrate the events which changed the world's diet forever by introducing processed vegetable fats in it.

Procter and Gamble researchers learned how to extract the oil, refine it, partially hydrogenate it (causing it to be solid at room temperature and thus mimic lard), and can it under nitrogen gas. It was cheaper, easier to stir into a recipe, and could be stored at room temperature for two years without turning rancid.

Procter and Gamble filed a patent application for the new creation in 1910, describing it as "a food product consisting of a vegetable oil, preferably cottonseed oil, partially hydrogenated, and hardened to a homogeneous white or yellowish semi-solid closely resembling lard.

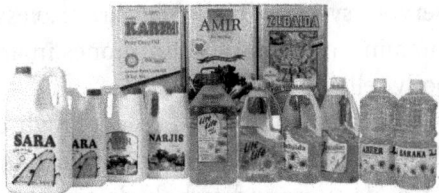

The special object of the invention is to provide a new food product for a shortening in cooking." They came up with the name Crisco, which they thought conjured up crispness, freshness, and cleanliness.

Convincing homemakers to swap butter (and lard) for a new fat created in a factory would be quite a task, so the new form of food needed a new marketing strategy. Never before had Procter and Gamble - or any company for that matter - put so much marketing support or advertising dollars behind a product.

It it came from a plant, eat it. It it was made in a plant, don't.
~ Michael Pollan

They hired the J. Walter Thompson Agency, America's first fullservice advertising agency staffed by real artists and professional writers. Samples of Crisco were mailed to grocers, restaurants, nutritionists, and home economists. Eight alternative marketing strategies were tested in different cities and their impacts calculated and compared.

Doughnuts were fried in Crisco and handed out in the streets. Women who purchased the new industrial fat got a free cookbook of Crisco recipes. It opened with the line, "The culinary world is revising its entire cookbook on account of the advent of Crisco, a new and altogether different cooking fat." Recipes for asparagus soup, baked salmon with Colbert sauce, stuffed beets, curried cauliflower, and tomato sandwiches all called for three to four tablespoons of Crisco.

Health claims on food packaging were then unregulated (and misleading, as they are now), and the copywriters claimed that cottonseed oil was healthier than butter for digestion. Advertisements in the Ladies' Home Journal encouraged homemakers to try the new fat and "realize why its discovery will affect every family in America."

The unprecedented product rollout resulted in the sales of 2.6 million pounds of Crisco in 1912 and 60 million pounds just four years later. It also helped usher in the age of margarine as well as low-fat foods.

Procter and Gamble's claims about Crisco touching the lives of every American proved eerily prescient. The substance (like many of its imitators) was 50 percent trans fat, and it wasn't until the 1990s

---

"While it is true that many people simply can't afford to pay more for food, either in money or time or both, many more of us can. After all, just in the last decade or two we've somehow found the time in the day to spend several hours on the internet and the money in the budget not only to pay for broadband service, but to cover a second phone bill and a new monthly bill for television, formerly free. For the majority of Americans, spending more for better food is less a matter of ability than priority."

~ Michael Pollan, In Defense of Food: An Eater's Manifesto

that its health risks were understood. It is estimated that for every two percent increase in consumption of trans fat (still found in many processed and fast foods) the risk of heart disease increases by 23 percent. As surprising as it might be to hear, the fact that animal fats like butter pose this same risk is not supported by science.

Around the same time, other innovations were taking place 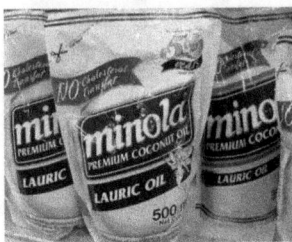 to radically altar our millennia old food habits. Soybeans, an exciting new crop from China arrived in the 1930s. Soy was protein-rich, with a medium viscosity oil. Henry Ford established a soybean research laboratory, developed soybean plastics and a soy-based synthetic wool, and built a car "almost entirely" out of soybeans.

By the 1950s and 1960s, soybean oil had become the most popular vegetable oil in the US.

In the mid-1970s, Canadian researchers developed a low-erucic-acid rapeseed cultivar. Because the word "rape" was not considered optimal for marketing, they coined the name "Canola" (from "Canada Oil low acid"). The U.S. Food and Drug Administration approved use of the canola name in January 1985, and U.S. farmers started planting large areas that spring. Today Canola is the beauty queen of the vegetable oil industry

Unscrupulous, All Powerful Food Lobby

According to the acclaimed author, Sally Fallon, vital researches in the 20th century by nutrition experts like Weston Price, Robert Mccarrison etc. remain largely forgotten because the importance of their findings, if recognized by the general populace, would bring down the world's largest industry--food processing and its three supporting pillars--refined sweeteners, white flour and vegetable oils. Representatives of this industry have worked behind the scenes to erect the huge edifice of the "lipid hypothesis"--the untenable theory that saturated fats and cholesterol cause heart disease and cancer.

All one has to do is look at the statistics to know that it isn't true. Butter consumption in America at the turn of the century, according to Sally Falon, was eighteen pounds per person per year, and the use of vegetable oils almost nonexistent. Yet cancer and heart disease were rare. Today butter consumption hovers just above four pounds per person per year while vegetable oil consumption has soared--and cancer and heart disease are endemic.

What the research really shows is that both refined carbohydrates and vegetable oils cause imbalances in the blood and at the cellular level that lead to an increased tendency to form blood clots, leading to myocardial infarction. This kind of heart disease was virtually unknown in America in 1900.

Today it has reached epidemic levels. Atherosclerosis, or the buildup of hardened plague in the artery walls, cannot be blamed on saturated fats or cholesterol. Very little of the material in this plaque is cholesterol. A 1994 study appearing in the Lancet showed that almost three quarters of the fat in artery clogs is unsaturated. The "artery clogging" fats are not animal fats but vegetable oils.

Built into the whole cloth of the lipid hypothesis is the postulate that the traditional foods of our ancestors - the butter, cream, cold pressed oils, that were necessary to produce "splendid physical development" in "primatives" - are bad for us.

A number of schemes have served to imbed this notion in the consciousness of the people, not the least of which was the National Cholesterol Education Program (NCEP), during which tax payers paid for a packet of "information" on cholesterol and heart disease to be sent to every physician in America.

In 1990, the National Cholesterol Education Program recommended a lowfat diet for all Americans above the age of two. The advantage of such a diet is supposed to be reduced risk of heart disease in later life--even though not a single study has shown such an hypothesis to be tenable.

What the scientific literature does tell us is that low fat diets for children, or diets in which vegetable oils have been substituted for healthy fats like natural butter, result in failure to thrive--failure to grow tall and strong--as well as learning disabilities, susceptibility to infection and behavioral problems. Teenage girls who adhere

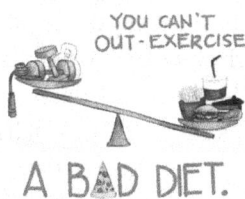

to such a diet risk reproductive problems. If they do manage to conceive, their chances of giving birth to a low birth weight baby, or a baby with birth defects, are high.

Compared to this folly, the wisdom of the so-called primitive in regards to ensuring the health of his children has inspired the awe of many experts. Tribal groups--especially those in Africa and the South Pacific--fed special foods to young men and women before conception, to women during pregnancy and lactation, and to children during their growing years.

For a future of healthy children--for any future at all--we must turn our backs on the dietary advice of sophisticated medical orthodoxy. We must return to the food wisdom of our so-called primitive ancestors, choosing traditional whole foods that are organically grown, minimally processed and above all not shorn of their vital lipid component.

The Process of Extracting Vegetable Oils

Vegetable oils look clean and bright on the grocers shelves, but a description of their processing reveals the true nature of these products. These poor oils go through 'more primping and processing than a dog at a Kennel Club show.'

According to Paul Hawken & Fred Rohe, one very basic difference between our way of looking at vegetable oils and the industrial oil technician's viewpoint should be understood. When he sees dark color, it represents the presence of "impurities" -- material that prevents the oil from being light colored, odorless and bland in taste. From our viewpoint, those "impurities" look desirable -- the things which impart color, odor and flavor are 'nutrients'.

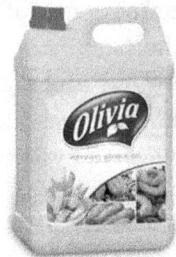

It is both tragic and ironic that the removal of nutrients should be equated with "purity".

Modern method of oil extraction called solvent extraction is described in the book 'The Lowdown on Edible Oils' as "definitely dangerous to health."

This process is not for the squeamish. Take a look at the steps and decide for yourself if this is a "food" you want to consume:

Oil seeds such as soybean, rapeseed, cotton, sunflower are gathered. Most of these seeds are from plants that have been genetically engineered or huge amounts of pesticides have been applied to them.

The seeds are husked and cleaned of dirt and dust, then crushed.

The crushed seeds are then heated to temperatures between 110 degrees and 180 degrees in a steam bath to start the oil extraction process.

The seeds are put through a high volume press which uses high heat and friction to press the oil from the seed pulp.

The seed pulp and oil are then put through a hexane solvent bath and steamed again to squeeze out more oil.

Hexane is produced by the refining of crude petroleum oil. It is a mild anesthetic. Inhalation of high concentrations produces first a state of mild euphoria, followed by sleepiness with headaches and nausea. Chronic intoxication from hexane has been observed in recreational solvent abusers and in workers in the shoe manufacturing, furniture restoration and automobile construction industries where hexane is used as a glue. The initial symptoms are tingling and cramps in the arms and legs, followed by general muscular weakness. In severe cases, atrophy of the skeletal muscles is observed, along with a loss of coordination and problems of vision. In 2001, the U.S. Environmental Protection Agency issued regulations on the control of emissions of hexane gas due to its potential carcinogenic properties and environmental concerns.

The big commercial edible oil processors and distributors tell us that if any of the solvent remains in the oils it is very little. But you know just how harmful these solvents may be. Pertinent here is an observation coming out of a symposium of cancer specialists organized by the International Union Against Cancer meeting in Rome in August 1956.

Among many things they observed 'Since various petroleum constitutents, including certain mineral oils and paraffin, have produced cancer in man and experimental animals, the presence of such chemicals in food appears to be objectionable, particularly when such materials are heated to high temperatures.'

Enough of hexane story. Now the seed/oil mixture is put through a centrifuge and phosphate is added to begin the separation of the oil and seed residues.

After solvent extraction, the crude oil is separated and the solvent is evaporated and recovered. The seed pulp residues are conditioned and reprocessed to make by-products such as animal feed.

The crude vegetable oil is then put through further refining techniques including degumming, neutralization and bleaching:

Water degumming: In this process, water is added to the oil. After a certain reaction period the hydrated phosphatides can be separated either by decantation (settling) or continuously by means of centrifuges. In this process step a large part of water soluble and even a small proportion of the non-water soluble phosphatides are removed. The extracted gums can be processed into lecithin for food, feed or for technical purposes.

Neutralization: Any free fatty acids, phospholipids, pigments, and waxes in the extracted oil promote fat oxidation and lead to undesirable colors and odors in the final products. These impurities are removed by treating the oil with caustic soda (sodium hydroxide) or soda ash (sodium carbonate). The impurities settle to the bottom and are drawn off. The refined oils are lighter in colour, less viscous, and more susceptible to oxidation.

Bleaching: The major purpose of bleaching is the removal of off colored materials in the oil. The heated oil is treated with various bleaching agents such as fuller's earth, activated carbon, or activated clays. Many impurities, including chlorophyll and carotenoid pigments, are absorbed by this process and removed by filtration. However, bleaching also promotes fat oxidation since some natural antioxidants and nutrients are removed along with the impurities.

Deodorization is the final step in the refining of vegetable oils. Pressurize steam at extremely high temps (500 degrees or more) is used to remove volatile compounds which would cause off odors and tastes in the final product.

The oil produced is referred to as "refined oil" and is ready to be consumed or for the manufacture of other products. A light solution of citric acid is often added during this step to inactivate any metals such as iron or copper present in the final product.

The process of refining vegetable oil damages the fats and makes the oils very unstable and prone to going rancid quite easily. Rancid oils in any form are particularly bad for your health because they introduce cancer causing free radicals into your body, without the benefit of including an antioxidant like vitamin E.

Author Sally Fallon adds a comment to this grim scenario:

"High-temperature processing causes the weak carbon bonds of unsaturated fatty acids, especially triple unsaturated linolenic acid, to break apart, thereby creating dangerous free radicals. In addition, antioxidants, such as fat-soluble vitamin E, which protect the body from the ravages of free radicals, are neutralized or destroyed by high temperatures and pressures. BHT and BHA, both suspected of causing cancer and brain damage, are often added to these oils to replace vitamin E and other natural preservatives destroyed by heat."

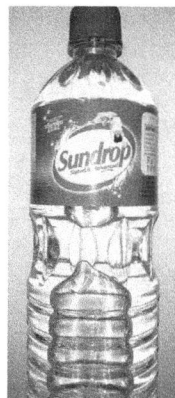

The process of refining oils is exactly analogous to the refining of whole wheat and whole sugar into white ones. In all cases, one takes a product full of natural vitamins, minerals, enzymes and other food factors and reduces the original natural food into a relative "nonfood" - devitalized, stripped.

Hydrogenated and Trans Fats

Even if you don't know much about hydrogenated fats or trans fats, you would probably agree that they sound like some kind of experiment gone awry in a science fiction movie. These fats seem like some experimental food produced in test tubes by evil scientists that come to life at night and start attacking everything in sight. Well, that's actually not far from the truth.

Hydrogenation is a process using high temperatures to change the structure of fat molecules from a liquid to a solid. The food industry benefits from this unnatural process because it prevents the oils from becoming rancid. People respond positively to the marketing campaigns that tell you the product will last longer.

But what is the human cost of this experimental food substance? Hydrogenation turns healthy fatty acids (cis-fatty acids) into harmful ones (trans fatty acids). Cis-fatty acids, which are sometimes called essential fatty acids, trigger healthy fat metabolism in the human body. They are critical to a healthy brain and nervous system, immune system, organs, tissues, and cells.

After a fat has been chemically altered to become a trans fatty acid, it no longer offers any of these benefits. Instead, the human body does not even recognize it as food. It treats trans fats as toxins and searches for dumping sites in the body fat stores. In some cases, trans fats get dumped into organs, like the liver, which usually cannot filter all of them over long periods of time.

Trans fats can also clog the liver and prevent healthy fatty acids from being absorbed from healthy foods. Trans-fatty acids can be referred to as '*plastic fats*' since they really do not resemble food any longer.

The melting point of trans-fatty acids found in todays margarines and most prepared and packaged foods is 46 degrees C. These fats do not melt or break down at body temperature (37 degrees C).

Stick margarine is up to 30 percent trans-fatty acids while shortening is up to 50 percent of these harmful fats. Most oils found on grocery store shelves contain trans fats as well. This is because of the high heat used to extract the oils from nuts and seeds during the manufacturing process.

Cooking oils to high temperatures, as in home cooking or industrial cooking, can cause the healthy fats to turn into trans fats. That includes most fried foods, potato chips, commercial salad dressings, baked goods, candy bars, breads, cookies, and chocolates, all of which can contain between 30 and 50 percent trans fats. If you check the ingredient list, you will typically find items such as partially hydrogenated oil or hydrogenated vegetable oil or shortening or vegetable oil shortening. These all indicate the presence of trans fats.

Cold-pressed oils or extra-virgin olive oil are better choices than commercial cooking oils, margarine, and shortening. Why bother with something so processed and unhealthy when there are umpteen other, better options out there?

Traditional Method

Traditional method of extracting vegetable oils from nuts, grains, beans, seeds or olives is by use of a hydraulic press. This is an ancient method and yields the best quality oil. The only two materials that will yield enough oil without heating them first are sesame seeds and olives. Therefore, sesame oil and olive oil from a hydraulic press are the only oils which could truly be called "cold pressed".

The term "virgin" for olive oil refers only to the first pressing by a hydraulic press without heat. The term "cold pressed" refers only to hydraulic pressing without heat. These oils are the closest possible to the natural state, therefore have the most color, odor and flavor - in a word, the most nutrition - but they will often be unavailable because these days, so little is produced this way.

If an oil which has been extracted by hydraulic press but has been heated prior to pressing, this will be referred to as 'pressed', not 'cold pressed'.

Expeller Method

This is the second method of oil extraction and it is much less violent than industrial refining. This process yields more oil compared to 'pressed' or 'cold pressed' methods.

This method by expeller is described in 'The Lowdown on Edible Oils' as follows: "This uses a screw or continuous press with a constantly rotating worm shaft. Cooked material goes into one end and is put under continuous pressure until discharged at the other end with oil squeezed out." Temperatures between 200 and 250 degrees are normal. Obviously, this type of extraction does not qualify as 'cold pressed'. Oil produced this way is referred to as 'expeller pressed.'

Unlike 'pressed' or 'cold pressed' method, 'expeller pressed' oil needs some refining after extraction, though not as massive as industrial refining.

Clogging The Arteries

Like all natural foods, natural fats are blessed with a natural 'life cycle', a period of optimum nutritional density during which they must be eaten, and after which they become toxic and degrade.

Hydrogenation forces natural fats into becoming molecularly "shelf" stable by accelerating the oxidation process with high temperatures and addition of heavy metal nickel catalyst to force the insertion of additional hydrogen atoms into the molecule, and the subsequent "refining" process removes the bad oxidation tastes and smells by further high heat steam sparging and deodorization.

In other words, all liquid vegetable oils that are packaged in clear glass or plastic bottles and displayed at room temperature on open shelves are stable because they are already oxidized and biologically dead and toxic.

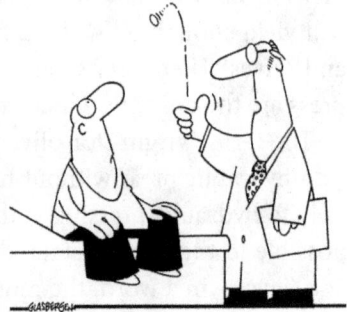

"Heads, you get a quadruple bypass. Tails, you take a baby aspirin."

There are too many individual parts to the story to post here, so for the rest of the story can be read in the Wikipedia articles about Hydrogenation, Trans vs. Cis molecules, and also the one about Essential Fatty Acids. It is very simple and easily understandable and there are even pictures of the molecules that will help you understand why industrially processed pre-oxidized and adulterated vegetable oils are a direct cause of arterial plaque formation (progressive atherosclerosis) and cancer.

In a nutshell it is because when vegetable oils are heated the molecules straighten out (trans vs. cis) and glue themselves together like straws, they polymerize and become a type of natural plastic which is not dissolvable by blood plasma and body fluids.

That is also why boiled linseed oil is used to make paints and varnishes.

Margarine - Trust A Cow More Than A Chemist

Margarine was originally manufactured to fatten turkeys. When it killed the turkeys, the people who had put their money into the research wanted a payback so they put their heads together to figure out what to do with this product.

It was a white substance with no food appeal, so they added the yellow colouring and sold it to people to use in place of butter.

How do you like it? Then they came out with some clever new flavourings.

During World War II, a shortage of butter and other fats gave a boost to popularity of margarine. Today it has become a major part of the Western diet and overtook butter in popularity in the mid-20th century. In the United States, for example, in 1930 the average person ate over 18 pounds (8.2 kg) of butter a year and just over 2 pounds (0.91 kg) of margarine. By the end of the 20th century, an average American ate around 5 lb (2.3 kg) of butter and nearly 8 lb (3.6 kg) of margarine.

Although a staple of the American diet, butter came under a great deal of scrutiny when its high levels of saturated fat were associated with increased heart disease risk. Many people accepted the demise of butter in stride, ruing the loss of its savory flavor but agreeing that its effect on the heart might be too high a price to pay. They dutifully switched to margarine, as researchers and nutritionists suggested.

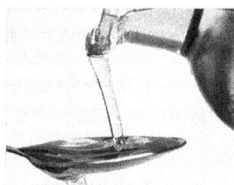

Then the hazards of margarine came to light. Its high levels of trans fats packed a double whammy for heart disease by raising levels of LDL (bad cholesterol) and lowering levels of HDL (good cholesterol). Many people felt betrayed or duped.

The truth is, there never was any good evidence that using margarine instead of butter cut the chances of having a heart attack or developing heart disease.

Margarine intake has been linked to a host of illnesses such as colitis and arthritis. The hardening agents used in the production

Sept. 2010 I stopped consumption of all vegetable oil and replaced them with olive oil and butter. I also stopped eating sugar (as much as possible). I shed 30 lbs. and have kept it off.

More than a year later, HDLs are up, LDLs about the same - HDL/LDL ratio MUCH better (and still <200), and triglycerides are down too. Oh, and I cut my BP meds in half, and I feel great at 60. I wish I had come across this information 10 years ago!

~ Brian, Tahiti

of margarine include nickel and cadmium. Nickel is a toxic metal that causes lung and kidney problems. Cadmium is among the most toxic of the heavy metals. It may contribute to serious diseases such as arteriosclerosis, high blood pressure and malignancy.

Process of Manufacture

Manufacturers cannot use liquid oils in baked goods or frying, and they are not spreadable. So to harden the liquid vegetable oils to make margarine and shortening, they put the oils through a process called partial hydrogenation. To make margarine or shortening, first the oil is extracted under high temperature and pressure, and with hexane solvents as we have already seen in detail.

These oils are then mixed with a nickel catalyst and put into a huge high-pressure, high-temperature reactor. What goes into the reactor is a liquid, but what comes out of that reactor is a semi-solid that looks like grey cottage cheese and smells terrible. Emulsifiers are mixed in to smooth out the lumps. The product is then steam cleaned a second time to get rid of the horrible smell. Then it is bleached to get rid of the grey color. At this point, the product can be used as vegetable shortening.

To make margarine, they add artificial flavors and synthetic vitamins. Then they add annatto or some other natural coloring. It is then packaged in blocks and tubs. Advertising promotes this garbage as a health food.

No Veggie Oil!

I stopped eating vegetable oils a few years ago and I immediately noticed a HUGE change in my body. I was suffering from constant burning mouth (it's an actual syndrome, believe it or not, and it's awful), fatigue, and cystic acne which, for a woman in her 30s, was distressing. As soon as I cut out vegetable oil in all forms, my symptoms literally disappeared within in a matter of days. If I slip and eat vegetable oil, they come right back! I've never had such a drastic response to a dietary change.

Thanks for sharing this information. I get some crazy looks when I tell people I can't eat vegetable oil, so I appreciate having this information to share with them.

~ Sharon, Oregon

Margarine is but one molecule away from being plastic and shares 27 ingredients with paint.

You can try this yourself: Purchase a tub of margarine and leave it open in your garage or shaded area. Within a couple of days you will notice a couple of things:

No flies, not even those pesky fruit flies will go near it. That should tell you something.

It does not rot or smell differently because it has no nutritional value; nothing will grow on it. Even those teeny weeny microorganisms will not a find a home to grow. Why? Because it is nearly plastic. Would you melt your Tupperware and spread that on your toast?

All of the margarines, shortenings, spreads, even low-trans spreads contain trans fats plus many other artificial ingredients. In the groceries stores there is just a little bit of space for the butter because all the high-profit margarine foods have totally invaded the food supply. Virtually all packaged or processed foods contain trans fatty acids. They're in all the chips and crackers, and they now use them for French fries.

It used to be that when you made desserts for your kids, at least these contained butter, cream and nuts and other healthy ingredients—all good wholesome foods. Now the industry can imitate the butter, cream and so many other things, so most desserts end up being mostly sugar, partially hydrogenated oils and a long list of artificial ingredients.

I usually buy Organic Valley's "Pasture Butter" or Kerry Gold. Why, because they are butters made from milk from cows that were grazing on green growing grass. If you compare the color of these butters with other butters, you will find that they are much yellower. The yellow color comes from the vitamin K in the grass. This is how most butter used to look and why, when margarine first came on the market, it was called "oleo" (which is the name of the yellow coloring added to make them look more like butter). Enjoy!

~ Lori Mel

Problems with Hydrogenated Oils

Many, many diseases have been associated with the consumption of trans fatty acids, such as heart disease, cancer, digestive disorders and degeneration of joints and tendons (which is why we have so many hip replacements today). Trans fats are associated with auto-immune disease, skin problems, growth problems in children and learning disabilities. The only reason that we are eating this stuff is because we have been told that the competing fats and oils—butter, cream, coconut oil etc.—are bad for us and cause heart disease. This message is nothing but industry propaganda to get us to buy substitutes.

The Low-Fat Craze

"Low-fat" everything has produced an epidemic of obesity, diabetes, hypoglycemia, and even some of the ADHD and perhaps cancers that are so common today. These diseases were not as prevalent before people began believing the lie that quality fats are bad for you.

What few people realize is that if you do not eat fats and oils, you must consume many more sugars or starches to obtain the calories you need. This easily exceeds most people's carbohydrate tolerance level and leads to many diseases.

Also, prepared foods that are low in fat usually contain many more chemicals in order to give the food the flavor that fats normally provide. Many of these chemical additives are of questionable safety.

> *I have suffered from IBS for years and tried everything EXCEPT what a naturalist doctor insisted would help me. In the end, in desperation - I did what he said : eliminated all refined oils from my diet ENTIRELY, and use only Virgin cold pressed Olive Oil, sesame oil and butter. Honest to God - my IBS vanished after a couple of weeks and has gone from my life. It is now years later and I feel good. Though anecdotal and of no statistical or scientific value - I truly believe sharing my story above can help some of you suffering from IBS. Give it a try.*
> *~ Jason Miller, Lewisville Texas*

Low-Fat Diet Does Not cut Cancer, Heart And Other Health Risks

By Gina Kolata, The New York Times, February 8, 2006

Following is a press report busting the myth of low fat diet. This myth has demonized traditional fats like butter and cream for almost a century.

The largest study ever to ask whether a low-fat diet reduces the risk of getting cancer or heart disease has found that the diet has no effect.

The $415 million federal study involved nearly 49,000 women ages 50 to 79 who were followed for eight years. In the end, those assigned to a low-fat diet had the same rates of breast cancer, colon cancer, heart attacks and strokes as those who ate whatever they pleased, researchers are reporting today.

"These studies are revolutionary," said Dr. Jules Hirsch, physician in chief emeritus at Rockefeller University in New York City, who has spent a lifetime studying the effects of diets on weight and health. "They should put a stop to this era of thinking that we have all the information we need to change the whole national diet and make everybody healthy."

"The study, published in today's issue of The Journal of the American Medical Association, was not just an ordinary study", said Dr. Michael Thun, who directs epidemiological research for the American Cancer Society. It was so large and so expensive, Dr. Thun said, that it was "the Rolls-Royce of studies." As such, he added, it is likely to be the final word.

"We usually have only one shot at a very large-scale trial on a particular issue," he said.

The results, the study investigators agreed, do not justify recommending low-fat diets to the public to reduce their heart disease and cancer risk. Given the lack of benefit found in the study, many medical researchers said that the best dietary advice, for now, was to follow federal guidelines for healthy eating, with less saturated and trans fats, more grains, and more fruits and vegetables.

The study found that women who were randomly assigned to follow a low-fat diet ate significantly less fat over the next eight years. But they had just as much breast and colon cancer and just as much heart disease. The women were not trying to lose weight, and their weights remained fairly steady. But their experiences with the diets allowed researchers to question some popular notions about diet and obesity.

Although all the study participants were women, the colon cancer and heart disease results should also apply to men, said Dr. Jacques Rossouw, the project officer for the Women's Health Initiative.

While cancer researchers said they were disappointed by the results, heart disease researchers said they were not surprised that simply reducing total fat had no effect, because they had moved on from that hypothesis.

Junk Cheese

Most cheese today is mass-produced in huge batches and many shortcuts are taken to make it ferment faster. For instance, many chemicals may be added to it, it is not aged naturally and preservatives and other chemicals are added or sprayed on later to make it keep longer.

As a result, most cheese is close to junk food status, unfortunately. This is what your child is eating when he or she eats most pizza, for example, or most Mexican dishes. It is especially the case in restaurants, where cutting costs is the primary consideration, and not your health.

The worst cheese is called "cheese food" or "processed cheese". Velveeta and Kraft make this fake food. Its ingredients don't let you know that it may be made from rejected milk and other dairy products that cannot

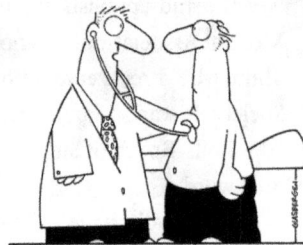

"It's easy to tell the difference between good cholesterol and bad cholesterol. Bad cholesterol has an evil laugh."

be sold fresh. Then many chemicals, colors, flavors and more, are added and even glue is added to give it "consistency". This is not really a food, but it is what is served in some schools, many restaurants and even in fancy establishments as well.

Cholesterol Myths

Dr. Lawrence Wilson, MD

Cholesterol is an essential fat compound manufactured in our livers that is needed to make all of the sex hormones and steroid hormones. It is mainly made in our bodies. However, a little, relatively speaking, is found in animal fats.

Odd as it sounds, I have seen a number of vegetarian patients with high serum cholesterol, although they ate no cholesterol at all. The reasons are explained below.

Saturated fat is not the same as cholesterol. Coconut and palm oil, for example, are quite saturated fats (solid at room temperature) but contain no cholesterol. This is because they are vegetable products and only animal fats contain any cholesterol at all.

Eating cholesterol does not necessarily raise blood cholesterol and does not automatically clog your arteries. In fact, the connection between elevated cholesterol and heart disease is much more tenuous and tentative than we are led to believe. Some studies show no correlation at all between high levels of cholesterol in the blood and coronary heart disease.

Refined vegetable oils

In the United States, during the 90-year period from 1909 to 1999, a striking increase in the use of vegetable oils occurred. Specifically, per capita consumption of salad and cooking oils increased 130%, shortening consumption increased 136%, and margarine consumption increased 410%. These trends occurred elsewhere in the world and were made possible by the industrialization and mechanization of the oil-seed industry.

The industrial advent of mechanically driven steel expellers and hexane extraction processes allowed for greater world-wide vegetable oil productivity, whereas new purification procedures permitted exploitation of nontraditionally consumed oils, such as cottonseed. New manufacturing procedures allowed vegetable oils to take on atypical structural characteristics. Margarine and shortening are produced by solidifying or partially solidifying vegetable oils via hydrogenation, a process first developed in 1897. The hydrogenation process produces novel trans fatty acid isomers (trans elaidic acid in particular) that rarely, if ever, are found in conventional human foodstuffs. Consequently, the large-scale addition of refined vegetable oils to the world's food supply after the Industrial Revolution significantly altered both quantitative and qualitative aspects of fat intake.

~ Emken EA. (Nutrition and biochemistry of trans and positional fatty acid isomers in hydrogenated oils)

It now appears that much better methods of monitoring the condition of your arteries are by testing for elevated homocysteine, C-reactive protein (which measures inflammation), and non-invasive tests such as an ultrasound or Doppler test for arterial blockage can also be done.

Minerals such as calcium, copper, iron, cadmium and others may also build up in the arteries and contribute to heart disease.

These can, at times, be revealed on a hair mineral analysis or perhaps with a 'urine metals challenge test' using EDTA. I believe these methods are much better than checking cholesterol if one suspects or wishes to prevent heart disease.

An elevated cholesterol level in the blood is not good, but of itself is not a serious problem. It is mainly a liver stress indicator. It will come down on its own, in my experience, as one's general health improves on a nutritional balancing healing program based on hair mineral testing.

Cholesterol-Lowering Drugs

Dr. Lawrence Wilson, MD

A recent medical nightmare is the widespread use of cholesterol-lowering drugs, often called "statin drugs". Their names include Crestor, Zocor, Lovastatin, Mevacor, Crestor and a dozen others from different companies. They are all basically similar to each other. The word "statin" is a misnomer as the drugs have nothing to do with stasis. It is just another lie of the pharmaceutical industry to increase sales of these quite awful drugs that kill people regularly.

These are now prescribed to millions of Americans and others worldwide. They have few benefits in most studies and are quite costly.

The adverse effects of the statin drugs are often much worse than the elevated cholesterol. In fact, one of the "adverse effects" of these drugs includes heart attacks, the very condition these drugs are supposed to prevent. So I advise everyone to avoid these drugs completely if you value your health at all.

If a doctor suggests that you take a drug to lower your cholesterol, here are my suggestions:

1. A mildly elevated cholesterol level is not a cause for concern in my opinion. It is usually a stress indicator and that is all.

2. Before considering dangerous drug therapy, which is the truth about the statin drugs, first try natural methods for lowering cholesterol. The most complete and reliable method is a nutritional balancing program.

However, simple, symptomatic remedies such as red rice yeast, chromium, or more fiber may help. I do not recommend any niacin, however, in any form. In doses above about 100 mg daily, it may build up in the liver, even if it controls cholesterol.

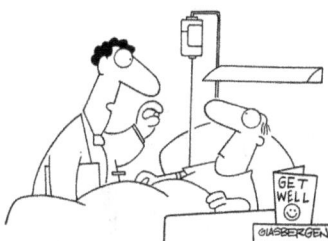

"We found a bunch of these clogging your arteries. They're cholesterol pills."

However, I don't recommend these remedies very much, as none of them correct the cause of the elevated cholesterol. Overall, the cholesterol debate has ruined the reputation of many wonderful fats like grassfed butter. This has been most unfortunate for the health of millions of people.

Mental Development And Brain Fats

Human beings are capable of much more than most people believe. Under the right circumstances, and by eating correctly, the brain actually grows larger and one can develop unusual abilities.

Fats and oils play a critical role in this type of development. They coat the nerves with myelin, an important fatty substance that is needed to conduct nerve impulses properly. Without enough quality fats and oils, human beings will simply not develop their minds as well as they could. One of the serious problems in the nations of Africa and some Asian nations is that the food supply is low in these "brain fats". People are forced to live on mainly starches such as grains, beans, fruits and some nuts. They do not have enough dairy products to nourish their brains properly, so they suffer mentally, as well as physically.

Only Irish coffee provides in a single glass all four essential food groups: alcohol, caffeine, sugar, and fat." - Alex Levine.

This is a critical benefit of eating high quality fats and oils every day.

Health authorities such as William Campbell Douglass, MD suggest that fats are one of the most important food groups. This is no doubt the case with growing children, whose brains and nervous systems absolutely require sufficient amounts of high-quality saturated fats for optimum brain development. It is also true of most adults, especially those who wish to have truly good health.

Dairy As A Source Of Healthy Fats

These include whole milk fat, fat in yogurt, cheeses, butter, and cream. Dairy fats are excellent if they are natural or raw, and not pasteurized or homogenized. This is important because pasteurization and homogenization damage the fat and other components of dairy products so they become much less healthful.

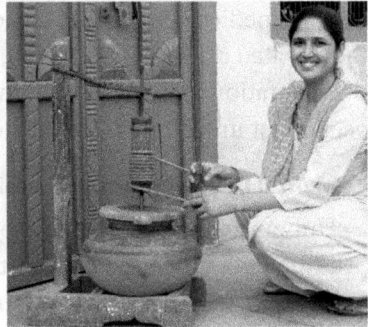

Most cows today are hybrids and their products are not as healthful as in the past. Many people these days are insisting on dairy products from traditional breeds of the cows.

In many parts of the world, goat, sheep, yak, camel and reindeer have been used as a source of milk and butter.

If one cannot find raw milk products, the next best appears to be organic dairy products. Regular pasteurized commercial dairy products are not nearly as good.

Children And Fats

Babies and children have a critical need for high quality fats for the development of their brain and nervous systems. It is most unfortunate when parents do not feed their children fat, for fear the children will become overweight. It is also unfortunate when children are fed poor quality, pasteurized dairy products and overcooked fried oils, and other inferior fats and oils.

Even worse, instead of giving their children quality milk, yogurt and other fat-containing foods, some parents substitute soymilk, artificial fruit juice and sugar-laden soda pop. These contain much more sugars, which tend to make children overweight and ill.

Another horror is most commercial baby formula that contains cheap soymilk or soy oil, when babies desperately need all the essential fatty acids for their brain development. Babies who cannot drink mother's milk, which is over 50% fat, often do well on unprocessed cow or goat milk.

Fats to avoid for everyone, particularly children, are French fries fried in vegetable oil, fast-food milk shakes, which are mostly chemicals, and other fried foods. Avoid grilled cheese sandwiches, cheese dips, and processed cheeses used in pizza and other dishes. These fats and oils are usually old, overheated and quite unhealthful.

One cannot emphasize enough that babies and children must have high-quality fats and oils every day to nourish their brains and avoid many kinds of developmental and behavioral problems.

Ghee

Ghee, also called clarified butter, is a product used extensively in India and some other nations. It is the age old cooking medium in these countries and it's been around for thousands of years. It is just butter with the milk solids removed. As a result, it is clear in color and has less of a buttery taste.

Ghee is made by gently heating butter just a little, until the white-colored milk solids separate. These are skimmed off, leaving ghee.

Ghee has certain advantages over butter, specifically for cooking. Without the milk solids, ghee will not burn as easily, and can be heated to a higher temperature as a result.

My friends in SW France had a Jersey cow for years, and there was always a surplus of fresh cream. Simply decanting the cream into a mason jar, and then shaking it for (what seemed like) ages, it would suddenly "turn" `and we would then just squeeze off the buttermilk with a pair of butter hands (wooden spatulas) and our weekly butter was ready!

So tasty, satisfying, and quite good exercise too!

More people should make butter like this. We wouldn't feel so guilty for eating a special and superb food if we'd made it ourselves!

Butter, in fact, has a few advantages over ghee. The milk solids contain some added nutrients, which are lost when one makes it into ghee. Ghee is considered an ambrosia in Indian Ayurvedic tradition. Even today, no household can do without it. Unfortunately in India, most of the commercially sold ghee is adulterated with lard or vegetable fats. Food cooked in ghee has an aroma and taste which is unlike anything else in the world.

Make Your Own Healthy, Delicious Oils At Home

There are many companies selling manual oil presses these days. With one such press, you can extract your own healthy oils, right in your own kitchen. These presses can extract oil from almost all kinds of seeds and nuts. These home made, cold pressed oils are superior to industrial oils in every conceivable way. Freshly pressed oils have unique, complex flavors that bottled oils can't match. And then there are added health benefits. These oils carry all the natural goodness of their respective seeds or nuts. Though most of these are hand operated, it doesn't take much time or effort to extract a bottleful of oil. For a small family, this arrangement is quite sufficient. Some of the brands can be ordered online.

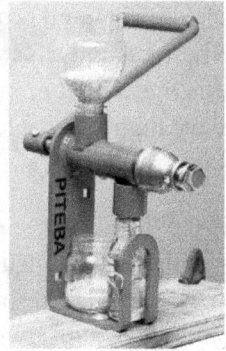

I remember my mother making butter with the full fat cream skimmed off the top of the gallon jars of fresh unpasteurized milk that was delivered to us, along with complimentary bible tracks, by an aging bachelor farmer whose octogenarian mother always accompanied him in the car. There's no place like home.

~ Mari, June 22, 2007

64.

Lowfat Diet "Scientifically and Morally Indefensible"

Cardiologist Recommends Grassfed Butter

By Sarah, The Healthy Home Economist

D r. Dwight Lundell MD is a cardiologist who beat the drum of lowfat diet and cholesterol lowering drugs to prevent heart disease for over 25 years.

He has performed over 5,000 open heart surgeries and trained with prominent "opinion maker" physicians who considered any deviation from the recommended therapy of severely limited fat intake and cholesterol lowering meds to reduce heart disease risk complete heresy that could possibly result in a malpractice lawsuit.

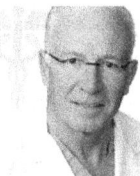

I did research on this doctor about a year ago. What I found was a highly qualified successful doctor who in his retirement spoke out against the low fat scam. As soon as he did this, the witch hunt began to discredit him. The medical board trumped up charges to have his medical license taken away even though he was already retired. If you speak out with the truth they will try to take you down. Thanks for the link Cyni.

~ Rebecca Handlon-Miller via Facebook December 3, 2012
Reply:
Yes, my own father who is an MD eats butter and doesn't buy the lowfat baloney. Also, Dr. Tom Cowan MD who practices in San Francisco agrees with Dr. Lundell as well. MANY other doctors do as well but they stay silent as speaking up gets you blackballed.
~ The healthy home economist via Facebook December 3, 2012

Dr. Lundell now admits that this long held notion is wrong. Not only is it completely and utterly wrong, it is also scientifically and morally indefensible.

Following the recommended mainstream diet low in saturated fat and high in grain based carbohydrates has created an epidemic of obesity and diabetes "the consequences of which dwarf any historical plague in terms of mortality, human suffering and dire economic consequences". **T H I N K** *before you* By following the recommended lowfat diet, Dr. Lundell says that people are **E A T** unknowingly causing "repeated injury to their blood vessels". This repeated injury, day in and day out, is what is causing rampant inflammation across all population groups which has resulted in the epidemic of heart disease, diabetes, and obesity.

Inflammation - The True Cause of Heart Disease

Dr. Lundell explains that a slow paradigm shift which identifies inflammation as the true cause of heart disease is occurring.

He goes on to say that the conventional lowfat diet which warns against saturated fats and promotes polyunsaturated vegetable oils as a healthier alternative is the biggest culprit in causing chronic and deadly inflammation.

Unless inflammation is present in the body, cholesterol is unable to accumulate in plaques in the blood vessels causing heart attacks and strokes. In an inflammation free body, cholesterol moves freely and causes no health problems.

That is a pretty strong statement...as a cardiac SURGEON (not a cardiologist) I believe he saved quite a few lives not ended them. I assume you do not work in the healthcare industry because if you did you would know that any recommendation made by a doctor must be in line with current best practice guidelines as put forth by organization like the American Heart Association, etc. unless otherwise contraindicated. So perhaps we should give MD's a break as this information about the dangers of the low fat was not understood by mainstream medicine until recently and is still widely unknown by most. Dr. Lundell is a pioneer to admit that medical community is wrong.

~Jeff Lee, Indianapolis

In other words, it is inflammation caused by a lowfat diet that causes cholesterol to become trapped in the body. Cholesterol lowering drugs have been a dismal failure to eliminate or reduce the problem as 25% of the population now takes statin drugs and yet more Americans than ever will die of heart disease this year.

How One Innocent Donut Causes Deadly Inflammation

Dr. Lundell explains the deadly 3 step process of how eating a simple donut or sweet roll causes a cascade of inflammation in the body:

Step One: Refined Grains and Sugar Consumption Spike Blood Sugar

"Imagine spilling syrup on your keyboard and you have a visual of what occurs inside the cell. When we consume simple carbohydrates such as sugar, blood sugar rises rapidly. In response, your pancreas secretes insulin whose primary purpose is to drive sugar into each cell where it is stored for energy. If the cell is full and does not need glucose, it is rejected to avoid extra sugar gumming up the works.

When your full cells reject the extra glucose, blood sugar rises producing more insulin and the glucose converts to stored fat.

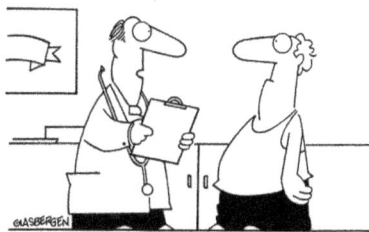

"An aspirin a day will help prevent a heart attack if you have it for lunch instead of a cheeseburger."

What does all this have to do with inflammation? Blood sugar is controlled in a very narrow range. Extra sugar molecules attach to a variety of proteins that in turn injure the blood vessel wall. This repeated injury to the blood vessel wall sets off inflammation. When you spike your blood sugar level several times a day, every day, it is exactly like taking sandpaper to the inside of your delicate blood vessels."

Step Two: Omega 6 Vegetable Oils Produce Cytokines

It's not just the refined grains and sugar in the donut causing spiking and crashing blood sugar that is the problem. Dr. Lundell continues by describing additional inflammation caused by the rancid omega 6, polyunsaturated oils (usually soybean) in the donut:

"That innocent looking goody not only contains sugars, it is baked in one of many omega-6 oils such as soybean. Chips and fries are soaked in soybean oil; processed foods are manufactured with omega-6 oils for longer shelf life. While omega-6s are essential -they are part of every cell membrane controlling what goes in and out of the cell — they must be in the correct balance with omega-3s.

If the balance shifts by consuming excessive omega-6, the cell membrane produces chemicals called cytokines that directly cause inflammation. "

Step Three: Excess Weight Pours Out Pro-Inflammatory Chemicals

The final nail in the coffin for producing exorbitant levels of inflammation when that innocent looking donut is consumed is the excess weight that most Americans are carrying:

"To make matters worse, the excess weight you are carrying from eating these foods creates overloaded fat cells that pour out large quantities of pro-inflammatory chemicals that add to the injury caused by having high blood sugar. The process that began with a sweet roll turns into a vicious cycle over time that creates heart disease, high blood pressure, diabetes and finally, Alzheimer's disease, as the inflammatory process continues unabated."

Ditch the Lowfat Diet and Get Off the Inflammation Freight Train

Dr. Lundell counsels that mainstream medicine has made "a terrible mistake" by advising people to avoid saturated fats in favor of vegetable oils. This flawed and dangerous recommendation is a direct contributor to the epidemic of inflammation that is plaguing the Western world in the form of obesity, diabetes, heart disease, and numerous other ailments.

Dr. Lundell advises to leave manufactured vegetable oils and other processed foods behind and return to the whole, unprocessed diet of our ancestors.

As for the ideal fats in the diet, Dr. Lundell recommends olive oil and grassfed butter. He says the science that saturated fat causes heart disease is non-existent and the science that saturated fat raises blood cholesterol as very weak.

Given that inflammation and not cholesterol causes heart disease, any concern about saturated fats in the diet is nothing short of "absurd" according to Dr. Lundell.

> *In the United States and most Western countries, diet-related chronic diseases represent the single largest cause of morbidity and mortality. These diseases are epidemic in contemporary Westernized populations and typically afflict 50–65% of the adult population, yet they are rare or nonexistent in hunter-gatherers and other less Westernized people. Although both scientists and lay people alike may frequently identify a single dietary element as the cause of chronic disease (eg, saturated fat causes heart disease and salt causes high blood pressure), evidence gleaned over the past 3 decades now indicates that virtually all so-called diseases of civilization have multifactorial dietary elements that underlie their etiology, along with other environmental agents and genetic susceptibility.*
>
> *Coronary heart disease, for instance, does not arise simply from excessive saturated fat in the diet but rather from a complex interaction of multiple nutritional factors directly linked to the excessive consumption of novel Neolithic and Industrial era foods (processed dairy products, refined cereals, refined sugars, refined vegetable oils, fatty meats, refined salt, and combinations of these foods).*
>
> *These foods, in turn, adversely influence proximate nutritional factors, which universally underlie or exacerbate virtually all chronic diseases of civilization: 1) glycemic load, 2) fatty acid composition, 3) macronutrient composition, 4) micronutrient density, 5) acid-base balance, 6) sodium-potassium ratio, and 7) fiber content.*
>
> *However, the ultimate factor underlying diseases of civilization is the collision of our ancient genome with the new conditions of life in affluent nations, including the nutritional qualities of recently introduced foods.*
>
> *~ Loren Cordain, S Boyd Eaton, Origins and evolution of the Western diet: health implications for the 21st century*

65.

Getting Some Culture

Does It Get Any Better Than Butter?

By Melissa Kronenthal

Yes butter, but not just any butter. Of course I'm not talking about the butter I grew up eating — or I should say, the butter I ate before the anti-butter scaremongering hit the media and my parents switched to some vile, purportedly heart-healthier substance. I honestly have no idea when I first tasted that butter, but it was probably long before I started making taste memories. I'm talking about the butter I discovered on my very first trip to France, at the home of the family friend who hosted me for a week and took it upon herself to introduce me to as many of France's gastronomic delights as humanly possible. Among the cheeses and patés and potages and pastries she stuffed me with, I had a taste of a butter so remarkable I couldn't stop thinking about it for years.

In my defence, it was amazing stuff. That butter possessed a creaminess beyond description, and a sweetly subtle, almost cheesy flavor. I had never had anything like it, and I slathered it on every surface I could find (including my naked fingers), probably consuming more in that week than in the totality of my life up to that point. What must they be feeding those French cows to get butter like this? I wondered. I imagined them lolling about in green fields, being hand-fed choice bits of tender spring stalks by doting farmers. Maybe they had regular massages à la Kobe cows, and perhaps soothing classical music was piped into their climate-controlled barns at night to help them sleep. I mean really, how else could you explain why this French butter was so good?

While I can't say for sure that none of that actually happens in France, I do know something now that I didn't know then. French butter is actually so delicious because the French routinely do something to their butter that Americans (and British, and most of the rest of the world) don't: they give it some culture.

Simply put, culturing butter consists of fermenting the cream before the butter is churned. Have you ever had crème fraîche? Then you've tasted cultured butter's parent. By introducing some dairy-friendly bacteria to the fresh cream, the sugars in the cream are converted to lactic acid; this, along with souring the cream, produces additional aroma compounds including diacetyl which make for a more complex and "buttery" taste. You wouldn't think that souring cream would necessarily have a positive impact on the butter made from it (I mean, the thought of sour butter doesn't exactly get your mouth watering, does it?), but surprisingly, it does: the butter absorbs just enough of the flavor compounds to acquire a subtle, mysterious and completely addictive tang.

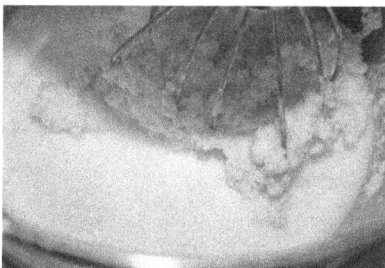

When I was in the U.S. last summer, I noticed that Americans' fascination with all things European has expanded to the dairy case, and cultured butter is now widely available. It was indeed delicious, but it was also obscenely expensive; I was almost glad that I don't live there and have to face decisions such as either indulging in cultured butter or paying my rent on a regular basis. At home I still scanned the butter aisle religiously, however, hoping

> My parents grew up on small farms a mile apart and my father grew up with cultured butter. If you just leave raw cream out till it sours that is the traditional way to make cultured butter. My father grew up eating it that way all the time. My mothers family always kept theirs in the fridge so it was sweet. My fathers family is much healthier than my mothers family and I do wonder if that approach to food is part of the reason why.
>
> ~Patty, Los Angeles

against hope that the cultured variety was about to catch on here in the UK, when lo and behold, I stumbled upon a completely unexpected piece of information. Did you know that cultured butter is actually a cinch to make at home? I certainly didn't, but I have since confirmed it myself: it is not only a cinch, it is spectacular. All it takes is a quart of the richest, freshest organic cream you can lay your hands on, a few spoonfuls of a fermented dairy product like yogurt or buttermilk, and a little bit of patience. In 24 hours, you can have as much fresh, cultured butter as your long-suffering tastebuds desire - at a cost so low you will be able to slather it on not only your toast every morning, but each and every one of your fingers too, and you'll still be able to pay your rent in the process.

Cultured Butter

I actually have reader and fellow blogger Dominic to thank for clueing me in to the fact that cultured butter can be made at home. I had no idea, but after reading his description, I got to work and have now made my own not once, not twice, but three times in the last week. Uh yeah, I know that's a lot of butter. But it's amazing stuff, and worth every luscious, calorie-laden bite. There's not much to tell you here that the recipe doesn't; the only thing I'll stress is the importance of getting yourself really good (preferably organic) cream, since tasty cream=tasty butter. But you could have probably figured that one out for yourself.

Yield: 12-14 ounces (340-400g) of butter, depending on the fat content of your cream (note that the recipe can easily be halved)

4 cups (1ltr) heavy or double cream (the best quality, and highest butterfat you can find)

> In India, we do it all the time - in practically every household that buys full-cream milk. Everyday the cream is skimmed off the top of the milk after it has boiled and cooled, and put out for a few hours in a clean bowl mixed with some yoghurt, till it is set (cultured!). Fresh cream is added to it everyday, mixed, and put back in the fridge till the bowl is full. Once full, it is turned into butter exactly as you have described. And buttermilk obtained this way is the ingredient for the best kadhi you can have!
>
> ~ Anita, Jaipur

1/3 cup (80ml) plain whole-milk yogurt, crème fraîche or buttermilk (check the ingredients to make sure these do not contain any gums or stabilizers)

Ice

Salt, to taste

Begin by culturing your cream (this is an overnight process, so plan accordingly). In a clean glass or ceramic container (bowl, jar, etc) combine the cream and yogurt, crème fraîche or buttermilk. Cover loosely and place it in a warmish part of the house - the ideal temperature is around 75F (23C), but anywhere in the range from 70-80F (20-26C) is okay.

After 12-18 hours, the cream should be noticeably thicker and should taste slightly tangy, i.e. like crème fraîche. If it's bubbling and gassy, some unwanted bacteria have gotten in there so discard your cream and start again (note that this has never happened to me). If it hasn't thickened yet, leave it alone for another few hours and eventually it will. When your cream has thickened, if you are not ready to make your butter right away, transfer the container to the fridge where you can leave it for up to another 24 hours.

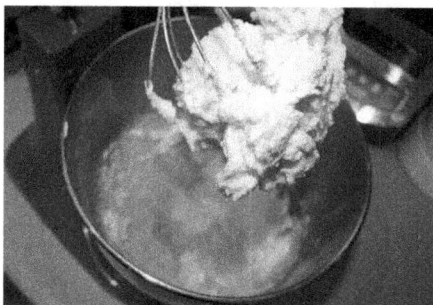

In order to churn properly, the cream needs to be at about 60F (15C). If you're taking it out of the fridge just let it warm up until it reaches this temperature; if you're making it from room temperature you'll need to place the bowl in a bath of ice water for a few minutes to cool it down. Also, fill a large bowl with water and ice cubes and keep it handy.

You can use any method you want to beat the cream; handheld electric beater, stand mixer, etc - even whisking by hand if you're

"These women trying to shape up in health spas -- they should churn butter and chant Hare Krishna. The Lord would be pleased, and they'd be in better shape than Jane Fonda."
~ Caranaravinda dasi

trying to pre-emptively burn off a few calories. Basically, just put the thickened cream in a clean, deep bowl and start beating as if you're making whipped cream. When the cream starts to form stiff peaks, reduce the speed to low. At this point watch carefully; first the peaks will start to look grainy, and a few seconds later the cream will break. When it does you'll know it - globules of yellow butterfat will be swimming in a sea of buttermilk, and if you're beating too fast you'll have buttermilk everywhere. Stop beating and carefully tilt the bowl over a cup, holding back the butter clumps as best you can, and drain away as much buttermilk as possible. You can use this just like commercial buttermilk, by the way, and it's delicious.

Now you have to wash the butter to get rid of all the residual buttermilk, which would cause it to spoil prematurely. Using a fork (my preferred implement) or a stiff rubber spatula, pour some of your reserved icewater over the butter, kneading and stirring it around vigorously. The water will turn whitish and the butter will firm up, making it cohere and knead more easily. Pour out the liquid and repeat as many times as needed until the water sloshing around in your bowl is completely clear. After you've poured off the last of the liquid, continue kneading for a few more minutes to get as much water as possible out of the butter. If you want salted butter, add your favorite salt now, to taste.

You've now got a generous supply of your very own cultured butter. Pack it into ramekins, roll it in waxed paper, or fill cute little molds with it before refrigerating; I recommend freezing some if you won't be able to finish what you've made within a week or so. Whether storing it in the fridge or freezer, though, keep it tightly covered, as butter is a sponge for other aromas.

66.

Why Butter Is Better

By Sally Fallon and Mary G. Enig, PhD

When the fabricated food folks and apologists for the corporate farm realized that they couldn't block America's growing interest in diet and nutrition, a movement that would ultimately put an end to America's biggest and most monopolistic industries, they infiltrated the movement and put a few sinister twists on information going out to the public. Item number one in the disinformation campaign was the assertion that naturally saturated fats from animal sources are the root cause of the current heart disease and cancer plague. Butter bore the brunt of the attack, and was accused of terrible crimes. The Diet Dictocrats told us that it was better to switch to polyunsaturated margarine and most Americans did. Butter all but disappeared from our tables, shunned as a miscreant.

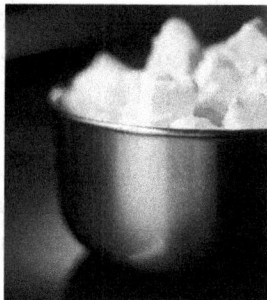

> *Processed dairy products, cereals, refined sugars, refined vegetable oils, and alcohol make up 72.1% of the total daily energy consumed by all people in the United States, these types of foods would have contributed little or none of the energy in the typical preindustrial diet. An impressive range of processed foods like cookies, cake, bakery foods, breakfast cereals, bagels, rolls, muffins, crackers, chips, snack foods, pizza, soft drinks, candy, ice cream, condiments, and salad dressings are dominating the typical US diet, apart from of course factory farmed meats.*
> *~Anna, Jan 14 2013*

This would come as a surprise to many people around the globe who have valued butter for its life-sustaining properties for millennia. When Dr. Weston Price studied native diets in the 1930's he found that butter was a staple in the diets of many supremely healthy peoples.[1] Isolated Swiss villagers placed a bowl of butter on their church altars, set a wick in it, and let it burn throughout the year as a sign of divinity in the butter. Arab groups also put a high value on butter, especially deep yellow-orange butter from livestock feeding on green grass in the spring and fall. American folk wisdom recognized that children raised on butter were robust and sturdy; but that children given skim milk during their growing years were pale and thin, with "pinched" faces.[2]

Does butter cause disease? On the contrary, butter protects us against many diseases.

Butter & Heart Disease

Heart disease was rare in America at the turn of the century. Between 1920 and 1960, the incidence of heart disease rose precipitously to become America's number one killer. During the same period butter consumption plummeted from eighteen pounds per person per year to four. It doesn't take a Ph.D. in statistics to conclude that butter is not a cause. Actually butter contains many nutrients that protect us from heart disease. First among these is vitamin A which is needed for the health of the thyroid and adrenal glands, both of which play a role in maintaining the proper functioning of the heart and cardiovascular system. Abnormalities of the heart and larger blood vessels occur in babies born to vitamin

Love the taste of butter and my "gut" just knew that it wasn't a "bad" thing. I leave a stick at a time out in a butter dish to easily slather on whenever. Been doing this for many years and never a problem with it going bad. It doesn't sit out too long because it's used regularly.

Satisfies those night time cravings....Wheat toast or english muffins with organic butter and a small glass of cold raw milk, then to bed.

I'm 60 and people think I'm 50 and I rarely get sick. Moderation, common sense, and listen to what the body tells you.(Mine wants butter!) I'm not a big meat eater at all, so that's how I justify it.

~ Anna, Ottawa, January 2013

A deficient mothers. Butter is America's best and most easily absorbed source of vitamin A.

Butter contains lecithin, a substance that assists in the proper assimilation and metabolism of cholesterol and other fat constituents.

Butter also contains a number of anti-oxidants that protect against the kind of free radical damage that weakens the arteries. Vitamin A and vitamin E found in butter both play a strong anti-oxidant role. Butter is a very rich source of selenium, a vital anti-oxidant--containing more per gram than herring or wheat germ.

Butter is also a good dietary source cholesterol. What?? Cholesterol an anti-oxidant?? Yes indeed, cholesterol is a potent anti-oxidant that is flooded into the blood when we take in too many harmful free-radicals--usually from damaged and rancid fats in margarine and highly processed vegetable oils.[3] A Medical

Pasteurization and its effects...

After a great deal of research about the effects pasteurization has on milk, I found that once this process is done, the nutritional value is destroyed and all that is left is a delicious sanitized liquid of oxidized fat that causes more health problems than the miraculous elixir of raw milk ever did. Simply put, the reasons why pasteurization regulations were put into law was because, as the demand for milk consumption increased so did the proper cleanliness of the cows and the milking plants. Reckless care in cleanliness within those milking plants, the cows, as well as the employees were not regulated and inspected like say, a restaurant is today. Food establishments are required to have the proper permits, pass inspections and employees must go through a procedure, get the proper education, and obtain a food-handler health card. Smart, common sense cleanliness and strict guidelines would allow the elixir of raw milk to once again be served as the miraculous nourishment it is in its natural state. But you must understand that the huge milk producers love the pasteurization process because rather than having to deal with strict guidelines of cleanliness and proper food-handling it's just more convenient and more profitable and safer (yeah, whatever) to cook the nutritional life out of it.

~Glenn, Ontario

Research Council survey showed that men eating butter ran half the risk of developing heart disease as those using margarine.[4]

Butter & Cancer

In the 1940's research indicated that increased fat intake caused cancer.[5] The abandonment of butter accelerated; margarine--formerly a poor man's food-- was accepted by the well-to-do. But there was a small problem with the way this research was presented to the public. The popular press neglected to stress that fact that the "saturated" fats used in these experiments were not naturally saturated fats but partially hydrogenated or hardened fats--the kind found mostly in margarine but not in butter. Researchers stated--they may have even believed it--that there was no difference between naturally saturated fats in butter and artificially hardened fats in margarine and shortening. So butter was tarred with the black brush of the fabricated fats, and in such a way that the villains got passed off as heroes.

Actually many of the saturated fats in butter have strong anti-cancer properties. Butter is rich in short and medium chain fatty acid chains that have strong anti-tumor effects.[6] Butter also contains

---

The Land Of Food Inventions.... And The Land Of The Sick

In the United States, chronic illnesses and health problems either wholly or partially attributable to diet represent by far the most serious threat to public health. Sixty-five percent of adults aged ≥20 years in the United States are either overweight or obese, and the estimated number of deaths ascribable to obesity is 280184 per year. More than 64 million Americans have one or more types of cardiovascular disease (CVD), which represents the leading cause of mortality (38.5% of all deaths) in the United States. Fifty million Americans are hypertensive; 11 million have type 2 diabetes, and 37 million adults maintain high-risk total cholesterol concentrations (>240 mg/dL). In postmenopausal women aged ≥50 y, 7.2% have osteoporosis and 39.6% have osteopenia. Osteoporotic hip fractures are associated with a 20% excess mortality in the year after fracture. Cancer is the second leading cause of death (25% of all deaths) in the United States, and an estimated one-third of all cancer deaths are due to nutritional factors, including obesity.

~ CDC figures

---

conjugated linoleic acid which gives excellent protection against cancer.[7]

Vitamin A and the anti-oxidants in butter--vitamin E, selenium and cholesterol--protect against cancer as well as heart disease.

Butter & the Immune System

Vitamin A found in butter is essential to a healthy immune system; short and medium chain fatty acids also have immune system strengthening properties. But hydrogenated fats and an excess of long chain fatty acids found in polyunsaturated oils and many butter substitutes both have a deleterious effect on the immune system.[8]

Butter & Arthritis

The Wulzen or "anti-stiffness" factor is a nutrient unique to butter. Dutch researcher Wulzen found that it protects against calcification of the joints--degenerative arthritis--as well as hardening of the arteries, cataracts and calcification of the pineal gland.[9] Unfortunately this vital substance is destroyed during pasteurization. Calves fed pasteurized milk or skim milk develop joint stiffness and do not thrive. Their symptoms are reversed when raw butterfat is added to the diet.

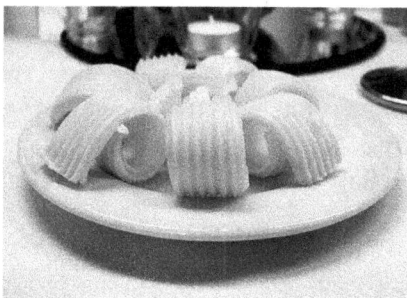

Butter & Osteoporosis

Vitamins A and D in butter are essential to the proper absorption of calcium and hence necessary for strong bones and teeth. The plague of osteoporosis in milk-drinking western nations may be due to the fact that most people choose skim milk over whole, thinking

> Doctor just told me to go back to eating butter. I laughed and he said he'd had it with all this food nonsense and recommended just eating natural foods ie. food from my farm! Ha, ha...
> ~James, Oregon, July 2012

it is good for them. Butter also has anti-cariogenic effects, that is, it protects against tooth decay.[10]

Butter & the Thyroid Gland

Butter is a good source of iodine, in highly absorbable form. Butter consumption prevents goiter in mountainous areas where seafood is not available. In addition, vitamin A in butter is essential for proper functioning of the thyroid gland.[11]

Butter & Gastrointestinal Health

Butterfat contains glycospingolipids, a special category of fatty acids that protect against gastro-intestinal infection, especially in the very young and the elderly. For this reason, children who drink skim milk have diarrhea at rates three to five times greater than children who drink whole milk.[12] Cholesterol in butterfat promotes health of the intestinal wall and protects against cancer of the colon.[13] Short and medium chain fatty acids protect against pathogens and have strong anti-fungal effects.[14] Butter thus has an important role to play in the treatment of candida overgrowth.

Butter & Weight Gain

The notion that butter causes weight gain is a sad misconception. The short and medium chain fatty acids in butter are not stored in the adipose tissue, but are used for quick energy. Fat tissue in humans is composed mainly of longer chain fatty acids.[15] These come from olive oil and polyunsaturated oils as well as from refined carbohydrates. Because butter is rich in nutrients, it confers a feeling of satisfaction when consumed. Can it be that consumption

---

The Rosickys had been at one accord not to hurry through life, not to be always skimping and saving. They saw their neighbours buy more land and feed more stock than they did, without discontent. Once when the creamery agent came to the Rosickys to persuade them to sell him their cream, he told them how much the Fasslers, their nearest neighbours, had made on their cream last year. "Yes," said Mary, "and look at them Fassler children! Pale, pinched little things, they look like skimmed milk. I'd rather put some colour into my children's faces than put money into the bank."~Passage from "Neighbor Rosicky", by American author Willa Cather

of margarine and other butter substitutes results in cravings and bingeing because these highly fabricated products don't give the body what it needs?.

Butter for Growth & Development

Many factors in butter ensure optimal growth of children. Chief among them is vitamin A. Individuals who have been deprived of sufficient vitamin A during gestation tend to have narrow faces and skeletal structure, small palates and crowded teeth.[16] Extreme vitamin A deprivation results in blindness, skeletal problems and other birth defects.[17] Individuals receiving optimal vitamin A from the time of conception have broad handsome faces, strong straight teeth, and excellent bone structure. Vitamin A also plays an important role in the development of the sex characteristics. Calves fed butter substitutes sicken and die before reaching maturity.[18]

The X factor, discovered by Dr. Weston Price (and now believed to be vitamin K2), is also essential for optimum growth. It is only present in butterfat from cows on green pasture.[19] Cholesterol found in butterfat plays an important role in the development of the brain and nervous system.[20] Mother's milk is high in cholesterol and contains over 50 percent of its calories as butterfat. Low fat diets have been linked to failure to thrive in children[21] -- yet low-fat diets are often recommended for youngsters! Children need the many factors in butter for optimal development.

I should add another reason for using butter - the nutrients in butter are essential for absorbing and utilizing the nutrients in vegetables, so butter those veggies!

Here in Australia I find that the battle is often lost to turn friends and family away from margarine mainly because of price. 250 grams of pasteurized butter can cost $1.97 up to $5 if it is "organic" whilst 1kg margarine is just $1.25 and the very few outlets for 'natural organic butter' charge around $12 a kilo.

However, we must keep on pointing out the truth, in the end the Truth will indeed set us free.

Doctors are the other problem

~ John, May 2010

Beyond Margarine

It's no longer a secret that the margarine Americans have been spreading on their toast, and the hydrogenated fats they eat in commercial baked goods like cookies and crackers, is the chief culprit in our current plague of cancer and heart disease.[22] But mainline nutrition writers continue to denigrate butter--recommending new fangled tub spreads instead.[23] These may not contain hydrogenated fats but they are composed of highly processed rancid vegetable oils, soy protein isolate and a host of additives. A glitzy cookbook called Butter Busters promotes butter buds, made from maltodextrin, a carbohydrate derived from corn, along with dozens of other highly processed so-called low-fat commercial products.

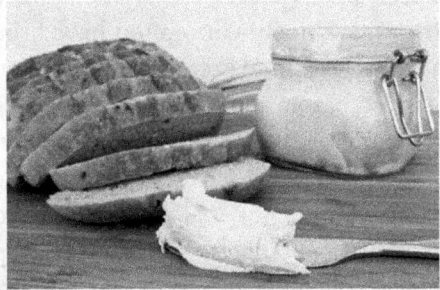

Who benefits from the propaganda blitz against butter? The list is a long one and includes orthodox medicine, hospitals, the drug companies and food processors. But the chief beneficiary is the large corporate farm and the cartels that buy their products--chiefly cotton, corn and soy--America's three main crops, which are usually grown as monocultures on large farms, requiring extensive use of artificial fertilizers and pesticides. All three--soy, cotton and corn--can be used to make both margarine and the new designer spreads. In order to make these products acceptable to the up-scale consumer, food processors and agribusiness see to it that they are promoted as health foods. We are fools to believe them.

> *I was raised milking the cows, waiting for cream then taking it to the guy that pasturized it - it was far better tasting milk and butter and some of the fondest memories of childhood include taking the cream by finger when no one was looking - I refuse to let ANY tub of fake lard soy crap in my house, Thank for the info.*
> *~Terry Evans, Denver*

Butter & the Family Farm

A nation that consumes butterfat, on the other hand, is a nation that sustains the family farm. If Americans were willing to pay a good price for high quality butter and cream, from cows raised on natural pasturage--every owner of a small- or medium-sized farm could derive financial benefits from owning a few Jersey or Guernsey cows. In order to give them green pasture, he would naturally need to rotate crops, leaving different sections of his farm for his cows to graze and at the same time giving the earth the benefit of a period of fallow--not to mention the benefit of high quality manure. Fields tended in this way produce very high quality vegetables and grains in subsequent seasons, without the addition of nitrogen fertilizers and with minimal use of pesticides.

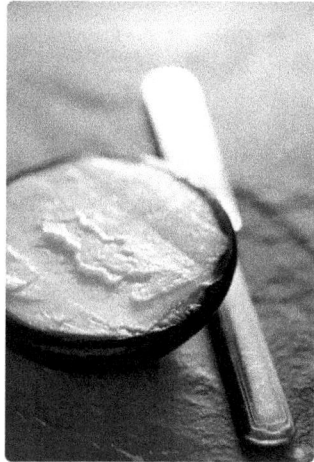

If you wish to reestablish America as a nation of prosperous farmers in the best Jeffersonian tradition, buy organic butter, cream, whole milk, whole yoghurt. These bring good and fair profits to the yeoman producer without concentrating power in the hands of conglomerates.

Ethnic groups that do not use butter obtain the same nutrients from things like insects, organ meats, fish eggs and the fat of marine animals, food items most of us find repulsive. For Americans--who do not eat bugs or blubber--butter is not just better, it is essential.

Notes

1. Price, Weston, DDS Nutrition and Physical Degeneration, 1945, Price Pottenger Nutrition Foundation, Inc., La Mesa, California

I stopped buying plastic maybe 1 1/2 year ago. We use ONLY butter. I leave some in the fridge and some in a butter dish for toast and such. You don't need as much and it tastes great, it adds a richness to our foods that many times you don't need to add dessert because you have already satisfied that area and you don't even realize it.
~ Sarah, Mar 02, 2010

2. "Neighbor Rosicky", by American author Willa Cather.

3. Cranton, EM, MD and JP Frackelton, MD, Journal of Holistic Medicine, Spring/Summer 1984

4. Nutrition Week Mar 22, 1991 21:12:2-3

5. Enig, Mary G, PhD, Nutrition Quarterly, 1993 Vol 17, No 4

6. Cohen, L A et al, J Natl Cancer Inst 1986 77:43

7. Belury, MA Nutrition Reviews, April 1995 53:(4) 83-89

8. Cohen, op cit

9. American Journal of Physical Medicine, 1941, 133; Physiological Zoology, 1935 8:457

10. Kabara, J J, The Pharmacological Effects of Lipids, J J Kabara, ed, The American Oil Chemists Society, Champaign, IL 1978 pp 1-14

11. Jennings, IW Vitamins in Endocrine Metabolism, Charles C. Thomas Publisher, Springfield, Ill, pp 41-57

12. Koopman, JS, et al American Journal of Public Health 1984 74(12):1371-1373

13. Addis, Paul, Food and Nutrition News, March/April 1990 62:2:7-10

14. Prasad, KN, Life Science, 1980, 27:1351-8; Gershon, Herman and Larry Shanks, Symposium on the Pharmacological Effect of Lipids, Jon J Kabara Ed, American Oil Chemists Society, Champaign, Illinois 1978 51-62

15. Levels of linoleic acid in adipose tissues reflect the amount of linoleic acid in the diet. Valero, et al Annals of Nutritional Metabolism, Nov/Dec 1990 34:6:323-327; Felton, CV et al, Lancet 1994 344:1195-96

16. Price, op cit

17. Jennings, op cit

18. DeCava, Judith Journal of the National Academy of Research Biochemists, September 1988 1053-1059

19. Price, op cit

20. Alfin-Slater, R B and L Aftergood, "Lipids", Modern Nutrition in Health and Disease, Chapter 5, 6th ed, R S Goodhart and M E Shils, eds, Lea and Febiger, Philadelphia 1980, p 131

21. Smith, MM, MNS RD and F Lifshitz, MD Pediatrics, Mar 1994 93:3:438-443

22. Enig, op cit

23. "Diet Roulette", The New York Times, May 20, 1994.

67.

Toxins on Your Toast

By Valerie James, BA

The latest buzzword in the food industry is "neutra-ceuticals," plant-derived substances added to foods to make them "healthier." This is the food industry's solution to the problem of sluggish growth and declining profit margins on processed foods.

There's more money in pills containing "phytonutrients" like indoles or isothiocyanates derived from broccoli, than in broccoli itself; and more profit from "functional foods" like "energy bars" with added soy isoflavones, touted as a panacea for everything from menopausal symptoms to osteoroposis, than from old-fashioned candy bars.

Recently the FDA allowed the industry the right to add plant-derived sterols to such pedestrian products as vegetable oil spreads, salad dressings, health drinks, health bars and yoghurt-type products. These phyto-sterols include beta-sitosterol, campesterol and stigmasterol, all estrogen-like compounds derived mostly from wood-pulp effluent.

NUTRACEUTICALS

Safety   Efficacy

Scientific Evidence

Nutritional Supplements   Pharmaceuticals

The products will carry a health label claiming cholesterol-lowering properties, thanks to FDA largesse, and consumers will pay highly inflated prices for the privilege of spreading these known toxins on their morning toast.

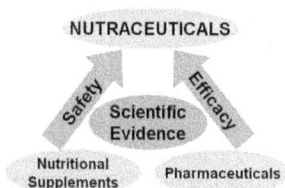

Advertising Blitz

"My father died young," says an earnest-looking man on a television commercial. "When I found out I had a cholesterol problem, I just thought, 'Well, I'm not waiting around for it to happen to me.' So I started using Flora ProActiv margarine which actually reduced my cholesterol absorption. With Flora ProActiv, I'm down from 6.5 to 4.5 in just three weeks. Now I can do anything I've been wanting to do for years."

Not all consumers watch television. In fact, those consumers most concerned about their health don't watch much television at all. Nutrition writers have been quick to comply with their advertisers' wishes with articles on the virtues of functional foods. And the National Heart, Lung and Blood Institute's "New Guidelines" for preventing heart disease recommend the consumption of cholesterol-lowering margarines and spreads providing 2 grams of sterols or stanols per day.

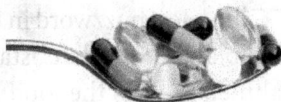

The cash registers are ringing up the dollars; cholesterol-lowering phytosterols are already big business. Recently, the pharmaceutical giant Novartis sold the licence for its phytosterol product, Reducol, to Forbes Meditech, Inc. of Canada for US $200 million despite the fact that these sterols are not even legal additives in Canada. Predictably, Forbes Meditech is now lobbying the Canadian government for permission to sell to Canadians, and on their website they say they are confident that they can soon build significant sales and can establish a wide and extensive customer base for these products.

Dangerous and Also Useless

In 1990, Dr Peter Skrabanek of Dublin University commented in the prestigious medical journal The Lancet on the dogma that cholesterol reduction could extend life.[1] He wrote: "There is not a scrap of evidence that it is capable of changing the risk of dying from coronary heart disease, but there is reasonable evidence that it does not. The oldest consensus among the vendors of health, and other traders along the valley of the shadow of death, is that people want to be deceived and should be pleased accordingly. In the past, mountebanks were distinguishable from their more respectable colleagues at least in appearance and manners, if not by the effectiveness of their cures. Nowadays, the convergence of medicine and its 'alternatives' is an ominous foretaste." Dr Skrabanek recommends that "people should temper their faith in experts--particularly when they see them coming in droves--with their own informed scepticism."

1. Skrabanek, "Nonsensus Consensus," The Lancet 1990 335:1446-1447.)

68.

WHO 'Infiltrated By Food Industry'

Sarah Boseley, The Guardian, Thursday 9 January 2003

British newspaper, The Guardian reveals the extent to which companies will exert influence and political power:

The food industry has infiltrated the World Health Organisation, just as the tobacco industry did, and succeeded in exerting "undue influence" over policies intended to safeguard public health by limiting the amount of fat, sugar and salt we consume, according to a confidential report obtained by the Guardian.

The report, by an independent consultant to the WHO, finds that:

- food companies attempted to place scientists favourable to their views on WHO and Food and Agricultural Organisation (FAO) committees.

- they financially supported non-governmental organisations which were invited to formal discussions on key issues with the UN agencies.

- they financed research and policy groups that supported their views.

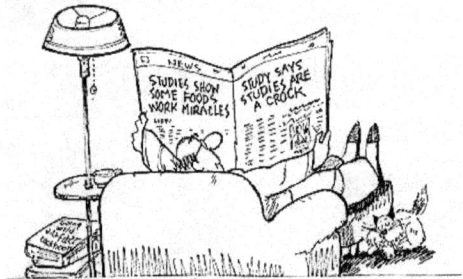

- they financed individuals who would promote "anti-regulation ideology" to the public, for instance in newspaper articles.

"The easy movement of experts - toxicologists in particular - between private firms, universities, tobacco and food industries and international agencies creates the conditions for conflict of interest," says the report by Norbert Hirschhorn, a Connecticut-based public health academic who searched archives set up during litigation in the US for references to food companies owned or linked to the tobacco industry.

"If it's advertised on TV, you probably shouldn't be eating it."

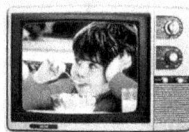

He finds that there is reasonable suspicion that undue influence was exerted "on specific WHO/FAO food policies dealing with dietary guidelines, pesticide use, additives, trans-fatty acids and sugar.

"The food industry is considerably engaged in genetically modified foods and the tobacco industry has studied the matter

> One should know, however, that all the necessities of life that the human society requires are supplied by the empowered agents of the Lord. No one can manufacture anything. Take, for example, all the eatables of human society. These eatables include grains, fruits, vegetables, milk, sugar, etc., for the persons in the mode of goodness, and also eatables for the nonvegetarians, like meats, none of which can be manufactured by men. Then again, take for example heat, light, water, air, etc., which are also necessities of life -- none of them can be manufactured by the human society. Without the Supreme Lord, there can be no profuse sunlight, moonlight, rainfall, breeze, etc., without which no one can live. Obviously, our life is dependent on supplies from the Lord. Even for our manufacturing enterprises, we require so many raw materials like metal, sulphur, mercury, manganese, and so many essentials -- all of which are supplied by the agents of the Lord, with the purpose that we should make proper use of them to keep ourselves fit and healthy for the purpose of self-realization, leading to the ultimate goal of life, namely, liberation from the material struggle for existence.
>
> ~ Srila Prabhupada (Bhagavad-gita 3.12)

closely with respect to its product; there is evidence the tobacco industry planned also to influence the debate over biotechnology."

The WHO and FAO need the scientific input of the food industry, says the report, but that input must be transparent and subject to open debate.

"One industry-led organisation, International Life Sciences Institute (ILSI), has positioned its experts and expertise across the

Stan Correy of the Australian Broadcasting Corporation (ABC) comments, "the days of an apple-a-day to keep the doctor away are over, because the food companies have to move on from apples to make new profits. To give credibility to these new products, they use scientists, doctors and people from the legal professions to speak for them."

Fortunately, not all government officials have bowed to the interests of the food conglomerates. Dr Mark Lawrence of Australia's Deakin University, formerly head of the Australian Food Standards Committee, resigned from his post last September largely because of his concerns about the aggressive targeting of public officials and consumers by functional food promotions. "The Food Standards Committee is not able to be vigilant enough because it is dominated by food industry representatives," he said. "I found the situation untenable. I and the other public health nutritionists could not feel confident that public health was going to take precedence over other dimensions." Later, on Radio New Zealand, he explained that the Food Standards Committee was basically dominated by food industry interests, and that they were relaxing any kind of control over functional foods.

Last September, ABC devoted a full program to "The Twilight Zone: Medicalizing the Food Supply," a program about the marketing of functional foods. Interviewer Stan Correy reported that the traditional food industry has "hit the proverbial brick wall. It simply cannot make extra profits by just selling plain grains, veggies and fruit; it has to find new ways to tempt consumers to their products. It is no longer credible for the food to be just delicious, especially if it is full of fat and bad things. There is nowhere to go but to make it full of supposedly good things... Think about it: fish oil in ice cream: it increases your memory; Brocco-bites, that's broccoli in a pill; wood chips or cholesterol-lowering plant phytosterols in margarine; all part of the wonderful 'healthy' world of functional food and neutriceuticals." And of corporate profit motivation.

~ Valerie James

whole spectrum of food and tobacco policies: at conferences, on FAO/WHO food policy committees and within WHO, and with monographs, journals and technical briefs."

A picturesque scene of green paddy fields enlivens the heart of the poor agriculturalist, but it brings gloom to the face of the capitalist who lives by exploiting the poor farmers.

With good rains, the farmer's business in agriculture flourishes. Agriculture is the noblest profession. It makes society happy, wealthy, healthy, honest, and spiritually advanced for a better life after death. The vaisya community, or the mercantile class of men, take to this profession. In Bhagavad-gita the vaisyas are described as the natural agriculturalists, the protectors of cows, and the general traders. When Lord Sri Krishna incarnated Himself at Vrndavana, He took pleasure in becoming a beloved son of such a vaisya family. Nanda Maharaja was a big protector of cows, and Lord Sri Krishna, as the most beloved son of Nanda Maharaja, used to tend His father's animals in the neighboring forest. By His personal example Lord Krishna wanted to teach us the value of protecting cows. Nanda Maharaja is said to have possessed nine hundred thousand cows, and at the time of Lord Sri Krishna (about five thousand years ago) the tract of land known as Vrndavana was flooded with milk and butter. Therefore God's gifted professions for mankind are agriculture and cow protection.

Trade is meant only for transporting surplus produce to places where the produce is scanty. But when traders become too greedy and materialistic they take to large-scale commerce and industry and allure the poor agriculturalist to unsanitary industrial towns with a false hope of earning more money. The industrialist and the capitalist do not want the farmer to remain at home, satisfied with his agricultural produce. When the farmers are satisfied by a luxuriant growth of food grains, the capitalist becomes gloomy at heart. But the real fact is that humanity must depend on agriculture and subsist on agricultural produce.

No one can produce rice and wheat in big iron factories. The industrialist goes to the villagers to purchase the food grains he is unable to produce in his factory. The poor agriculturalist takes advances from the capitalist and sells his produce at a lower price. Hence when food grains are produced abundantly the farmers become financially stronger, and thus the capitalist becomes morose at being unable to exploit them.

~ Srila Prabhupada, (Light of Bhagavata, verse 10)

Some of the strongest criticism in the report is levelled against the ILSI, founded in Washington in 1978 by the Heinz Foundation, Coca-Cola, Pepsi-Cola, General Foods, Kraft (owned by Philip Morris) and Procter & Gamble. Until 1991 it was led by Alex Malaspina, vice-president of Coca-Cola.

Dr. Malaspina established ILSI as a non-governmental organisation "in official relations" with the WHO and secured its "specialised consultative status" with the FAO.

Eileen Kennedy, global executive director of ILSI, said that the funding of its regional groups came exclusively from industry, while the central body received money from the branches, from government and from an endowment set up by Dr. Malaspina. Nonetheless, she said, ILSI regarded itself as an independent body.

The man that brought you monsanto's genetically engineered bovine growth hormone (bgh) is now america's food safety czar.

Michael Taylor became the senior advisor to the commissioner of the FDA. He is now America's food safety czar.

If GMOs are indeed responsible for massive sickness and death, then the individual who oversaw the FDA policy that facilitated their introduction holds a uniquely infamous role in human history. That person is Michael Taylor. He had been Monsanto's attorney before becoming policy chief at the FDA.

69.

Ready for breakfast?

Story Of Packaged Cereals

By Sally Fallon

Dry breakfast cereals are produced by a process called extrusion. Cereal makers first create a slurry of the grains and then put them in a machine called an extruder. The grains are forced out of a little hole at high temperature and pressure. Depending on the shape of the hole, the grains are made into little o's, flakes, animal shapes, or shreds (as in Shredded Wheat or Triscuits), or they are puffed (as in puffed rice). A blade slices off each little flake or shape, which is then carried past a nozzle and sprayed with a coating of oil and sugar to seal off the cereal from the ravages of milk and to give it crunch.

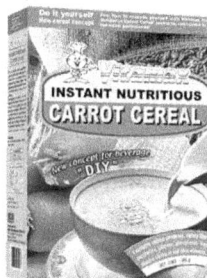

In his book Fighting the Food Giants, Paul Stitt tells us that the extrusion process used for these cereals destroys most of the nutrients in the grains. It destroys the fatty acids; it even destroys the chemical vitamins that are added at the end. The amino acids are rendered very toxic by this process. The amino acid lysine, a crucial nutrient, is especially denatured by extrusion. This is how all the boxed cereals are made, even the ones sold in the health food stores. They are all made in the same way and mostly in the same factories. All dry cereals that come in boxes are extruded cereals.

The only advances made in the extrusion process are those that will cut cost regardless of how these will alter the nutrient content of the product. Cereals are a multi-billion dollar business, one that has created huge fortunes.

With so many people eating breakfast cereals, you might expect to find some studies on the effect of extruded cereals on animals or humans. Yet, there are no published studies at all in the scientific literature.

The Rat Experiments

Let me tell you about two studies which were not published. The first was described by Paul Stitt who wrote about an experiment conducted by a cereal company in which four sets of rats were given special diets. One group received plain whole wheat, water and synthetic vitamins and minerals. A second group received puffed wheat (an extruded cereal), water and the same nutrient solution. A third set was given only water. A fourth set was given nothing but water and chemical nutrients. The rats that received the whole wheat lived over a year on this diet. The rats that got nothing but water and vitamins lived about two months. The animals on water alone lived about a month. But the company's own laboratory study showed that the rats given the vitamins, water and all the puffed wheat they wanted died within two weeks—they died before the rats that got no food at all. It wasn't a matter of the rats dying of malnutrition. Autopsy revealed dysfunction of the pancreas, liver and kidneys and degeneration of the nerves of the spine, all signs of insulin shock.

Results like these suggested that there was something actually very toxic in the puffed wheat itself! Proteins are very similar to certain toxins in molecular structure, and the pressure of the puffing process may produce chemical changes, which turn a nutritious grain into a poisonous substance.

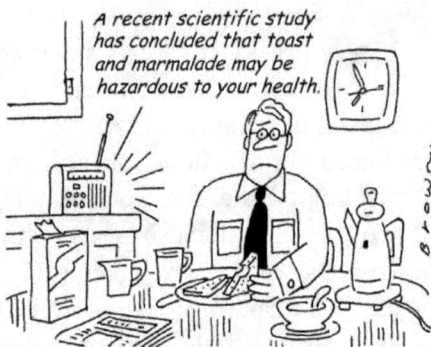

A recent scientific study has concluded that toast and marmalade may be hazardous to your health.

Another unpublished experiment was carried out in the 1960s. Researchers at University of Michigan were given 18 laboratory rats. They were divided into three groups: one group received corn flakes and water; a second group was given the cardboard box that the corn flakes came in and water; the control group received rat chow and water. The rats in the control group remained in good health throughout the experiment. The rats eating the box became lethargic and eventually died of malnutrition. But the rats receiving the corn flakes and water died before the rats that were eating the box! (The last corn flake rat died the day the first box rat died.)

But before death, the corn flake rats developed schizophrenic behavior, threw fits, bit each other and finally went into convulsions. The startling conclusion of this study is that there was more nourishment in the box than there was in the corn flakes.

This experiment was actually designed as a joke, but the results were far from funny. The results were never published and similar studies have not been conducted.

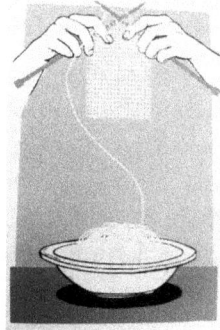

Most of America eats this kind of cereal. In fact, the USDA is gloating over the fact that children today get the vast majority of their important nutrients from the nutrients added to these boxed cereals.

Cereals sold in the health food stores are made by the same method. It may come as a shock to you, but these whole grain extruded cereals are probably more dangerous than those sold in the supermarket, because they are higher in protein and it is the proteins in these cereals that are so denatured by this type of processing.

We have got nice kitchen. We can prepare varieties of foodstuff by mixing so many eatables. Because we have got intelligence, we can do. The animals cannot do.

~*Srila Prabhupada (Srimad-Bhagavatam 5.5.3 -- Stockholm, September 9, 1973)*

There are no published studies on the effects of these extruded grains on animals or humans, but I did find one study in a literature search that described the microscopic effects of extrusion on the proteins. "Zeins," which comprise the majority of proteins in corn, are located in spherical organelles called protein bodies. During extrusion, these protein bodies are completely disrupted and deformed. The extrusion process breaks down the organelles, disperses the proteins and the proteins become toxic. When they are disrupted in this way, you have absolute chaos in your food, and it can result in a disruption of the nervous system.

Old-Fashioned Porridge

So what are you going to have for breakfast? We need to go back to the old fashioned porridges. These porridges should be soaked overnight in an acid medium to get rid of the anti-nutrients. Soaking will neutralize the tannins, complex proteins, enzyme inhibitors and phytic acid. You soak the grains in warm water with one tablespoon of something acidic like whey, yoghurt, lemon juice or vinegar. The next morning, the porridge cooks in about a minute. Of course, you eat your porridge with butter or cream like our grandparents did. The nutrients in the fats are needed to absorb the nutrients in the grains. That was one of the great lessons of Weston Price, that without the vitamins present in animal fats (vitamins A and D), you cannot assimilate minerals and other vitamins. You can be taking mineral supplements, drinking green juices or eating organic food until it comes out your ears, but you cannot absorb the minerals in your food without vitamins A and D that are exclusively found in the animal fats like butter and cream.

70.

Processed Milk

By Sally Fallon

The minute you start to process your milk, you destroy Mother Nature's perfect food. You can live exclusively on raw milk, especially milk from nature's sacred animal, the cow. We have no sense of the sacredness of our animals today. Instead, we have an industrial system of agriculture that puts our dairy cows inside on cement all their lives and gives them foods that cows are not designed to eat—grain, soy, citrus peel cake and bakery waste. These modern cows produce huge amounts of watery milk which is very low in fat.

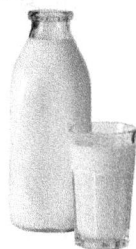

Milk from these industrial cows is then shipped to a milk factory. Emily Green wrote an excellent article in the LA Times, August 2000 about milk processing. Milk processing plants are big, big factories where visitors are not allowed. Lots can go wrong in these factories. The largest milk poisoning in American history occurred in 1985 where more than 197,000 people across three states were sickened after a "pasteurization failure" at an Illinois bottling plant.

Inside the plants all you can see is stainless steel. Inside that machinery, milk shipped from the farm is completely remade. First it is separated in centrifuges into fat, protein and various other solids and liquids. Once segregated, these are reconstituted to set levels for whole, low-fat and no-fat milks; in other words, the milk is reconstituted to be completely uniform.

Of the reconstituted milks, whole milk will most closely approximate original cow's milk. The butterfat left over will go into butter, cream, cheese, toppings and ice cream. The dairy industry loves to sell low fat milk and skim milk because they can make a lot more money from the butterfat when consumers buy it as ice cream. When they remove the fat to make reduced fat milks, they replace the fat with powdered milk concentrate, which is formed by high temperature spray drying. All reduced-fat

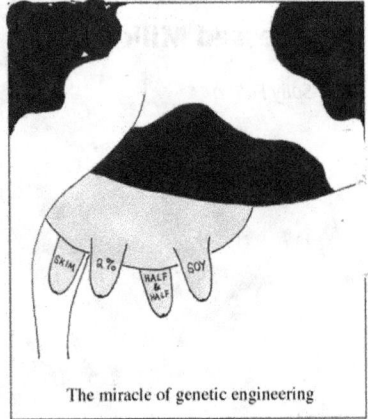

The miracle of genetic engineering

milks have dried skim milk added to give them body, although this ingredient is not usually on the labels. The result is a very high-protein, lowfat product. Because the body uses up many nutrients to assimilate protein—especially the nutrients contained in animal fat—such doctored milk can quickly lead to nutrient deficiencies.

The milk is then pasteurized at 161 degrees F by rushing it past superheated stainless steel plates. If the temperature is 200 degrees the milk is called ultrapasteurized. This will have a distinct cooked milk taste but it is sterile and can be sold on the grocery shelf. In

Nalini-kanta: The scientists are saying that milk is the major cause for heart attack. Milk is a very harmful food. It causes heart attack.

Prabhupada: Just see. Milk is the miracle food, and they are condemning by a scientific process.

And from the milk we can make hundreds of vitaminous foodstuff, hundreds. They're all palatable. So such a nice animal, faithful, peaceful, and beneficial. After taking milk from it, if we kill, does it look very well? Even after the death, the cows supply the skin for your shoes. It is so beneficial. You see. Even after death. While living, he gives you nice milk. You cannot reject milk from the human society. As soon as there is a child born, milk immediately required. Old man, milk is life. Diseased person, milk is life. Invalid, milk is life. So therefore Krishna is teaching by His practical demonstration how He loves this innocent animal, cow.

~ Srila Prabhupada (Lecture, Los Angeles, December 4, 1968)

other words, they don't even have to keep it cool. The bugs won't touch it. It does not require refrigeration. As it is cooked, the milk is also homogenized by a pressure treatment that breaks down the fat globules so the milk won't separate. Once processed, the milk will last for weeks, not just days.

Milk Allergies

Many people, particularly our children, cannot tolerate the stuff that we are calling milk that is sold in the grocery shelves. And you can see why. It starts with cows in confinement, cows fed feed that cows are not designed to digest, and then it goes into these factories for dismantlement and reconfiguration.

The protein compounds in milk have many important roles, including protection against pathogens, enhancement of the immune system and carrier systems for nutrients. However, like the proteins in grains, the proteins in milk are complex, three-dimensional molecules that are very fragile. The pasteurization process deforms and denatures these proteins. When we drink pasteurized milk, the body mounts an immune response instead of deriving instant nourishment.

Numerous animal studies in the 1930s and 1940s showed the superiority of raw milk over pasteurized in building strong bone, healthy organs and a strong nervous system.

Fortunately what we call real milk, that is full-fat milk from pasture-fed cows, milk that is not pasteurized, processed or homogenized, is becoming more available. Parents are discovering

The whole world is coming to like that. And it is said in the sastra, gradually this condition of human civilization will deteriorate to such extent that no more rice will be available, no more wheat will be available, no more sugar will be available. Everything will be... No more milk will be available. Finished. Simply you have to eat the seeds of the... There is not fruit, only seed. Just like in the mango, there is one seed and pulp. The pulp will not be available, only seed will be available. These are already foretold. No fruits will be available, no grains will be available, no milk will be available.

~ Srila Prabhupada (Srimad-Bhagavatam, 5.5.3 -- Stockholm, September 9, 1973)

just how healthy and happy their children can be when they drink raw milk instead of pasteurized.

Powdered Milk

A note on the production of skim milk powder: liquid milk is forced through a tiny hole at high pressure, and then blown out into the air. This causes a lot of nitrates to form and the cholesterol in the milk is oxidized. Those of you who are familiar with my work know that cholesterol is your best friend; you don't have to worry about natural cholesterol in your food; however, you do not want to eat oxidized cholesterol. Oxidized cholesterol contributes to the buildup of plaque in the arteries, to atherosclerosis. So when you drink reduced-fat milk thinking that it will help you avoid heart disease, you are actually consuming oxidized cholesterol, which initiates the process of heart disease.

71.

Orange Juice

By Sally Fallon

Now let's turn to the orange juice in this supposedly healthy breakfast. It is quite shocking what turns up in a literature search on orange juice processing.

A quote from Processed and Prepared Foods states that "a new orange juice processing plant is completely automated and can process up to 1,800 tons of oranges per day to produce frozen concentrate, single strength juice, oil extracted from the peel, and cattle feed."

In the processing, the whole orange is put into the machine. Enzymes are added to get as much oil as possible out of the skin. Oranges are a very heavily sprayed crop. These sprays are cholinesterase inhibitors, which are real neurotoxins. When they put the oranges in the vats and squeeze them, all those pesticides go into the juice.

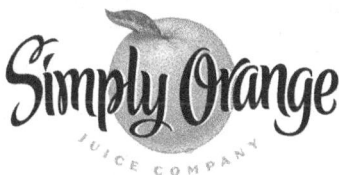

What about the orange peel used for cattle feed? The dried left-over citrus peel is processed into cakes which are still loaded with cholinesterase inhibitors and organophosphates. Mark Purdey in England has shown these neurotoxins are correlated with "Mad Cow Disease" (Bovine Spongiform Encephalitis or BSE). The use of organophosphates either as a spray on the cows or in their feed is one of the causes of the degeneration of the brain and nervous system in the cow and if these components are doing this to the nervous system of the cow, there's a possibility they are doing this to you also. In fact, a study carried out in Hawaii found that consumption of fruit and fruit juices was the number one dietary factor for the development of Alzheimer's disease. The researchers speculated that the real culprit was the pesticides used in fruit—and concentrated in the juices due to modern processing techniques.

The FDA has decreed that we can no longer buy raw juice, because it might be a source of pathogens. But it might surprise you to know that they have found fungus that is resistant to pressure and heat in the processed juices. One study found that 17% of Nigerian packages of orange juice and 20% of mango and tomato juices contained heat resistant fungi. They also found E. coli in the orange juice that was pressure resistant and had survived pasteurization. So there is plenty of danger from contamination from pasteurized juices.

In one study, heat-treated and acid-hydrolyzed orange juice was tested for mutagenic activity. The authors hypothesized that the heating process produces intermediate products, which under test conditions, give rise to mutagenicity, and cytotoxicity. In other words you have got cancer-causing compounds in your orange juice. In another study, gel filtration and high performance liquid chromatography were used to obtain mutagenic fractions from heated orange juice.

Another study shows just how toxic and damaging these juices are to teeth. They found that rats had more tooth decay from these commercial juices than they did from soda pop, which is loaded with sugar.

One more thing about processed orange juice. Have you ever wondered why processed orange juice stays cloudy, why the solids do not settle? This is because soy protein combined with soluble pectin is added, and this keeps the juice permanently cloudy. It might be interesting to know, for those of you who are allergic to soy.

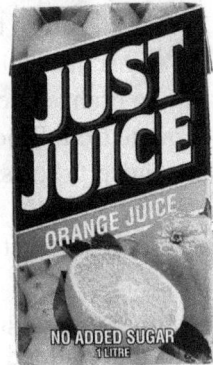

Why '100% Orange Juice' Is Still Artificial

The Huffington Post, July 29, 2011

Technically, '100% orange juice is "not from concentrate," but it's not really 100% orange juice either, according to a report at Civil Eats.

The process is rather depressing. Gizmodo explains part of the process:

Once the juice is squeezed and stored in gigantic vats, they start removing oxygen. Why? Because removing oxygen from the juice allows the liquid to keep for up to a year without spoiling. But! Removing that oxygen also removes the natural flavors of oranges. Yeah, it's all backwards. So in order to have Orange Juice actually taste like oranges, drink companies hire flavor and fragrance companies, the same ones that make perfumes for Dior, to create these "flavor packs" to make juice taste like, well, juice again.

Any taste difference in say Minute Maid versus Tropicana is therefore due to the specific flavor pack the company uses. Since these flavor packs are made from orange byproducts, they don't have to be considered an ingredient, and therefore are not required to appear on food labels. This is despite the fact they are chemically altered.

Perhaps its time to take the juicer out of that dusty corner in the garage.

UPDATE: Karen Mathis, the Public Relations Director of the Florida Department of Citrus wrote HuffPost Food the following letter that offers the citrus industry's description of the process, without disputing any of the above:

Dear Ms. Polis,

On behalf of the Florida Department of Citrus, I am writing in response to the article on HuffPost Food, entitled "Why 100% Orange Juice is Still Artificial." Please allow me to share further information.

Purchased by nearly 70 percent of American households, people choose 100 percent orange juice for its great taste and nutrition benefits. Both "from concentrate" and "not from concentrate" orange juice are healthy options that provide a variety of nutrients. By utilizing state-of-the-art technology, Florida is able to provide a consistent supply of high quality, nutritious orange juice year round.

By law, 100 percent orange juice is made only from oranges. The basic principle of orange juice processing is similar to how you make orange juice at home. Oranges are washed and the juice is extracted by squeezing the oranges. Seeds and particles are strained out. Orange juice is pasteurized to ensure food safety

During processing, natural components such as orange aroma, orange oil from the peel, and pulp may be separated from the orange juice. After the juice is pasteurized, these natural orange components may be added back to the orange juice for optimal flavor.

72.

Artificial Flavorings, Hydrolyzed Protein, and MSG

By Sally Fallon

Following the Second World War food companies discovered monosodium glutamate (MSG), a food ingredient the Japanese had invented in 1908 to enhance food flavors, including meat-like flavors. Humans actually have receptors on the tongue for glutamate—it is the protein in food that the human body recognizes as meat. Unfortunately, the free glutamic acid in MSG has a very different effect in the body than the natural glutamic acid in food, one that is harmful, especially to the nervous system. Any protein can be hydrolyzed to produce a base containing MSG, but the usual source is soy. When the industry learned how to make the flavor of meat in the laboratory using inexpensive proteins from grains and legumes, the door was opened to a flood of new products including bullion cubes, dehydrated soup mixes, sauce mixes, TV dinners, and condiments with a meat-flavored base.

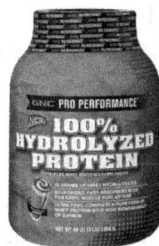

The fast food industry could not exist without MSG and other artificial meat flavors to make secret sauces and spice mixes that beguile the consumer into eating bland and tasteless food. The sauces in processed foods are basically MSG, water, thickeners and emulsifiers and some caramel coloring. Your tongue is tricked into thinking that it is getting something nutritious when it is getting nothing at all except some very toxic substances. Even the dressings, the Worcestershire sauce, rice mixes, dehydrated soups, all of these and anything that has a meat-like taste has MSG in it. Almost all canned soups and stews contain MSG, and the "hydrolyzed protein" bases often contain MSG in very large amounts. Trade names of monosodium glutamate include Ac'cent, Aji-No-Moto, and Vetsin.

So-called "homemade soup" in most restaurants is usually made by adding water to a powdered soup-base or soup cubes and then adding chopped vegetables, etc. Even things like lobster bisque and sauces in the seafood restaurants are full of these artificial flavors. It's all profit based. The industry even finds it too costly to just use a little onion and garlic for flavoring, so they are using the artificial flavors instead.

Most of the vegetarian foods are loaded with these flavorings. The list of ingredients in vegetarian hamburgers, hot dogs, bacon, baloney, etc. may include hydrolyzed protein and other "natural" flavorings. Soy foods contain large amounts of MSG as it is formed during processing. MSG is also formed during the spray drying of milk, so it is in reduced-fat milk because spray dried milk is added to these products.

MSG Labelling

As I point out in my various workshops, the three most toxic additives in our food supply are MSG, hydrolyzed protein, and aspartame, and the first two are in all of these secret sauces with "natural flavors." Anything that you buy that says "spices" or "natural flavors" contains MSG! The industry avoids putting MSG on the label by putting MSG in spice mixes, and if the mix is less than 50% MSG, manufacturers don't have to put it on the label. You may have noticed that that phrase "No MSG" has actually disappeared. That's because MSG is in all the spice mixes. Even Bragg's "Liquid Aminos" had to take "No MSG" off their label.

Health Problems with MSG

The industry has known about the health problems caused by MSG for a long time. In 1957 scientists found that mice became blind and obese when MSG was administered by feeding tube. In 1969, MSG-induced lesions were found in the hypothalamus region of the brain. Subsequent studies all pointed in the same direction.

MSG is a neurotoxic substance that causes a wide range of reactions, from temporary headaches to permanent brain damage. We have a huge increase in Alzheimer's, brain cancer, seizures, multiple sclerosis, and diseases of the nervous system, and one of the chief reasons is these flavorings in our food. MSG is also associated with violent behavior.

Most surprisingly, MSG causes obesity! In laboratory experiments on obese rats, scientists induce obesity by feeding the animals MSG!

Ninety-five percent of processed foods contain MSG, and as you may know, in the late 1950s it was added to baby food. After some congressional hearings on this subject, the industry told us they had taken it out of the baby food, but they didn't really remove it. They just called it by another name—hydrolyzed protein. I recommend that everyone read the book Excitotoxins, by Dr. Russell Blaylock. He describes how the nerve cells either disintegrate or shrivel up in the presence of free glutamic acid, that is, MSG, if it gets past the blood-brain barrier. The glutamates in MSG are absorbed directly from the mouth to the brain. Some investigators believe that the great increase in violence in this country is due, not to sugar, but to the huge increase in the use of MSG in the food which began in the late 1950's, and particularly because it was put in baby food in very large amounts.

73.

GMO 'Food" - The Last Nail in Our Food's Coffin

A Ticking Time Bomb, A Disaster Waiting To Happen

A genetically modified organism (GMO) is an organism whose genetic material has been altered using genetic engineering techniques. Organisms that have been genetically modified include micro-organisms such as bacteria and yeast, insects, plants, fish, and mammals. Few health topics are more hotly debated than the GM food issue and for good reason.

Genetic modification involves the insertion or deletion of genes. When genes are inserted, they usually come from a different species, which is a form of horizontal gene transfer.

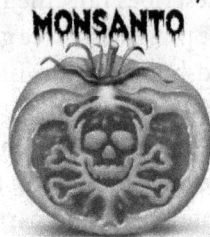

Scorpion Genes In Your Corn

The scorpion toxin gene put into corn and oilseed rape allows the plant to make its own pesticide. Caterpillars eating this corn die of the toxin. And what happens when pests become resistant to the in-bred toxin?

Of course it doesn't stop there. Genetic experiments are being carried out all over the world. Frog genes have been put into potatoes to help them resist infection. Human genes have been

> "Seeds have the power to preserve species, to enhance cultural as well as genetic diversity, to counter economic monopoly and to check the advance of conformity on all its many fronts."
> ~Michael Pollan, Second Nature: A Gardener's Education

put into pigs and fish to make them grow faster. Pigs are also being bio-engineered to provide organs for transplanting into humans. The list goes on and on and on.

Monsanto - Playing With Life On The Planet

Monsanto is heading up this sinister biotechnological revolution. They created Agent Orange used in the Vietnam war. Among other things, they've developed 'round-up ready soy' which is resistant to their own herbicide 'round-up'. So, farmers can now destroy all plant-life on a field except the soy. The impact on wildlife is disastrous. This is a nightmare vision of mono culture... a landscape of human crops devoid of all other life. Whilst these companies can spin their compassionate message of how they are helping poor people with their products, the truth is that third world farmers are getting locked into deals with the powerful companies. Once they're in, they can't get out.

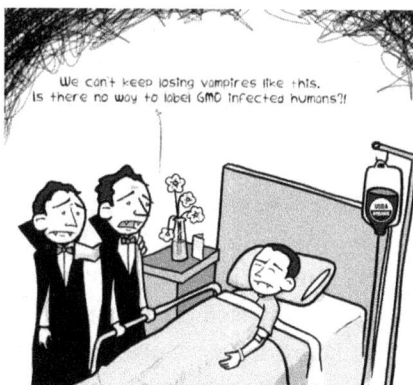

Monsanto - A Humanitarian Organization?

Companies like Monsanto proudly justify their dangerously insane schemes. Their publicly stated aim is 'to feed an ever growing population with limited arable land...'

Only a brain dead person will buy into their ridiculous humanitarian justifications. They are merchants of death and their motivation is money and destruction.

> *"Half of all broccoli grown commercially in America today is a single variety- Marathon- notable for it's high yield. The overwhelming majority of the chickens raised for meat in America are the same hybrid, the Cornish cross; more than 99 percent of turkeys are the Broad-Breasted Whites."*
>
> *~Michael Pollan, In Defense of Food: An Eater's Manifesto*

It's truly frightening to see the lengths some organisations will go in the name of profit.

The most authoritative evaluation of agriculture, the International Assessment of Agricultural Knowledge, Science and Technology for Development, determined that the current GMO's have nothing to offer towards the goals of reducing hunger and poverty, improving nutrition, health and rural livelihoods, and facilitating social and environmental sustainability.

The report was a three-year collaborative effort with 900 participants and 110 countries, and was co-sponsored by all the majors, e.g. the World Bank, FAO, UNESCO, WHO. In reality, GMO's reduce yield, increase farmers' dependence on multinationals, reduce biodiversity, increase herbicide use, and take money away from more successful and appropriate methods.

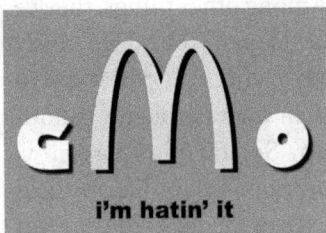

i'm hatin' it

In Developing Nations, GMO's Can Be Catastrophic.

In India, for example, Monsanto convinced hundreds of thousands of farmers to take out high interest loans to pay for expensive GM cotton seeds and associated chemicals. Inconsistent yields left desperate farmers unable to even pay back their loans. In last 10 years, more than 2,50,000 farmers have committed suicide.

Playing God Is Not An Option

Unbelievably, crops are purposely being developed that don't produce viable seeds. These are called the 'Terminator Genes.' This prevents farmers using the traditional methods of saving some seed for next years sowing. How is this 'helping' feed the world? Folks really wanting to help feed the world would be pushing with all their might for sustainable farming. *In any case, starving populations are about governments, politics and distribution, not actual lack of food.*(Mike Kinnaird)

Higher Residues Of Poisonous Herbicide

The primary reason crops are engineered is to allow them to drink poison. They're called herbicide tolerant, and are inserted with bacterial genes that allow them to survive otherwise deadly doses of toxic herbicide.

Biotech companies sell the seed and herbicide as a package. Monsanto sells Roundup Ready crops and Roundup herbicide. Bayer CropScience sells Liberty Link crops and Liberty herbicide.

Between 1996 and 2008, US farmers sprayed an extra 383 million pounds of herbicide on these poison drinking GMO's.

Because weeds are becoming resistant to the overused herbicide, farmers are spraying considerably more each year.

Nutrition Facts
None of Your Business
INGREDIENTS: You don't have a right to know. We will only be confused or alarmed by the labels.

WHAT IF EVERYTHING WAS LABELED LIKE GENETICALLY ENGINEERED FOODS?

The last 2 years of the 13-year study alone accounted for 46 percent of the increased herbicide use.

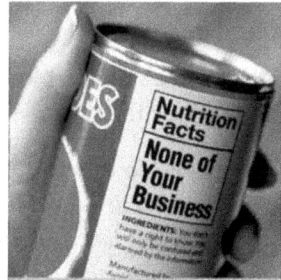

Your Intestinal Bacteria Into Living Pesticide Factories

GM genes can convert your intestinal bacteria into living factories that continuously produce pesticides or other harmful products.

The ONLY published GMO human feeding study (that's right, there's only one) confirmed that genes transfer from GM soybeans into the DNA of bacteria living inside our small intestines and continue to function. [Netherwood et al, "Assessing the survival of transgenic plant DNA in the human gastrointestinal tract]

Human subjects that ate Roundup Ready soybeans ended up with "Roundup Ready gut bacteria"—unkillable with Roundup. If

saka-mulamisa-ksaudra-
phala-puspasti-bhojanah
anavrstya vinanksyanti
durbhiksa-kara-piditah

Harassed by famine and excessive taxes, people will resort to eating leaves, roots, flesh, wild honey, fruits, flowers and seeds. Struck by drought, they will become completely ruined.

~ Srimad Bhagavatam 12.2.9

the pesticide-producing Bt gene in corn chips were also to transfer, it could turn your intestinal flora into living pesticide factories—possibly for the long term. (Jeffrey M. Smith)

Gaining Ground

America's supermarkets are awash in genetically modified foods. Over the past decade, biotech companies have dominated

Grow More Food

"Many countries have invested quite heavily in plans to bring back into use land abandoned for hundreds of years, or land that has never been used at all. They have brought all kinds of heavy earth moving tractors and machines for land development and introduced new forms of power into their agriculture. In many cases tractors, machines and implements have been brought in without taking into account the position of the cultivator, of the man who works on the land and who must ultimately make these things pay. And frequently they have been purchased before sufficient training and maintenance facilities were available. Of course, there are also exceptions and some land development and mechanisation projects have proved successful from their inception."

The above is a quotation from 'UNESCO' Food and Agriculture organisation. The enthusiasm for tractors over other implements has not always proved successful and on many cases, as we have personal experience of some places in U.P., it has often meant false starts on scheme that on paper looked so promising and easy.

The transcendentalist however will not agree with that tractors and other agricultural implements only can solve the problem of grow more food and inadequate living standard. Besides the tractor, implements, the man who will work on the land of cultivation, there is another supreme hand in the successful termination of the productive enthusiasm. This ultimate cause is called "Daiva" or the unseen power of God inconceivable by human brain. This power can ultimately make all things null and void and conquer over all other enthusiasm and ability of the human being. In the Bhagvad Gita we have this information as follows:-

adhisthanam tatha karta
karanam ca prthag-vidham
vividhas ca prthak cesta
daivam caivatra pancamam
(Bg. 18.14)   (Continued on next page...)

dinner tables with crops like corn, soybeans and canola modified to survive lethal doses of herbicides, resulting in increased herbicide use, a surge in herbicide-resistant weeds, and the contamination of organic and conventional crops. According to the Center for Food Safety, more than half of all processed food in U.S. grocery

---

(.....continued from previous page)

To effect successful result in the attempt of agricultural enthusiasm there are five causes namely the situation of the land, the man who works in the field, the instruments or implements applied in the enterprise and above all the hidden hand natural forces, known as Daiva.

Whatever is attempted and done in this world physically or mentally by any man, which may be right or wrong in the estimation of the public, must have all the above mentioned five causes behind the attempt. Nobody should therefore see only the visible causes for effective result but must look into the invisible cause called the Daiva.

Above all other causes the Daiva cause is the most powerful. This Daiva cause or the Supreme cause is the ultimate control of physical nature which is the external energy of Godhead. The land, implements, the worker, the attempt all depend on the ultimate cause called 'Daiva.' It is also known as 'Prakriti.' Everything is done by the 'Prakriti' but egoistic fools think that the work is performed by them. In spite of good tilling of the land and the expert tiller, good tractors or other implements and the most sincere and accurate plan of the work it is quite possible that the whole attempt may be frustrated for want of sufficient rains. Without rains all other arrangement will stand null and void due to the reaction of the Daiva cause. This Daiva cause is made effectively favourable by the process of 'Yajna' described elsewhere in this issue.

Along with the creation of the 'Prajas' or the living being, the 'Yajnas' or sacrifices on account of Vishnu the Supreme Being was also created. By the performance of 'Yajnas' the controlling deities, who supply us light, air, heat, water etc. which are all essential factors in the matter of grow more food campaign, are satisfied. By their satisfaction only everything is produced nicely, sufficiently. When there is sufficient production by the mercy of Daiva the inadequate standard of living is mitigated. Otherwise every attempt becomes futile.

~ Srila Prabhupada (Handwritten note under the title: "add with Geeta Nagari)

stores—items like cereals, corn dogs and cookies—contain GMO ingredients.

"This technology is a one-trick pony," says George Kimbrell, an attorney at the Center for Food Safety. "They don't help us feed the world, they don't fight climate change, and they don't help us better the environment. They just increase pesticides and herbicides. That's what they do."

Companies like Syngenta, Bayer and Dow are trying hard to catch up with Monsanto and they have all created their own herbicide tolerant seeds, modified to withstand the company's corresponding herbicide treatment.

This is a vast subject and we have only given a few glimpses of a grave crisis.

74.

Soft Drinks : The World's Other Drinking Problem

An American Case Study

By Judith Valentine, PhD, CNA, CNC

The addict feels low. His body needs a boost. He reaches into his pocket and finds a dollar bill. He slides it into the machine and a can rolls out. He opens the can and guzzles. He feels his energy return. His fix will last a couple of hours, enough to keep him alert for the rest of the morning.

The addict is twelve years old and his drug is a soft drink, purchased from a vending machine in his school. This addict and thousands like him will attend special classes, sponsored by his school, to warn him about the dangers of drugs, tobacco and alcohol. But no one will tell him about America's other drinking problem.

According to the National Soft Drink Association (NSDA), consumption of soft drinks is now over 600 12-ounce servings (12 oz.) per person per year. Since 1978, soda consumption in the US has tripled for boys and doubled for girls. Young males age 12-29 are the biggest consumers at over 160 gallons per year—that's almost 2 quarts per day. At these levels, the calories from soft drinks contribute as much as 10 percent of the total daily caloric intake for a growing boy.

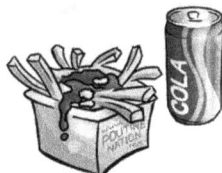

Targeting The Young

Huge increases in soft drink consumption have not happened by chance—they are due to intense marketing efforts by soft drink corporations. Coca Cola, for example, has set the goal of raising consumption of its products in the US by at least 25 percent per year. The adult market is stagnant so kids are the target. According to an article in Beverage, January 1999, "Influencing elementary school students is very important to soft drink marketers."

Since the 1960s the industry has increased the single-serving size from a standard 6-½-ounce bottle to a 20-ounce bottle. At movie theaters and at 7-Eleven stores the most popular size is now the 64-ounce "Double Gulp."

Soft drink companies spend billions on advertising. Much of these marketing efforts are aimed at children through playgrounds, toys, cartoons, movies, videos, charities and amusement parks; and through contests, sweepstakes, games and clubs via television, radio, magazines and the internet. Their efforts have paid off. Last year soft drink companies grossed over $57 billion in sales in the US alone, a colossal amount.

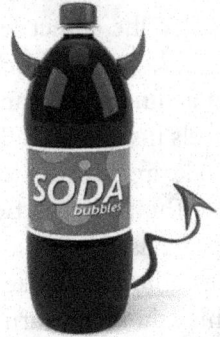

In 1998 the Center for Science in the Public Interest (CSPI) warned the public that soft drink companies were beginning to infiltrate our schools and kid clubs. For example, they reported that Coca-Cola paid the Boys & Girls Clubs of America $60 million to market its brand exclusively in over 2000 facilities. Fast food companies selling soft drinks now run ads on Channel One, the commercial television network with programming shown in classrooms almost every day to eight million middle, junior and high school students.

In 1993, District 11 in Colorado Springs became the first public school district in the US to place ads for Burger King in its hallways and on the sides of its school buses. Later, the school district signed a 10-year deal with Coca-Cola, bringing in $11 million during the life of the contract. This arrangement was later imitated all over Colorado. The contracts specify annual sales quotas with the result that school administrators encourage students to drink sodas, even in the classrooms. One high school in Beltsville, Maryland, made nearly $100,000 last year on a deal with a soft drink company.

While our children are exposed to unremitting publicity for soft drinks, evidence of their dangers accumulates. The consumption of soft drinks, like land-mine terrain, is riddled with hazards. We as practitioners and advocates of a healthy life-style recognize that consuming even as little as one or two sodas per day is undeniably connected to a myriad of pathologies. The most commonly associated health risks are obesity, diabetes and other blood sugar disorders, tooth decay, osteoporosis and bone fractures, nutritional deficiencies, heart disease, food addictions and eating disorders, neurotransmitter dysfunction from chemical sweeteners, and neurological and adrenal disorders from excessive caffeine.

Early Warnings

Warnings about the dangers of soft drink consumption came to us as early as 1942 when the American Medical Association's (AMA) Council on Food and Nutrition 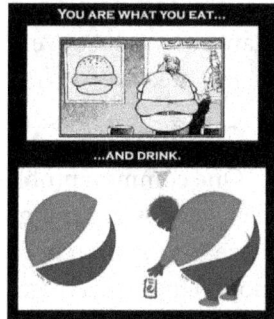 made the following noble statement: "From the health point of view it is desirable especially to have restriction of such use of sugar as is represented by consumption of sweetened carbonated beverages and forms of candy which are of low nutritional value. The Council believes it would be in the interest of the public health for all practical means to be taken to limit consumption of sugar in any form in which it fails to be combined with significant proportions of other foods of high nutritive quality."

Since that time the first notable public outcry came in 1998, 56 years later, when the CSPI published a paper called "Liquid Candy" blasting the food industry for "mounting predatory marketing campaigns [especially] aimed at children and adolescents." At a press conference, CSPI set up 868 cans of soda to represent the amount of soda the average young male consumed during the prior year. For additional shock effect, CSPI displayed baby bottles with soft drink logos such as Pepsi, Seven-Up and Dr. Pepper, highlighting a study that "found that parents are four times more likely to feed their children soda pop when their children use those logo bottles than when they don't."

In "Liquid Candy" CSPI revealed that even though, over a period of fifty years, soft drink production increased nine times and by 1998 "...provided more than one-third of all refined sugars in the diet,... the AMA and other health organizations [remained] largely silent." How could the medical community and we as responsible citizens concerned with health policy have been apathetic for a half a century? Considering this question makes me feel like a tired old guard dog that knows he is ignoring his responsibilities, but is too worn down to do anything about them. Even if inertia were not a problem, the money and effort required to launch a public interest campaign to stand up to the soft drink industry would be Herculean if not impossible. In the meantime, the relentlessly ambitious and wealthy soft drink companies with their very hip life-style ads manage to seduce ever increasing numbers of consumers, most of them our kids.

GI Distress

One common problem I have seen over the years, especially in teenagers, is general gastrointestinal (GI) distress. This includes increased stomach acid levels requiring acid inhibitors and moderate to severe gastric inflammation with possible stomach lining erosion. The common complaint I hear is chronic "stomach ache." In almost every case, when the client successfully abstains from sodas and caffeine, the symptoms will go away.

What causes these symptoms? We know that many soda brands contain caffeine and that caffeine does increase stomach acid levels. What we may not be aware of is that sodas also contain an array of chemical acids as additives, such as acetic, fumaric, gluconic and phosphoric acids, all of them synthetically produced. That is why certain sodas work so well when used to clean car engines. For human consumption, however, the effects are much less satisfying and quite precarious. Drinking sodas, especially on an empty stomach, can upset the fragile acid-alkaline balance of the stomach and other gastric lining, creating a continuous acid environment. This prolonged acid environment can lead to inflammation of the stomach and duodenal lining which becomes quite painful. Over the long term, it can lead to gastric lining erosion.

Another problem with sodas is that they act as dehydrating diuretics, much like tea, coffee and alcohol. All of these drinks can inhibit proper digestive function. It is much healthier to consume herbal teas, nutritional soups and broths, naturally lacto-fermented beverages and water to supply our daily fluid needs. These fluids support, not inhibit, digestion.

Sports Drinks

Students are now being given "electrolyte" drinks called "ergogenic aids" to replace electrolytes that are allegedly depleted during workouts. There are three problems with using these drinks as a rehydration solution. First, most soft drinks are diuretics, meaning they squeeze liquids out of the body, thus exacerbating dehydration instead of correcting it. Second, most people actually lose few electrolytes during exercise. After exercise the body is usually in an electrolyte load having lost more fluids than electrolytes. If sweating has been profuse, electrolytes can be replaced by drinking a lacto-fermented beverage or pure mineral water, which contains a proper ratio of minerals (electrolytes), and by eating a healthy diet containing Celtic sea salt. Third, when we give sugar-laden drinks to dehydrated kids, the high sugar content requires that blood be sent to the stomach to digest it. This fluid shift can lower the blood volume in other parts of the body making them more susceptible to cramps and heat-related illnesses.

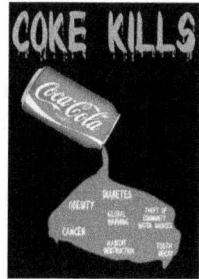

Stimulant Soft Drinks And Violence

The industry has begun to market so-called stimulant soft drinks, which usually consist of higher-than-usual levels of caffeine, along with other compound stimulants. According to an article published in The Lancet, December 2000, the Irish government ordered "urgent research" into the effects of so-called "functional energy" or stimulant soft drinks after the death of an 18-year-old who died while playing basketball. He had consumed three cans of "Red Bull," a stimulant soft drink. The article noted there have been reports of a rise in aggressive late-night violence occurring when people switch to these drinks while drowsy from too much alcohol. The resulting violence was so pervasive that some establishments in Ireland have refused to sell stimulant drinks. The entire European community has taken the problem seriously enough to ask the EU's scientific community to examine stimulant sodas and their effect on food and health safety, but no such outcry has been heard in the US.

Bone Fractures

Over the last 30 years a virtual tome of information has been published linking soft drink consumption to a rise in osteoporosis and bone fractures. New evidence has shown an alarming rise in deficiencies of calcium and other minerals and resulting bone fractures in young girls. A 1994 report published in the Journal of Adolescent Health summarizes a small study (76 girls and 51 boys) and points toward an increasing and "strong association between cola beverage consumption and bone fractures in girls." High calcium intake offered some protection. For boys, only low total caloric intake was associated with a higher risk of bone fractures. The study concluded with the following: "The high consumption of carbonated beverages and the declining consumption of milk are of great public health significance for girls and women because of their proneness to osteoporosis in later life."

A larger, cross sectional retrospective study of 460 high school girls was published in Pediatrics & Adolescent Medicine in June 2000. The study indicated that cola beverages were "highly associated with bone fractures." In their conclusion the authors warned that, ". . . national concern and alarm about the health impact of carbonated beverage consumption on teenaged girls is supported by the findings of this study."

Phosphoric Acid And Tooth Rot

Now that soft drinks are sold in almost all public and private schools, dentists are noticing a condition in teenagers that used to be found only in the elderly—a complete loss of enamel on the teeth, resulting in yellow teeth. The culprit is phosphoric acid in soft drinks, which causes tooth rot as well as digestive problems and bone loss. Dentists are reporting complete loss of the enamel on the front teeth in teenaged boys and girls who habitually drink sodas. Normally the saliva is slightly alkaline, with a pH of about 7.4. When sodas are sipped throughout the day, as is often the case with teenagers, the phosphoric acid lowers the pH of the saliva to acidic levels. In order to buffer this acidic saliva, and bring the pH level above 7 again, the body pulls calcium ions from the teeth. The result is a very rapid depletion of the enamel coating on the teeth.

When dentists do cosmetic bonding, they first roughen up the enamel with a chemical compound—that chemical is phosphoric acid! Young people who must have all their yellowed front teeth cosmetically bonded have already done part of the dentist's job, by roughening up the tooth surface with phosphoric acid.

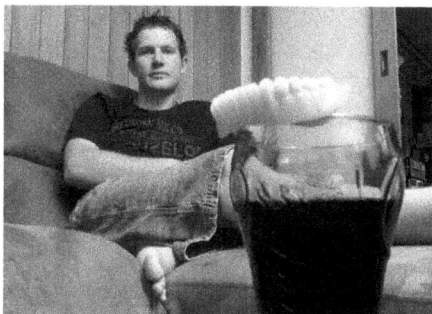

Recently the National Institutes of Health held a conference on dental decay worldwide. The speakers discussed many possible causes and solutions, but not one mentioned the known effects of phosphoric acid in soft drinks!

The Battle Ahead

The dangers of society's other drinking problem have recently been in the news. Senator Christopher Dodd and Representative George Miller have commissioned a study on the uses and oversight of school vending machines. Pending legislation in the State of Maryland would turn school soda vending machines off during the school day. Senator Patrick Leahy has introduced a bill requiring the USDA to rule within 18 months on banning or limiting the sale of soda and junk food in schools before students have eaten lunch.

The soft drink industry has fought back by funding four studies on soft drink consumption at the Georgetown Center for Food and Nutrition Policy. Predictably, these studies found that there was nothing wrong with soft drinks. In fact, researchers said they found a positive relationship between soft drink consumption and exercise. All this means is that those children participating in sports programs drank more sodas.

The National Association of Secondary School Principals (NAASP) says that decisions about soda sales should be made at the local level and not by the federal government. School administrators are caught between demands of a few parents for a saner food policy and the need for more funds in the face of dwindling school budgets.

One good idea comes from the Philippines, a country where malnutrition is an ominous health threat. A recently devised plan there would allow citizens to cash in on the country's "junk food diet" by taxing every liter bottle of carbonated soft drink sold. If the US taxed soft drink sales, the new income stream generated could then be distributed to declining school budgets. Is this not a better idea than forcing our schools to sell their souls to soft drink companies under the titanic sink of fiscal degradation?

The alarm has been sounded! Are you listening? I strongly encourage all who are concerned about the health of their families to consider the debilitating consequences of drinking soft drinks.

How many more studies and reports need to be published before we notice the tsunami lurking ahead? In the 1970s, we finally recognized the risks of smoking. In the 1990s, the problem of teenage drinking became widely known. The new millennium is the time for awakening to the risks of soda consumption—America's other drinking problem.

References

"Soft Drinks Hard Facts," The Washington Post /Health, February 27, 2001.

"Schools Hooked on Junk Food," The Washington Post, February 27, 2001.

"Coke to Dilute Push in Schools For Its Products," The New York Times, March 14, 2001.

National Soft Drink Association. Web Site, www.thesodafountain.com.

"Some Nutritional Aspects of Sugar, Candy and Sweetened Carbonated Beverages," Journal of the American Medical Association, 1942;120:763-5.

Liquid Candy, How Soft Drinks are Harming Americans' Health, M. Jacobson, PhD.

Web Site, CSPI.com.

"Soft Drinks Undermining Americans' Health: Teens Consume Twice as Much 'Liquid Candy' as Milk," CSPI Press Release, Oct. 21, 1998.

Food Surveys Research Group – What We Eat in America. USDA Web Site.

"Relationship Between Consumption of Sugar-Sweetened Drinks & Childhood Obesity: AProspective and Observational Analysis," The Lancet, 2001. 357:505-08.

"The Cariogenicity of Soft Drinks in the United States," Journal of the American Dental Association, Aug. 1984 109(2):241-5.

"How Sugar-Containing Drinks Might Increase Adiposity in Children," The Lancet, 2001. 357; 9225.

"Junk Food Boost for Health in the Philippines," The Lancet, 1997. 350; 9087.

"Teenaged Girls, Carbonated Beverage Consumption, and Bone Fractures," Pediatrics & Adolescent Medicine, June 2000. 154(6).

"Carbonated beverages, dietary calcium, the dietary calcium/phosphorus ratio, and bone fractures in girls and boys," Journal of Adolescent Health, May 1994. 15(3): 210-5.

"Soft drink consumption among US children and adolescents: nutritional consequences," Journal of the American Dietetic Association,. April 1999. (4): 436-41.

"Irish concerned about health effects of stimulant soft drinks," The Lancet, December 2000; 356; 9245.

The Diet Cure, Julia Ross. 1999. Penguin Books, NY, NY.

Eating for A's. Alexander Schauss, Barbara Friedlander Meyer, Arnold Meyer. 1991: NY Pocket Books.

The Encyclopedia of Nutrition & Good Health. Robert Ronzio.1997. Facts on File, NY.

Fast Food Nation. Eric Schlosser. 2001. Houghton Mifflin.

Nourishing Traditions. Sally Fallon, with Mary Enig, PhD. NewTrends Publishing, Washington, DC.

75.

Pepsi, Coke Double Up As Pesticides

Even Pesky Pests Can't Handle Them

What are Coke and Pepsi good for besides cleaning rust off the bumper of your car? If you're a farmer in India, they're also good as pesticides.

Hundreds of farmers in Andhra Pradesh and Chhattisgarh areas have discovered that spraying their cotton and chilly crop with world famous beverages works out cheaper than many expensive pesticides.

Gotu Laxmaiah, a farmer from Ramakrishnapuram, says he was delighted with his new cola spray, which he applied this year to several hectares of cotton. "I observed that the pests began to die after the soft drink was sprayed on my cotton," he said.

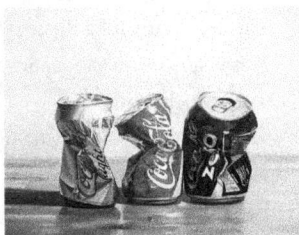

Laxmaiah and others say their cola sprays are invaluable because they are safe to handle, do not need to be diluted and, mainly, because they are so cheap. One litre of highly concentrated Avant, Tracer or Nuvocron -- three popular Indian pesticides -- costs around Rs 10,000 (£120). A litre-and-a-half of locally made Coca-Cola costs just Rs 30.

Its becoming a bit hard to swallow for the soft drink manufacturers. A spokesman for Coca-Cola in Atlanta, USA, said: "We are aware of one isolated case where a farmer may have used a soft drink as part of his crop management routine. But soft drinks do not act in a similar way to pesticides when applied to the ground or crops. There is no scientific basis for this and the use of soft drinks for this purpose would be totally ineffective."

Anupam Verma, Pepsi sales manager in Chhattisgarh, admits that sales figures in rural areas of the state have increased by 20%.

According to Mike Adams, there's something in the sodas that may deters pests. Phosphoric acid, for example, is highly acidic and may function as a pest deterrent. Or perhaps it's the aspartame in the diet soda. Since aspartame is well known to promote neurological side effects in humans, it is conceivable that it may function as a neurotoxic pesticide when sprayed on crops.

In addition to be useful as pesticides when sprayed on crops, Coke and Pepsi are also very good at cleaning up blood stains from concrete due to their carbonation effect. They can clean toilet bowls, car bumpers and garage floors, too.

Oh, and if you really want to, you can also drink Coke and Pepsi, although that's not advisable unless you really want a stomach full of high-fructose corn syrup and phosphoric acid.

76.

Ingredients In Soft Drinks—A Witch's Brew

High Fructose Corn Syrup, now used in preference to sugar in sodas, is associated with poor development of collagen in growing animals, especially in the context of copper deficiency. All fructose must be metabolized by the liver. Animals on high-fructose diets develop liver problems similar to those of alcoholics.

Aspartame, used in diet sodas, is a potent neurotoxin and endocrine disrupter.

Caffeine stimulates the adrenal gland without providing nourishment. In large amounts, caffeine can lead to adrenal exhaustion, especially in children.

Phosphoric acid, added to give soft drinks "bite," is associated with calcium loss.

Citric acid often contains traces of MSG, a neurotoxin.

Artificial Flavors may also contain traces of MSG.

Water may contain high amounts of fluoride and other contaminants.

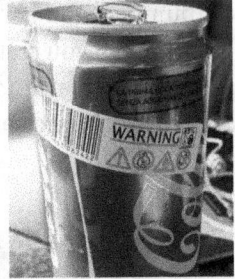

Cola Drinks Lead To Gestational Diabetes

Drinking too much sugar-sweetened cola a week prior to pregnancy may increase risk of developing gestational diabetes, according to a new study.

The study was conducted by researchers from LSU Health Sciences Center New Orleans School of Public Health, Eunice Kennedy Shriver National Institute of Child Health and Human Development (NICHD), Harvard School of Public Health, Brigham and Women's Hospital, and Harvard Medical School.

The research team studied a group of 13,475 women from the Nurses' Health Study II. During 10 years of follow-up, 860 incident GDM cases were identified.

After adjustment for known risk factors for GDM including age, family history of diabetes, parity, physical activity, smoking status, sugar-sweetened beverage intake, alcohol intake, pre-pregnancy BMI, and Western dietary pattern, intake of sugar-sweetened cola was positively associated with the risk of GDM.

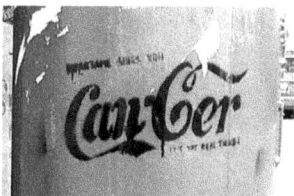

"Compared with women who consumed less than 1 serving per month, those who consumed more than 5 servings per week of sugar-sweetened cola had a 22 percent greater GDM risk," said Liwei Chen, Assistant Professor of Epidemiology at LSU Health Sciences Center New Orleans School of Public Health, and the lead author of the paper.

The study was published in the December 2009 issue of Diabetes Care .

Fruit Juices

Consumers often drink commercial fruit juices in the belief that they are healthier than soft drinks. However, the manufacture of fruit juices is a highly industrialized process as seen in earlier chapters. Although the juice is pasteurized under high temperatures and pressures, pressure-resistent and temperature-resistant fungi and molds can remain in the juice. Many mutagenic factors have been detected in commercial orange juice. A compound made of soy protein and pectin is added to orange juice so that it remains opaque and doesn't settle.

Other fruits, such as grapes, present additional problems because of the large amounts of fluoride-containing pesticides used on the crops.

Packaged fruit juices are very high in unhealthy sugars and have actually been more detrimental to the teeth of test animals than sodas!

If you want to drink fruit juice, buy a juicer and make your own with organic fruit.

77.

Refined Table Salt

Taste That Kills

Pure sea salts contain as many as 92 essential minerals; however, refined common table salts contain only 2 elements, sodium and chloride. In June of 2006, citing increased risk of hypertension, heart diseases and stroke, the American Medical Association issued a call to have salt removed from the "generally recognized as safe" food ingredient list. But what the AMA is too dim-witted to say is that it is the highly processed table salts that are poisonous to human health, not real whole sea salt with all the minerals still intact.

The truth is that table salt is not healthy not because of all the sodium but because it's presented for consumption without the normal mineral balance. Refined cocoa is cocaine; refined poppy is heroine, all three create addictions. Excessive salt is a learned taste, not a natural one.

Whole sea salts have those important minerals such as potassium and magnesium still intact. The synergistic effect of all the minerals in whole, unrefined salt helps the body to stay in balance. It is best to use natural sea salts (gray, pink, course, fine, etc.) in moderation for one's salt needs. Common table salt unfortunately contains aluminum used as an anti-caking agent. Aluminum is a toxic metal that has been linked to Alzheimer's disease and has no place in a healthy diet. Many brands are now using silica coating as an anti-caking agent. This trashes kidneys in just few years. This is one of the factors responsible for the chronic kidney disease epidemic around the globe.

Sodium is crucial for maintaining the health of the human system. It permeates the fluid between cells. Besides being a component of extracellular fluid that bathes every living cell, sodium is important in our blood and our lymphatic fluid. It is also necessary for the production of hydrochloric acid, the digestive enzyme secreted by the stomach in order to digest protein. Along with potassium, sodium is required for the proper functioning of our nerves and the contraction of our muscles. (The heart, as you may know, is our hardest - working muscle.) Finally, sodium is necessary to maintain several kinds of equilibrium - fluid balance, electrolyte balance and pH (acid/alkaline) balance - which are all of the utmost importance to the body.

Unrefined salt does not cause high blood pressure whereas regular refined salt does. All the scientific studies that have been done showing that salt "causes" high blood pressure were done on people, who took regular, refined salt. In the early 1980s, one Harvard researcher studied the blood pressure of people who follow the macrobiotic diet. He found that macrobiotic people, despite eating a fairly salty diet with generous amounts of miso, shoyu, salty pickles, etc, had very healthy blood pressure levels of about 10 points below the national average.

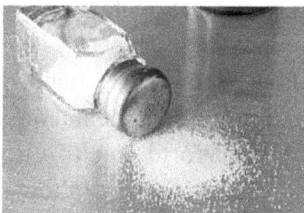

All the minerals processed out of white foods are important. Minerals provide the spark for most of the body's cellular processes and keep them running efficiently. Inorganic mineral nutrients are also essential in the structural composition of hard and soft body tissues and are necessary in processes such as the action of enzyme systems, the contraction of muscles, nerve reactions and the clotting of blood. Humans need a wide range of minerals to maintain good health and we need them in the right amounts and relations to each other (co-action). Small variations in established minerals levels can cause pathological states to occur.

Our body relies on ionic minerals and trace minerals to conduct and generate billions of tiny electrical impulses every second of our existence.

Mineral nutrients consist of two classes: the major elements such as calcium, phosphorus, magnesium, iron, iodine, and potassium; and trace elements such as copper, cobalt, manganese, fluorine, zinc and many others. All of these must be supplied in our diet because the body is unable to manufacture its own, and can only maintain its mineral balance for short periods of time. When the intake of minerals in our system becomes depleted, it draws from stores laid down in the muscles, the liver and bones.

Refined Salt Intake Linked To Stroke

The association between high salt intake and high blood pressure is well established, and it has been suggested that a population-wide reduction in dietary salt intake has the potential to substantially reduce the levels of cardiovascular disease. Reducing refined sodium intake should be a major public health priority for governments and nongovernmental organizations.

The World Health Organization recommended level of salt consumption is 5 g (about one teaspoon) per day at the population level.

In a study, Professor Pasquale Strazzullo at the University of Naples, Italy and Professor Francesco Cappuccio at the University of Warwick, UK, analysed the results of 13 published studies involving over 170,000 people that directly assessed the relationship between levels of habitual salt intake and rates of stroke and cardiovascular diseases. Differences in study design and quality were taken into account to minimise bias. Their analysis shows unequivocally that a difference of 5 gms a day in habitual salt intake is associated with a 23 per cent difference in the rate of stroke and a 17 per cent difference in the rate of total cardiovascular disease.

Based on these results, the authors estimate that reducing daily refined salt intake by 5 gms at the population level could avert one and a quarter million deaths from stroke and almost three million deaths from cardiovascular disease each year.

Reduce Refined Salt For A Healthier Life

In another study published in the Canadian Medical Association Journal, a diet high in sodium has been linked to high blood pressure, vascular and cardiac damage, stomach cancer, osteoporosis, and other diseases. Almost 1 billion adults worldwide have hypertension, and 17-30 percent of these cases can be attributed to excessive sodium consumption.

In developed countries, almost 80 percent of sodium intake is from processed food.

The researchers led by Dr. Kevin Willis, at Canadian Stroke Network, have said that the regulation of the food industry by the government will bring about the most effective change, although immediate voluntary action is desired.

"A population-wide reduction in sodium intake could prevent a large proportion of cardiovascular events in both normotensive and hypertensive populations. For example, a population-wide decrease of 2 mm Hg diastolic blood pressure would be estimated to lower the prevalence of hypertension by 17 percent, coronary artery disease by 6 percent and the risk of stroke by 15 percent, with many of the benefits occurring among patients with normal blood pressure," wrote Willis.

The researchers recommend that national public health policy be focused on reformulating processed food, educating consumers, labelling food clearly, and setting timelines to meet these targets.

Non-governmental groups should lobby the food industry to change practice and partner with governments to mount public education campaigns.

Besides, health care professionals should counsel patients about healthy choices in reducing sodium consumption. Training to do this should be incorporated into curricula.

Misconceptions About Salt

There is urgent need to bring back whole sea salts and ban the refined free flowing salts. Their usage is making entire nations sick.

Salt is required. Unless you're told specifically by a qualified specialist about limiting or stopping your salt intake, it should not be done so because it can cause terrible weakness, drowsiness, depression, convulsions, and even coma.

Interventional Cardiologist from India, Dr. Shantanu Deshpande says that salt is essential for maintaining homeostasis in our bodies. "The normal requirement is just 500 mg per day. Normally excessive salt intake is excreted in the urine. But in almost 50 per cent of individuals, the kidneys are not able to handle this excess of sodium. Excess of salt in your blood stream retains more water resulting in a rise in blood volumes and blood pressure. It also results in hypertrophy of heart and blood vessel musculature resulting in permanent rise in blood pressure. These effects are more pronounced in the elderly and diabetics. Reducing salt intake in your diet reduces blood pressure. A low salt diet containing less than 5 gm of salt per day is recommended for high blood pressure patients who should avoid items like junk food.

Senior Interventional Cardiologist Dr Rajiv Bhagwat says, "Reduction of refined salt is one of the most important and effective life style modifications to reduce blood pressure. A 2 mm reduction in historic blood pressure reduces stroke mortality by 10 per cent and seven per cent reduction in mortality from coronary diseases. Besides reducing blood pressure, salt reduction also reduces Left Ventricular Sickness (Hyper Trophy), reduces protein loss in urine, reduces osteoporosis and bone mineral loss with age, protects against stomach cancer, asthma and possibly against cataracts as well. Increase your intake of potassium, which is found in plenty in fruits, legumes, nuts and vegetables. Their intake is an effective mean to reduce blood pressure."

78.

SAD - Standard American Diet

By Ninja Guru

L ook what the Standard American Diet spells when you put it all together. It spells SAD and how appropriate that title is when you think about it. In a span of over thirty years (in my lifetime) the rate of obesity has skyrocketed exponetially. Also, the rate of people getting adult-onset diabetes (type 2), stroke, hypertension, cancer and other obesity related diseases has increased dramatically. The statistics tell the whole story. According to the CDC (Center for Disease Control and Prevention), obesity in adults has increased by 60% in the last twenty years and obesity in children has tripled in the past thirty years. A staggering 33% of American adults are obese and obesity-related deaths have climbed to more than 300,000 a year, second only to tobacco-related deaths. Why are so many Americans so fat. This is the problem of overabundance and convenience.

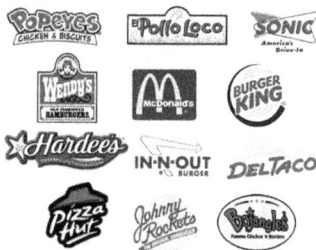

> In this age, Kali-yuga, gradually food grains will be reduced. It is stated in the Srimad-Bhagavatam, Twelfth Canto. No rice, no wheat, no milk, no sugar will be available. One has to eat meat. This will be the condition. And maybe to eat the human flesh also. This sinful life is degrading so much so that they will become more and more sinful.
> ~ Srila Prabhupada (Lecture, Bhagavad-gita 2.6, London, August 6, 1973)

485

The Age Of Convenience

After World War II the modern American housewife was searching for an easy and convenient way to feed her family efficiently and affordably. The answer came in the form of the now famous T.V. dinners. Coupled with this was the building of America's national highway system. This meant that American's were on the move. Diner's dotted along the highways provided travellers with a quick and affordable meal on the go. The emphasis was on convenience. Eventually, these diners gave way to the modern fast-food chain, McDonald's being one of the first. As the economy of the 50's and 60's kept humming so did the stagnant American lifestyle. American's were increasingly relying on fast-food as the main staples of their diet. This, in addition to processed foods, refined sugars and inactive lifestyle has lead to the modern obesity epidemic.

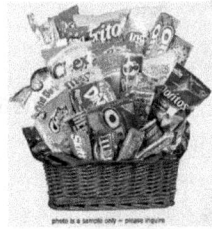

And we have seen even in our childhood that poor men, the laborer class, servant, they came from village in the town. We were residents of town, Calcutta, The servants class, they would come... Everywhere, not in Calcutta, everywhere. The villagers would come, and the small salary. Even in our young days, we were paying salaries to the servants, twelve rupees, fourteen rupees, without any food. And still they would save at least ten to twelve rupees out of that. And this money, the servant would send to his wife at home, and as soon as there is two hundred rupees, he'll purchase a piece of land. And in this way, when he has got sufficient land for producing food for the whole family, then he would no more come to city for working. We have seen it.

That means as soon as one has a land sufficient to produce, he is safe. His food problem—that is the real problem—is solved. So people are not being trained up to... In America, I have seen. Now the farmers, the father is working on the farm, and the sons, they do not come. They live in the city. This is the tendency all over the world. They are not producing food grains. Therefore there is scarcity. There is scarcity of...

So anyway, the whole world situation is degrading, that people are not producing their own food. This is the problem, real problem. Ksetra-ksetra-jna. This example is given. As every man must possess a piece of land... ~ Srila Prabhupada

79.

Junk Food

Dangerous And Addictive As Drugs

A British study suggests that a diet of burgers, chips and cake programmes your brain to crave even more for foods that are high in sugar, salt and fat content - just like drugs.

Over the years, junk food can become a substitute for happiness and can lead bingers to become addicted.

Paul Kenny, a neuro scientist, carried out the research which shows how dangerous high fat and high sugar foods can be to our health. "You lose control. It's the hallmark of addiction," he said.

Researchers believe it is one of the first studies to suggest brains may react in the same way to junk food as they do to drugs, reports the Telegraph.

"This is the most complete evidence till date that suggests obesity and drug addiction have common neuro-biological foundations," said Paul Johnson, Kenny's work colleague.

Kenny, who began his research at Guy's Hospital in London, but now works at Florida's Scripps Research Institute, divided rats into three groups for his research.

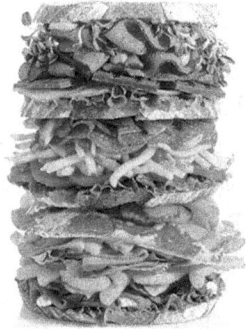

The beauty of making food at home is knowing exactly what goes into it!

One got normal amount of healthy food to eat. Another lot was given restricted amount of junk food and the third group was given unlimited amount of junk, including cheesecake, fatty meat products, and cheap sponge cakes and chocolate snacks.

There were no adverse effects on the first two groups but the rats who ate as much junk food as they wanted became, very fat and started bingeing.

When researchers electronically stimulated the part of the brain that feels pleasure, they found that the rats on unlimited junk food needed more and more stimulation to register the same level of pleasure as animals on healthier diets.

3 Burgers A Week Enough To Invite Asthma

Children who love junk food and eat at least three burgers in a week are inviting asthma, says a latest research.

The study which was conducted on 50,000 children across 20 countries revealed that the risk of asthma, because of improper diet, is highest of all in better-off countries, express.co.uk reports.

The findings showed that youngsters who enjoy a healthy diet rich in fruit and vegetables have the lowest risk to get affected by the disease.

When compared between rich and poor countries, it was found that a diet high in fish protected children against wheeze in well-off countries, while a diet rich in cooked vegetables guarded youngsters in poor countries.

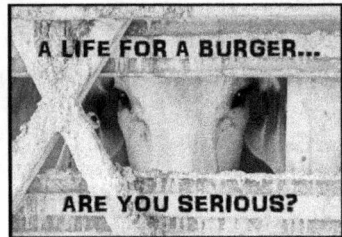

A LIFE FOR A BURGER... ARE YOU SERIOUS?

Elaine Vickers, of Asthma UK has advised children to "eat a healthy, balanced diet and get plenty of exercise".

Junk Food Ups Diabetes In Kids

A group of more than 100 diabetes experts has called for laws to ban ads of junk food that target children.

The experts from Royal College of Physicians of Edinburgh said that this was the best alternative for combating the rising cases of Type 2 diabetes amongst youngsters – which is caused by obesity.

They said that these ads should not just be banned in print, but in billboards and TV too.

The group also called for tighter regulations of the food, drink and catering industry following their recent meeting.

"Rates of obesity and diabetes are increasing at alarming rates and pose one of the most serious health challenges of this time," says Dr Scott Ramsay.

In response to this, diabetes experts from across the UK have come together to call on the Scottish and UK governments to demonstrate greater leadership in tackling this crisis.

"In particular we believe that the lessons from effective legislation on smoking should be used to promote healthier diets, increased physical activity and to inform transport and planning policy."

"This should involve tighter regulation of the food and drink industry and the extension of restrictions on 'less healthy' food and drink advertising in children"'s television programmes to all forms of advertising aimed at children," Ramsay adds.

However, Ian Barber of the Advertising Association says there is little evidence that advertising is a main driving factor behind obesity. "Advertising might influence which brand you choose, but there is very little evidence that it drives consumption," he adds.

Instant Noodles May Lead to Chronic Illness

By Althea Chang

> *They are now killing animal, but animal lives on this grass and grains. When there will be no grass, no grains, where they will get animal? They'll kill their own children and eat. That time is coming. Nature's law is that you grow your own food. But they are not interested in growing food. They are interested in manufacturing bolts and nuts.*
> *-Srila Prabhupada (Morning Walk — June 22, 1974, Germany)*

Ramen noodles could be putting college students and frugal eaters at greater risk of developing chronic illness, according to a recent study.

The instant noodles have long been a staple for the cash-strapped, but they could be putting their fans at risk of further nutritional deficits already caused by a lack of affordable and fresh fruits and vegetables, suggests a study presented at a meeting of the Dietitians Association of Australia.

According to the study, conducted by Australian researchers Danielle Gallegos and Kai Wen Ong, one in four college students reported insecurity about being able to afford food.

Of those students, two-thirds said they ate two or less servings of fruit per week, suggesting that money spent on more-filling but sodium- and MSG-laden Ramen noodles and fast food takes away from funds that could be spent on healthy but less-filling fruits and vegetables.

Those who relied on instant noodles and other cheap food with little nutritional content were at greater risk of chronic diseases including cancer, diabetes and heart disease, the researchers found.

While the study was based in Australia, results seem to reflect conditions among college kids and low-income individuals across the world.

Pets, Like Humans, Are Victims Of Junk Food

The junk food and poor eating habits affecting humans is also killing their four-legged pals, say veterinary surgeons and experts.

Allergies and obesity are reducing the life expectancy of Lassies and Mittens nourished worldwide on industrial foodstuffs, says Gerard Lippert, a Belgian acupuncturist for animals who has just completed a study on the diets of 600 dead dogs.

Of the 600 furry corpses he examined "those fed on processed foods died three years earlier than those fed on food made in the home."

The day is coming when a single carrot, freshly observed, will set off a revolution.
  -Paul Cezanne

Rippert said he was increasingly called on to heal skin, motor and digestive problems.

"Dry dog food and cat food croquettes are over-heated, which destroys vitamins, trace elements and other basic nutritional

---

yata-yamam gata-rasam
puti paryusitam ca yat
ucchistam api camedhyam
bhojanam tamasa-priyam (Bhagavad Gita 17.10)

Food prepared more than three hours before being eaten, food that is tasteless, decomposed and putrid, and food consisting of remnants and untouchable things is dear to those in the mode of darkness.

The purpose of food is to increase the duration of life, purify the mind and aid bodily strength. This is its only purpose. In the past, great authorities selected those foods that best aid health and increase life's duration, such as milk products, sugar, rice, wheat, fruits and vegetables. These foods are very dear to those in the mode of goodness. Some other foods, such as baked corn and molasses, while not very palatable in themselves, can be made pleasant when mixed with milk or other foods. They are then in the mode of goodness. All these foods are pure by nature. They are quite distinct from untouchable things like meat and liquor. Fatty foods, as mentioned in the eighth verse, have no connection with animal fat obtained by slaughter. Animal fat is available in the form of milk, which is the most wonderful of all foods. Milk, butter, cheese and similar products give animal fat in a form which rules out any need for the killing of innocent creatures. It is only through brute mentality that this killing goes on. The civilized method of obtaining needed fat is by milk. Slaughter is the way of subhumans. Protein is amply available through split peas, dal, whole wheat, etc.

Foods in the mode of passion, which are bitter, too salty, or too hot or overly mixed with red pepper, cause misery by reducing the mucus in the stomach, leading to disease. Foods in the mode of ignorance or darkness are essentially those that are not fresh. Any food cooked more than three hours before it is eaten (except prasadam, food offered to the Lord) is considered to be in the mode of darkness. Because they are decomposing, such foods give a bad odor, which often attracts people in this mode but repulses those in the mode of goodness.

~ Srila Prabhupada

elements," he says. "We don't know the origin of the proteins in the foods," he adds. "And there's an excessive amount of cereal, often genetically modified, and very little vegetables."

Laurence Colliard, a veterinary surgeon and nutritionist located in the Paris suburbs says, "I'm seeing an increasing number of allergies, diarrhea, vomitting, skin dermatitis as well as cases of obesity, specially amid cats because of the excessively high energy content in industrially-produced cat foods."

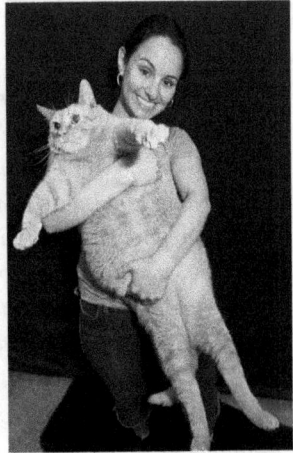

The pet food industry was born in England where James Spratt produced the world's first dog biscuits in 1860. Some 150 years later, many Internet sites are calling for a return to natural foods for pets.

It's only in the last 100 years pet owners have been led to believe that pets cannot survive without packaged food. They are told it would be harmful if they were to give them the scraps from their own home cooked meals.

Food grains or vegetables are factually eatables. The human being eats different kinds of food grains, vegetables, fruits, etc., and the animals eat the refuse of the food grains and vegetables, grass, plants, etc. Human beings who are accustomed to eating meat and flesh must also depend on the production of vegetation in order to eat the animals. Therefore, ultimately, we have to depend on the production of the field and not on the production of big factories. The field production is due to sufficient rain from the sky, and such rains are controlled by demigods like Indra, sun, moon, etc., and they are all servants of the Lord. The Lord can be satisfied by sacrifices; therefore, one who cannot perform them will find himself in scarcity -- that is the law of nature. Yajna, specifically the sankirtana-yajna prescribed for this age, must therefore be performed to save us at least from scarcity of food supply.

~ Srila Prabhupada (Bhagavad-gita 3.14)

80.

Why Quick, Cheap Food Is Actually More Expensive

By Mark Hyman, MD, For The Huffington Post

The odd paradox is that junk food is cheaper than healthy. I was in a grocery store yesterday. While I was squeezing avocados to pick just the right ones for my family's dinner salad, I overheard a conversation from a couple that had also picked up an avocado.

"Oh, these avocados look good, let's get some."

Then looking up at the price, they said, "Two for five dollars!" Dejected, they put the live avocado back and walked away from the vegetable aisle toward the aisles full of dead, boxed, canned, packaged goods where they can buy thousands of calories of poor-quality, nutrient-poor, factory-made, processed foods filled with sugar, fat, and salt for the same five dollars. This is the scenario millions of Americans struggling to feed their families face every day.

The odd paradox is that food insecurity—not knowing where the next meal is coming from or not having enough money to adequately feed your family—leads to obesity, diabetes and chronic disease. Examining this paradox may help us advocate for policies that make producing fresh fruits, vegetables, and whole other foods cheaper, while rethinking the almost $300 billion in government subsides that support the production of cheap, processed food derived from corn and soy.

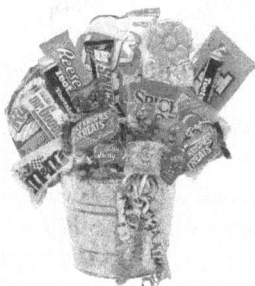

At the same time, a Food Revolution, along the lines of that advocated by Jamie Oliver, a radical chef, can help Americans

There is enough place for producing food. I have seen Africa, Australia. Enough place. If the foodstuff is produced there, ten times of the population can be well fed. But they are: "Don't enter. Don't come here." The Africans will say to the Indians, "Don't come here. Go out." What is this? Therefore Krishna consciousness is so nice. We say, "Everything belongs to Krishna. We are all sons of Krishna. Let us live peacefully and utilize Krishna's property." This is the best philosophy. But the so-called politicians and leaders, they are saying "No, you cannot enter here," immigration. America has got enough place to produce food. But they will, although they have gone to the United Nation, UNESCO, they could not find out any solution. Although there is possibility of producing ten times of the requisites of the whole population of the world, they will not allow. They will not allow. On God's side, this unit, this planet, purnam idam purnam adah purnat purnam udacyate [Isopanisad, Invocation] -- everything is complete. You require water. They save three times water than the land. And the water is distributed over the land, parjanyad anna-sambhavah so there will be sufficient food grains. And annad bhavanti bhutani [Bg. 3.14]. And if there is sufficient to eat, have sufficient eatables to the animals and to the men, then everything is prosperous. So where is that arrangement? There is enough land, enough possibility, enough water. Now utilize them and produce food grain, eat nicely and live peacefully and chant Hare Krishna and go back to home, back to Godhead. This is our philosophy. Why there should be industry? You want to eat after all. Instead of eating this flesh, killing poor animals, why don't you produce food grains, fruits, flowers, food grain, and take milk from the animals and produce milk products, all nutritious food, all nice food, and be happy and remember God for His kindness. This is civilization. What is this nonsense civilization? Now there is petrol problem. I see so many buses, and not a single man, one or two men. And for two men a big huge bus is being run, and so much petrol is consumed unnecessarily. I have seen. They are creating simply, the so-called advancement of civilization, creating problems, that's all. And that is due to these rascal leaders. Andha yathandhair upaniyamanas te 'pisa-tantryam uru-damni baddhah [SB 7.5.31]. They do not know what is the ideal of life, what is the aim of life. They are creating hodge-podge civilization and putting the mass of people in chaotic condition. This is the sum and substance. I do not know whether you'll agreed with me, but this is my study of the whole situation.

~ Srila Prabhupada (Room Conversation with Richard Webster, chairman, Societa Filosofica Italiana -- May 24, 1974, Rome)

take back their table and their health from a food industry that has driven us to eat more than 50 percent of our meals out of the home compared to less than 2 percent 100 years ago. And most of those meals eaten at home are produced in plants, not grown on plants, are from a food chemist's lab, not a farmer's field. Cooking and eating whole fresh foods at home, can be cheaper, more fun, and simpler than most people think.

One of the principal offenders amongst food additives is monosodium glutamate, commonly known as MSG. Researchers at Monash University have called for manufacturers to stop adding MSG to food. The use of this toxic chemical to artificially enhance the flavor of tinned food is so widespread that it is difficult to find any type of canned or processed food that does not contain it. It is commonly used in fast food outlets, the restaurant trade and is particularly favored by Chinese restaurants. Also it is used in the manufacture of hamburgers, pizzas and sausages. People who experience a reaction to MSG can suffer such symptoms. as tightening of the facial muscles, visual disturbances, headache, gastrointestinal pain, fainting, irritability, tiredness, dry mouth and disturbed sleep. These symptoms can be either immediate or delayed. It is now known that MSG slows learning ability, especially when given during the first few weeks of life. (Many tinned baby foods, in the past, have contained MSG). High doses can cause visible brain lesions, whilst low doses upset brain chemistry by triggering nerves which are not meant to be triggered.

Don't bring all rotten. In the market you cannot get fresh. All three hundred years old. Anything fresh, that is full of vitamin. Grow fresh, take fresh. In India there is no system to purchase three-hundred-years-old bread and eat. It must be freshly made. Wife is preparing in the simple oven, husband is eating, children are eating. You know Yasodamayi calling Krishna? "Come back! Your father is waiting!" You remember this? That is Indian system. The father and the children, they sit down, mother will bring fresh dal, rice and capati, and distribute, and they eat. We used to do that. Along with father we shall sit down for eating, separately. There was no need of table -- on the ground. And mother will distribute, cook. No servant; mother personally, wife personally.

~ Srila Prabhupada (Paris, August 3, 1976: Room Conversation at New Mayapura Farm)

81.

McDonald's Happy Meal - Is It biodegradable?

Shows No Sign Of Decomposing After Six Months

By Daily Mail Reporter, 21st October 2010

Looking almost as fresh as the day it was bought, this McDonald's Happy Meal is in fact a staggering six months old.

Photographed every day for the past half a year by Manhattan artist Sally Davies the kids meal of fries and burger is without a hint of mould or decay.

In a work entitled The Happy Meal Project, Mrs Davies, 54, has charted the seemingly indestructible fast food meals progress as it refuses to yield to the forces of nature.

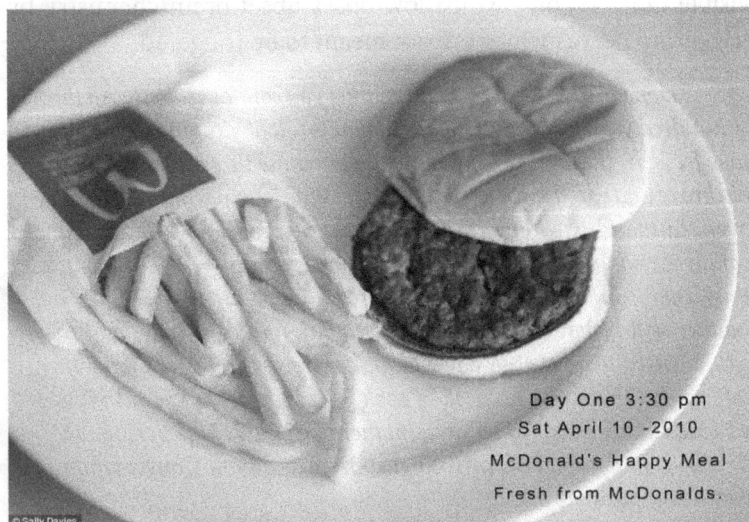

Day One 3:30 pm
Sat April 10 -2010
McDonald's Happy Meal
Fresh from McDonalds.

Expecting the food to begin moulding after a few days, Mrs Davies' surprise turned to shock as the fries and burger still had not shown any signs of decomposition after two weeks.

'It was then that I realised that something strange might be going on with this food that I had bought,' she explains.

'The fries shrivelled slightly as did the burger patty, but the overall appearance of the food did not change as the weeks turned to months.

'And now, at six months old, the food is plastic to the touch and has an acrylic sheen to it.

'The only change that I can see is that it has become hard as a rock.

Prabhupada: From an economic point of view, if one man has a cow and four acres of land he has no economic problem. That we want to start. He can independently live in any part of the world. Simply he must have one cow and four acres of land. So let the people be divided in four acres of land and a cow and there will be no economic question. All the factories will be closed. [everyone laughs]

[At this point, Allen and some of the New Vrindaban members discuss some of the problems of farming.]

Prabhupada: There is a proverb that agriculture is the noblest profession. Is it not?

Allen: Yes.

Prabhupada: And Krishna was a farmer, cowherd boy. Yes, and in Vedic literature you will find that the richest man is estimated by the possession of grains and cows. If he has sufficient quantity of grains, then he is rich. And actually that is a fact. Keep cows and have sufficient grains and the whole economic problem is solved. As for eating and sleeping ... you can take some wood and four pillows. Of course in your country it is cold, but in India all year they are lying under the sky.

Allen: Men lived this way for 20,000-30,000 years. Till the 19th Century.

Prabhupada: We have to think, "Plain living, high thinking." The necessities of this bodily existence should be minimized -- not unhealthy, but healthy to keep oneself fit. But the time should be utilized to develop Krishna Consciousness, spiritual life. Then his whole problem is solved.

(A.C. Bhaktivedanta Swami Prabhupada and poet Allen Ginsberg Conversations)

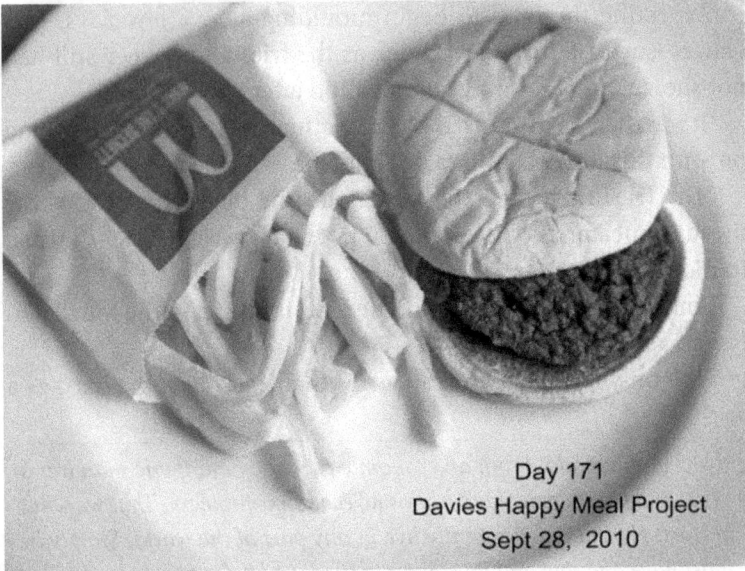

Day 171
Davies Happy Meal Project
Sept 28, 2010

Even though she is a vegan, Mrs Davies' experiment has brought her some fear.

Just like this Western civilization has created so may slaughterhouse for eating purposes. But wherefrom they are getting? From mahi, from the land. If there is no pasturing ground, grazing ground, wherefrom they will get the cows and the bulls? That is also... Because there is grass on the land and the cows and bulls eat them, therefore they grow. Then you cut their throat, civilized man, and eat, you rascal civilized man. But you are getting from the mahi, from the land. Without land, you cannot. Similarly, instead of cutting the throat of the cows, you can grow your food.

Why you are cutting the throat of the cows? After all, you have to get from the mahi, from the land. So as they are, the animal which you are eating, they are getting their eatables from the land. Why don't you get your eatables from the land? Therefore it is said, sarva-kama-dugha mahi. You can get all the necessities of your life from land. So dugha means produce. You can produce your food. Some land should be producing the foodstuff for the animals, and some land should be used for the production of your foodstuffs, grains, fruits, flowers, and take milk. Why should you kill these innocent animals? You take. You keep them muda, happy, and you get so much milk that it will moist, it will make wet the ground. This is civilization. This is civilization.

~ Srila Prabhupada

'I would be frightened at seeing this if I was a meat eater. Why hasn't even the bun become speckled with mould? It is odd.'

When asked if their food was not biodegradable, McDonald's spokeswoman Danya Proud said: 'This is nothing more than an outlandish claim and is completely false.'

It comes after Denver grandmother Joann Bruso left a Happy Meal to decay for a year to highlight the nutritional dangers of fast food.

Morgan Spurlock also made the film Super Size Me in 2004 charting the changes to his body eating just fast food for 28 days.

Richard Webster: Do you think it's worse now than it used to be? Can you say that it is worse, the condition of the world is worse now than it used to be or is it relatively the same or...?

Prabhupada: Oh, yes, yes. Worse now in these days because people cannot eat even. The facility which is given to the birds and beasts... They have no problem of eating. But you have created such a civilization that people are facing the problem so acutely that they have no means to eat. Do you think it is progress?

Richard Webster: Well, I would tend to doubt it very much.

Prabhupada: Yes, that is the problem.

82.

Biscuits, Cakes Up 'Womb Cancer' Risk

The Daily Mail, Aug 23, 2011

Women beware. Eating biscuits, buns or cakes three times a week could give you womb cancer, says a new study.

The 10-year study from the Karolinska Institute in Sweden looked at the eating habits of more than 60,000 women and found that those who gave themselves such a treat regularly were 33 per cent more likely to suffer the disease.

And for those who indulge more than three times a week, the risk jumps to 42 per cent.

The Swedish scientists wanted to see if there was a direct link between the amount of sweet foods eaten and the onset of cancer.

They studied data from thousands of women who, between 1987 and 1990, had answered dozens of questions on diet, lifestyle, weight and general health.

Ten years later, those still alive answered an even more extensive battery of questions on their eating habits.

In 2008, the researchers matched up the women's answers with their medical records, specifically looking for diagnoses of endometrial cancer – the most common form of womb cancer. They found 729 cases out of the 61,226 women studied.

> *Every man should produce his own food. That is Vedic culture. So this example is given: idam sariram ksetram. That means to own a certain piece of land is the basic civilization. Everyone must have a portion of land to produce his food. There will be no economic problem.*
> ~ *Srila Prabhupada*

Their findings were published in the journal Cancer Epidemiology, Biomarkers and Prevention

Why One Cookie Is Never Enough

Ever wondered why munching one cookie is not enough to satisfy your taste buds? Well, researchers have found the answer for you: the culprit is glucose-fructose syrup .

Research shows processed snack foods often contain glucose-fructose syrup, an ingredient that makes your brain think you need to eat more.

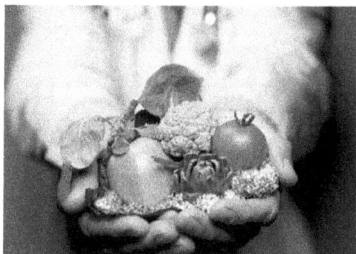

Glucose-fructose syrup is a type of sugar based on one found in fruit that is used to add bulk and moisture to foods. It's a common ingredient in processed snack foods, cereals, yogurt and fizzy drinks.

Dr Carel Le Roux, a consultant in metabolic medicine at Imperial College London, told the Daily Mail that fructose can scramble messages to the brain about being full.

"When we eat sugar, our body releases insulin which tells the brain that we have had enough to eat."

"High insulin levels are one of the factors that dampen the appetite," she said.

The expert added: "But fructose doesn't trigger as much of an insulin response as regular sugar, so the brain won't get the message that you are full."

We thought this was a good and very telling post from the LiveWell Wellness Centers. This is their 2-year old "fast food" display. The word "food" is most definitely questionable, seeing as what the fast food industry refers to as "food", has not molded or spoiled in any way. Insects don't even want it. Definitely think twice about giving this to your children. We truly are what we eat, so what does that say about today's society? ~ Briana Rognlin

83.

Chemicals, Chemicals, Everywhere

Floating Around In An Ocean Of Chemicals

In all of recorded history, humanity has never been engaged in a battle as significant as the one we face today. Never has our future been threatened as severely as it is now. The enemy is not a terrorist organization or a rogue nation seeking global domination; it is the environment we have created, the air we breathe, the water we drink, and the food we consume. We have taken the gifts of life presented to us and poisoned them.

Over the last two centuries, the human race has radically altered this planet and in so doing has radically reduced its own capacity to deal with toxic exposure.

Very, very large tract of land was lying vacant, nobody is producing any food. They are producing coffee.

How they will be happy? It is not possible. Most sinful activities. You produce your food. The bull will help you. And the cows will supply you milk. They are considered to be father and mother. Just like father earns money for feeding the children, similarly, the bulls help producing, plowing, producing food grains, and the cow gives milk, mother. And what is this civilization, killing father and mother? This is not good civilization. It will not stay. There will be catastrophe, waiting. Many times it has happened, and it will happen because transgressing the law of nature, or laws of God, is most sinful. That is sinful. Just like you become criminal by transgressing the law of state, similarly, when you transgress the law of God, then you are sinful.

~Srila Prabhupada

The human body possesses an incomprehensible wisdom that we have yet to fully grasp, a wisdom that enables us to heal from a multitude of injuries, illnesses, and traumas. However, our bodies were not designed to manage the magnitude of toxicity we expose them to every day. The result is an epidemic of cancer, respiratory and heart disease, diabetes, allergies, and a multitude of other environmental and physical illnesses. Detoxification, on both a global and a personal level, has become a necessity in our modern world.

Toxins are substances that disrupt the normal healthy flow within our bodies. Literally thousands of toxins and harmful synthetic chemicals lurk in our food, air, water, clothes, homes, and workplaces.

The very things that should nourish our bodies or comfort us are often making us ill. They take the form of foods, cleaning products, beauty and hygiene products, cooking oils, food additives, pesticides and herbicides, industrial chemicals in our air, damaging emotions, sugar, and much more.

Chemical Allergies And Modern Foods

An additional source of chemicals, which is still not generally appreciated by the medical profession and others, is the widespread use of pesticides and insecticides. These not only add toxic residues to fruits, vegetables

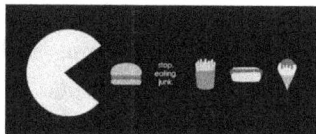

"But perhaps the most alarming ingredient in a Chicken McNugget is tertiary butylhydroquinone, or TBHQ, an antioxidant derived from petroleum that is either sprayed directly on the nugget or the inside of the box it comes in to "help preserve freshness." According to A Consumer's Dictionary of Food Additives, TBHQ is a form of butane (i.e. lighter fluid) the FDA allows processors to use sparingly in our food: It can comprise no more than 0.02 percent of the oil in a nugget. Which is probably just as well, considering that ingesting a single gram of TBHQ can cause "nausea, vomiting, ringing in the ears, delirium, a sense of suffocation, and collapse." Ingesting five grams of TBHQ can kill."

~ Michael Pollan, The Omnivore's Dilemma: A Natural History of Four Meals

and other food crops, but also contaminate meat and milk. Thus, another burden of toxicity is added to our already overloaded systems, resulting in allergic responses and a hastening of the degenerative disease process.

With thousands of varieties of pesticides in common use, what chance has the human body, when even fresh food is loaded with chemicals before reaching the table!

If you think negative, stressful thoughts much of the time, your body will create stress hormones that send messages throughout your body to divert its energy into protecting you from danger even if that danger is really self-imposed. These stress hormones are beneficial in truly stressful life-and-death situations, but when they are released over long periods of time, they damage your body.

You are exposed to many different toxins in an average day. The food and beverages you eat and drink are often full of sugar, synthetic chemicals, and hydrogenated fats. You may be eating excessive amounts of trans fats or animal protein that have a negative impact on your kidneys. The soap, skin-care and hair-care products, and perfumes and colognes you use are typically loaded with toxic chemicals you absorb through your skin or lungs.

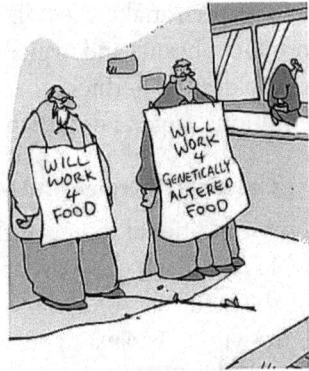

If you are frequently stressed out, your body secretes hormones that wreak havoc on your body over time. If you use pharmaceutical or over-the-counter medications, they often contain chemical fillers, heavy metals, and substances that have to be filtered by your body's detoxification systems. Depending on your lifestyle, you may be adding further toxins to an already overloaded system. These may include household cleaning products, building and furnishing materials in your home, cigarette smoke, recreational drugs, or excessive alcohol consumption.

Our bodies have developed sophisticated detoxification mechanisms over many thousands of years to eliminate most of the naturally produced toxins they encounter on a regular basis. The

Industrial Revolution and its resulting synthetic chemicals found in places such as food, water, soil, air, household and workplace materials, and medicine have created a new dilemma for the human body. Our bodies simply cannot handle the onslaught of synthetic chemicals we throw at them. We may be able to handle some of these toxins but over time, the large amount consumed, drunk, inhaled, or absorbed by the average person greatly exceeds his or her body's capacity.

You Are What You Eat And Drink

Lets say that you just bought a beautiful new vehicle. It looks fabulous and you are so proud to own it. What would happen if you used poor-quality gasoline as fuel? It contains residue and useless by-products of the drilling and refining processes. Over time, that gorgeous new vehicle would get poorer and poorer gas mileage, it might start having engine knock and excessive wear, and eventually the engine would likely malfunction. Your body is similar to a vehicle in that it requires high-quality fuel to function properly. By high quality, I am referring to food that Nature provides that is loaded with plentiful amounts of vitamins, minerals, fibre, enzymes, and many other building blocks to great health. These are the things holistic health practitioners are talking about when they refer to nutrition.

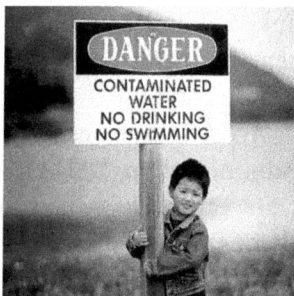

North American diet is increasingly replacing traditional diet all over the world. This diet has been rightly referred to as no-trition. The average person eats large amounts of fatty foods; animal protein; sugar; and packaged, prepared, or fast foods.

Imagine if every day you poured bacon fat down the drain of your kitchen sink. The drainage pipes were designed to handle water and small particles of food. If you keep pouring bacon fat into the

"Modern agriculture is the use of land to convert petroleum into food. Without Petroleum we will not be able to feed the global population." ~Professor Albert Bartlett

drain, it will clog and become ineffective at allowing water through the very substance it was designed to handle.

The same is true of your body. It was never designed to handle the artificial chemicals used by the food-processing industry. *You may be surprised to learn that more than three thousand additives and preservatives are found in our food supply today[1] before that food reaches your table.* It is inundated with artificial colours, flavours, flavour enhancers, bleach, texture agents, conditioners, acid/base balancers, ripening gases, waxes, firming agents, nutrient enrichers, preservatives, heavy metals, and other chemicals that find their way into your food.

Even before that food is processed, your food has been sprayed with pesticides, herbicides, and fungicides, most of which are linked to health problems in humans. An apple a day might have kept the doctor away prior to the industrialization of food growing and preparation.

According to research compiled by the United States Drug Administration (USDA) Agricultural Marketing Service, Pesticide Data Program, todays apple contains residue of many toxic chemicals used during the growing process. In only one category of chemicals, known as organophosphate insecticides, this federal government agency found residue of many different neurotoxins: azinophos, methyl chloripyrifos, diazinon, dimethoate, ethion, omethioate, parathion, parathion methyl, phosalone, and phosmet.

That doesnt sound too appetizing, does it? Neurotoxins are substances that medical research has proven to be toxic to the brain and nervous system of humans. You may be thinking, Well, in minute amounts maybe pesticides are okay. Think again. The average apple is sprayed with pesticides seventeen times before it is harvested. A study by the United States Environmental Protection Agency (EPA) identified more than fifty-five pesticides that can leave cancer-causing residues in food[2].

According to the Natural Resource Defense Council, the use of pesticides has risen more than tenfold since the 1940s. Currently, over 1.2 billion pounds of pesticides are used in agriculture every year in the United States alone.[3]

Dr. Patricia Fitzgerald cites a study by the Pesticide Action Network in her book The Detox Solution, showing that more than fifty million pounds of fungicides, herbicides, insecticides, and soil fumigants were applied to farmland in California alone in 1998.[4] Every year over 2.5 billion pounds of pesticides are dumped on crop lands, forests, lawns, and fields.[5]

Pesticides are not water-soluble. That means they are not easily washed off apples or any other food. The same is true once they are in your body, they are hard to eliminate. Fat-soluble pesticides are actually attracted to the fat stores in your body. Don't have much fat? Your body will start to hold fat to prevent these toxins from running rampant throughout your bloodstream. In your body's innate wisdom, it recognizes that these substances cause damage if they travel through your blood so it attaches them to fat in your body. That spells weight gain and difficulty losing weight at best. At worst, these dangerous neurotoxins attack your body's organs, tissues, brain, and nervous system.

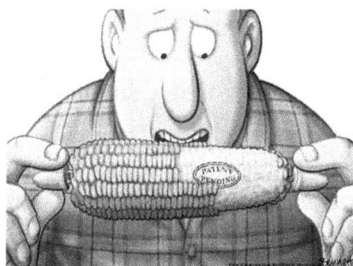

Consider one well-known pesticide that was banned in Canada and the United States three decades ago, DDT. It is still being manufactured and exported around the world to appear in our foods.[6] According to Dr. Fitzgerald, Each year, the EPA performs a study of the chemicals found in human fat tissue samples. DDT continues to be found in 100% of the tissue examined.[7]

Dr. Jozef Krop, a leading environmental medicine physician in Canada, asks a poignant question in his book Healing the Planet One Patient at a Time: When the food we eat is grown in nutrient-poor soil, watered with acid rain, sprayed with pesticides, and treated with food additives, and when the water we drink and the air we breathe are also contaminated, is it any wonder that chemicals have been detected in human blood and fat tissue?

Not only is today's apple not adequate to keep the doctor away, it is more likely to keep the doctor on call. Virtually every food item that is grown using commercial (non-organic) farming techniques contains these or other neurotoxins.

And what if that apple is processed into a frozen apple pie or the fast-food apple pies we consume in droves? There is a good chance that this apple will transform from a nutritious food into a toxic food-like substance we call food. Any of several thousand chemicals will be added to this apple during the many stages of processing.

Have you ever noticed that the incidence of food allergies and sensitivities seems to be higher than ever? I believe that many people are reacting to the potentially thousands of chemicals used in the growing and processing of foods, rather than the foods themselves.

Of course, some people are reacting to the food. But, considering that the average person eats 124 pounds of food additives every year,[8] toxic chemicals definitely play a role in our health. Farmed fish, particularly salmon, is one source of an especially nasty group of chemicals: PCBs. You may have read about the high amounts of polychlorinated biphenyls (more commonly known as PCBs) found in salmon.

Salmon isn't the only culprit. PCBs have shown up in other types of fish and in chicken, beef, pork, eggs, and even milk. This is quite an alarming discovery because research showed that PCBs were (and still are) powerful carcinogens and as a result were banned in the 1970s in both Canada and the United States.

Some government organizations claim that trace amounts of PCBs are fine. But one organization's trace amounts are another's poison. Consider that Health Canada and the United States Food and Drug Administration argue that foods with less than two thousand parts per billion (ppb) of PCBs are fine to eat. On the other side of the coin, the United States Environmental Protection Agency states that levels as low as fifty parts per billion are associated with an increased risk of cancer. Yikes!

Recent research shows that food colourings cross the blood-brain barrier.[9] There is a lock-and-key type of mechanism in your brain that allows some substances (such as nutrients) to go into the brain while preventing damaging substances from attacking the brain. This is referred to as the blood-brain barrier.

The term barrier creates a false sense of security, because chemicals such as food dyes trick the brain into allowing their entry, putting them in a position to do harm to perhaps the most delicate organ in your body. Consider one very common and well-known food additive: monosodium glutamate, better known as MSG. This pervasive chemical is added to food to enhance its flavour. It is frequently found in Chinese food, as well as in the following food ingredients, so don't be surprised if you don't see it labelled as MSG on ingredient lists:

Autolyzed yeast

Calcium caseinate

Gelatin

Glutamate

Glutamic acid

Hydrolyzed protein

Hydrolyzed soy protein

Monopotassium glutamate

Sodium caseinate

Yeast extract

Yeast food

Yeast nutrient

Many people react within forty-eight hours of ingesting even a small amount of MSG, making it sometimes difficult to trace back to the originating food item. Symptoms commonly suffered include headaches, dizziness, nausea, diarrhea, burning sensation of the skin, changes in heart rate, and difficulty breathing. According to Dr. Patricia Fitzgerald, ingesting MSG over the years has also been linked with Parkinsons and Alzheimers.[10]

Source: Michelle Schoffro Cook

References

1. Patricia Fitzgerald, The Detox Solution (Santa Monica, CA: Illumination Press, 2001), p. 70.

2. Fitzgerald, The Detox Solution, p. 28.

3. Fitzgerald, The Detox Solution, p. 29.

4. Fitzgerald, The Detox Solution, p. 28.

5. "Th e Importance of Detoxifi cation." Informational Brochure. Advanced Nutrition Publications, Inc., 2002.

6. Fitzgerald, The Detox Solution, p. 28.

7. Fitzgerald, The Detox Solution, p. 28.

8. "The Importance of Detoxifi cation."

9. Jacqueline Krohn Frances Taylor, Natural Detoxifi cation: A Practical Encyclopedia. (Port Roberts, WA: Hartley & Marks Publishers, Inc., 2000), p. 115.

10. Fitzgerald, The Detox Solution, p. 73.

84.

Mental Illness

Linked to Modern Diet

Mental illness is reaching epidemic levels. The World Health Organization claims that mental health problems "are fast becoming the number-one health issue of the 21st century". Clinical depression is the biggest international health threat after heart disease. At the same time, there is a growing dissatisfaction with the drug treatments available. In the UK, the number of prescriptions for antidepressants has more than doubled in 10 years, with 80% of GPs admitting they over-prescribe drugs such as Prozac because of the lack of alternative forms of treatment.

While medical science pins mental health problems on a combination of factors, including age, genetics and environmental influence, research reveals there might be a link between the modern diet and mental health problems.

In the last section, we have seen how a dentist, Dr. Weston A. Price traveled round the world studying cultures still eating their traditional foods, and compared their health with those members of the same

"The fast-food hamburger has been brilliantly engineered to offer a succulent and tasty first bite, a bite that in fact would be impossible to enjoy if the eater could accurately picture the feedlot and slaughterhouse and the workers behind it or knew anything about the 'artificial grill flavor' that made the first bite so convincing. This is a hamburger to hurry through, no question.

To eat slowly, then, also means to eat deliberately, in the original sense of the word: 'from freedom' instead of compulsion. "

~ Michael Pollan

culture eating western foods. Those continuing to eat traditional diets enjoyed excellent physical and emotional health. But those who had changed to a western diet high in white flour, sugar, and canned goods suffered from a range of physical and mental health problems and were prone to infectious diseases. This huge deterioration occurred after just one generation of exposure to processed foods. Our food affects not only the body but mind as well.

A recent study in the UK by food campaigners, 'Sustain and the Mental Health Foundation' has also linked the increasing incidence of mental ill-health to changes in our diet. They say the last 50 years have witnessed significant changes in the way food is produced. In a nutshell, modern food production has altered the balance of key nutrients we consume, and this may hold the key to preventing (or at least delaying) mental health problems, including depression and Alzheimer's disease.

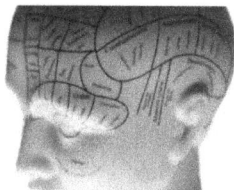

For example, chickens reach their slaughter weight twice as fast as they did 30 years ago, increasing the saturated fat content from 2% to 22%. The diet they are fed has also altered the balance of vital omega-3 and -6 fatty acids in chickens, which has a negative impact on our brain functioning.

Increase in Autism Linked to Modern Diet

Autism is another mental problem that has reached epidemic proportions. Bernard Rimland, PhD, founding director of the Autism Research Institute, estimates that there are now a minimum of 250,000 autistic children in America, a 10 to 15-fold increase in the past 50 or so years. Dr. Rimland has publicly stated that the current childhood vaccine programs are one of the major causes for the current epidemic of autism.

Dr. Mary Megson, a fellow of the American Academy of Pediatrics, agrees. She suggests that autism may be caused by inserting a G-alpha protein defect, the pertussis toxin found in the D.P.T. vaccine, into genetically at-risk children. This depletes the children of their existing supply of vitamin A.

She has treated over 2,000 children for autism by adding natural vitamin A (milk fat is a good source) to their diet. The majority of Dr. Megson's subjects come out of the autistic spectrum within six months — some within weeks, she says. She has seen children making eye contact for the first time in their lives after just three days of treatment.

Soda Consumption Linked to Teen Violence, Study Finds

By Jonathan Benson for Natural News, 26 Oct 2011

A new study has found that teenagers who consume high amounts of sugary soda appear to be more prone towards violence than teenagers who consume less or no sugary soda. The more soda a teenager consumes, in other words, the more likely he or she is to show violent aggression towards classmates, a significant other, and even family members.

David Hemenway, a professor at Harvard University's School of Public, and his colleagues instructed a group of 1,878 public school students from inner-city Boston to fill out questionnaires about how much soda they had consumed in the previous seven days. The questionnaires also asked the students how often they carried weapons, consumed alcohol, smoked, and had a violent interaction with another person.

The students, who ranged in age between 14 and 18, also answered other background questions about how often they ate meals with their families, and their race. After compiling the data and accounting for other outside factors, the research team discovered that soda intake was directly proportional to violence levels.

"What we found was that there was a strong relationship between how many soft drinks that these inner-city kids consumed and how violent they were, not only in violence against peers but also violence in dating relationships, against siblings," said Hemenway. "It was shocking to us when we saw how clear the relationship was."

The results showed that students who drank one or no cans of sugary soda a week were nearly half as likely as students who drank 14 cans a week to carry a gun or knife to school. The one or no soda group was also about half as likely to commit violence against a partner, or show violent aggression against peers, compared to the high-consumption group.

85.

Plastic - Everywhere, In Every Thing

Even In Your Food

Plastic has made a lot of things possible in the past century, proving so durable and versatile that people were soon taking it everywhere with them. In fact, there's a good chance you have some plastic in you right now.

In addition to creating safety problems during production, many chemical additives that give plastic products desirable performance properties also have negative environmental and human health effects. These effects include:

- Direct toxicity, as in the cases of lead, cadmium, and mercury
- Carcinogens, as in the case of diethylhexyl phthalate (DEHP)
- Endocrine disruption, which can lead to cancers, birth defects, immune system supression and developmental problems in children.

Chemical Migration From Plastic Packaging Into Contents

People are exposed to these chemicals not only during manufacturing, but also by using plastic packages, because some chemicals migrate from the plastic packaging to the foods they contain. Examples of plastics contaminating food have been reported with most plastic types, including Styrene from polystyrene, plasticizers from PVC, antioxidants from polyethylene, and Acetaldehyde from PET.

Among the factors controlling migration are the chemical structure of the migrants and the nature of the packaged food. In studies cited in Food Additives and Contaminants, LDPE, HDPE, and polypropylene bottles released measurable levels of BHT, Chimassorb 81, Irganox PS 800, Irganix 1076, and Irganox 1010 into their contents of vegetable oil and ethanol. Evidence was also found that acetaldehyde migrated out of PET and into water.

Activist groups such as Greenpeace and government agencies such as the United States Department of Agriculture (USDA) and the Centers for Disease Control and Prevention (CDC) are closely watching some of these chemicals. Unfortunately, no long-term studies have been conducted on the effects of plastic exposure on humans, even though it remains the most widely used packaging material in the world.

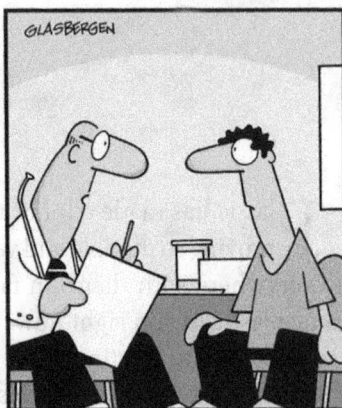

"You gave up fast food and lost 100 pounds. The bad news is, you've developed a styrofoam deficiency."

Dozens of animal studies conducted in the last few years demonstrate that many of these plasticizers are harmful to pregnant mice and their babies. One plasticizer in particular, bisphenol-A (BPA), is linked to chromosomal (that is, genetic) abnormalities.

It is by ignorance that people think that by opening factories they will be happy. Why should they open factories? There is no need. There is so much land, and one can produce one's own food grains and eat sumptuously without any factory. Milk is also available without a factory. The factory cannot produce milk or grains. The present scarcity of food in the world is largely due to such factories. When everyone is working in the city to produce nuts and bolts, who will produce food grains? Simple living and high thinking is the solution to economic problems. Therefore the Krishna consciousness movement in engaging devotees in producing their own food and living self-sufficiently so that rascals may see how one can live very peacefully, eat the food grains one has grown oneself, drink milk, and chant Hare Krishna.

~ Srila Prabhupada (Teaching of Queen Kunti, 18: Liberation from Ignorance and Suffering)

According to research reported by Leslie Crawford, exposure to the chemical, which creates hormonal imbalances, resulted in everything from high rates of spontaneous abortions to decreased sperm counts in male mice and early onset of puberty in female mice.

According to Ned Groth, a senior scientist for Consumers Union, in Yonkers, New York, when plastic is exposed to high heat or harsh soaps or when plastics are simply used repeatedly over time they can degrade and make their way into our food.

Polycarbonate is used for clear plastic baby bottles, five-gallon water jugs, clear plastic sippy cups for babies and children, and clear plastic cutlery. Many plastics of this kind contain unknown plastic ingredients that are linked with hormone disruption. According to some experts, all the studies that show plastic is safe for use in the food industry have been conducted by the plastic industry itself. If you are unsure, go with glass containers.

Recommendations

Find alternatives to plastic products whenever possible. Some specific suggestions:

- Buy food in glass or metal containers; avoid polycarbonate drinking bottles.

- Avoid heating food in plastic containers, or storing fatty foods in plastic containers or plastic wrap.

- Do not give young children plastic teethers or toys

- Use natural fiber clothing, bedding and furniture

- Avoid all PVC and Styrene products

Plastic	Common Uses	Adverse Health Effects
Polyvinyl chloride (#3PVC)	Food packaging, plastic wrap, containers for toiletries, cosmetics, crib bumpers, floor tiles, pacifiers, shower curtains, toys, water pipes, garden hoses, auto upholstery, inflatable swimming pools	Can cause cancer, birth defects, genetic changes, chronic bronchitis, ulcers, skin diseases, deafness, vision failure, indigestion, and liver dysfunction

Phthalates (DEHP, DINP, and others)	Softened vinyl products manufactured with phthalates include vinyl clothing, emulsion paint, footwear, printing inks, non-mouthing toys and children's products, product packaging and food wrap, vinyl flooring, blood bags and tubing, IV containers and components, surgical gloves, breathing tubes, general purpose labware, inhalation masks, many other medical devices.	Endocrine disruption, linked to asthma, developmental and reporoductive effects. Medical waste with PVC and pthalates is regularly incinerated causing public health effects from the release of dioxins and mercury, including cancer, birth defects, hormonal changes, declining sperm counts, infertility, endometriosis, and immune system impairment.
Polycarbonate, with Bisphenol A (#7)	Water bottles	Scientists have linked very low doses of bisphenol A exposure to cancers, impaired immune function, early onset of puberty, obesity, diabetes, and hyperactivity, among other problems (Environment California)
Plastic	Common Uses	Adverse Health Effects
Polystyrene	Many food containers for meats, fish, cheeses, yogurt, foam and clear clamshell containers, foam and rigid plates, clear bakery containers, packaging "peanuts", foam packaging, audio cassette housings, CD cases, disposable cutlery, building insulation, flotation devices, ice buckets, wall tile, paints, serving trays, throw-away hot drink cups, toys	Can irritate eyes, nose and throat and can cause dizziness and unconsciousness. Migrates into food and stores in body fat. Elevated rates of lymphatic and hematopoietic cancers for workers.

Plastic	Common Uses	Adverse Health Effects
Polyethelyne (#1 PET)	Water and soda bottles, carpet fiber, chewing gum, coffee stirrers, drinking glasses, food containers and wrappers, heat-sealed plastic packaging, kitchenware, plastic bags, squeeze bottles, toys	Suspected human carcinogen
Polyester	Bedding, clothing, disposable diapers, food packaging, tampons, upholstery	Can cause eye and respiratory-tract irritation and acute skin rashes
Urea-formaldehyde	Particle board, plywood, building insulation, fabric finishes	Formaldehyde is a suspected carcinogen and has been shown to cause birth defects and genetic changes. Inhaling formaldehyde can cause cough, swelling of the throat, watery eyes, breathing problems, headaches, rashes, tiredness
Plastic	Common Uses	Adverse Health Effects
Polyurethane Foam	Cushions, mattresses, pillows	Bronchitis, coughing, skin and eye problems. Can release toluene disocyanate which can produce severe lung problems
Acrylic	Clothing, blankets, carpets made from acrylic fibers, adhesives, contact lenses, dentures, floor waxes, food preparation equipment, disposable diapers, sanitary napkins, paints	Can cause breathing difficulties, vomiting, diarrhea, nausea, weakness, headache and fatigue
Tetrafluoro-ethelyne	Non-stick coating on cookware, clothes irons, ironing board covers, plumbing and tools	Can irritate eyes, nose and throat and can cause breathing difficulties

Sources:

Centers for Disease Control Report, "National Report on Human Exposure to Environmental Chemicals," 2001.

Dadd, Debra, Home Safe Home, Penguin Putnam, New York, 1997.

Ecology Center Plastic Task Force Report, Berkeley, CA, 1996.

Goettlich, Paul, "What are Endocrine Disruptors?," 2001

National Resources Defense Council website, "Endocrine Disruptors FAQ," 2001.

86.

India

Horrors Of Food Adulteration

India has become a hub of food adulteration and unscrupulous trade practices. There is no other place in the world where conditions are as serious. There are no government regulations and whatever little controls exist, they are openly flouted. Corrupt police force, judiciary and government officials ensure that the culprits go scot free.

Situation is so serious that in just one state Maharashtra, more than 10,000 cases of food adulteration are pending in courts since last ten years.

Krishna says, annad bhavanti bhutani [Bg. 3.14]. Anna. Anna means food grains, eatables. You must produce sufficient food grains. Why you are producing tire tube instead of food grains? And just entering your Delhi from Vrndavana, a big Goodyear factory, very big factory. You are producing tire tube, then iron, Goodyear and this and that. Where is food grain? And both sides, the field is vacant. Nobody is going to grow food grain. Then why you'll not starve? It is your fault. You are producing tire tube and iron instrument. You are neglecting agriculture. Then why you shall not suffer for want of food grain? And you are pleading, "Indians are starving." Well, why shall not starve if they do not follow Bhagavad-gita? They are thinking, "By increasing industry in America..." They have got industry, at the same time food grains also. But you are taking to industry without taking care of growing food grains.

~ Srila Prabhupada (Conversation with News Reporters, March 25, 1976, Delhi)

From vegetables, pulses and spices to chocolate, milk and energy drinks, nothing is contamination-proof. Consumers may be oblivious to the dangers, but tainted items are heightening the risk of conditions like cancer, paralysis and liver and heart damage.

Its a common practice to repackage expired goods and sell them in supermarkets along with the fresh goods. Thousands of establishments are raided every year by Food And Drug Administration (FDA) and spurious food items worth millions are seized but the practice continues unabated.

Melamine is added in chocolates which multiplies the risk of bladder cancer. Branded energy drinks may contain nearly 500 percent more caffeine than the legal limit which may cause cancer. Almost all the fruits are ripened with chemicals like calcium carbide, which can affect the nervous system and may contaminate the fruit with phosphorous and arsenic.

Spices are laced with toxic colours and heavy metals. While lead can cause anaemia, paralysis and the risk of abortion, colours can cause mental retardation in infants and increase the risk of cancers. Malachite is used to brighten green vegetables and can increase the risk of lung tumour.

J.S.Pai, executive director of the Protein Foods and Nutrition Development Association of India says, "Food adulteration in the short term may cause diarrhoea, food poisoning and gastrointestinal problems but in the long term toxic materials accumulate in the body with serious health implications." Most at risk are those who

---

If your energy is all engaged in manufacturing tires and wheels, then who will go to the... Actually I have seen in your country. Now the farmers' son, they do not like to remain in the farm. They go in the city. I have seen it. The farmers' son, they do not like to take up the profession of his father. So gradually farming will be reduced, and the city residents, they are satisfied if they can eat meat. And the farmer means keeping the, raising the cattle and killing them, send to the city, and they will think that "We are eating. What is the use of going to..." But these rascals have no brain that "If there is no food grain or grass, how these cattle will be...?" Actually it is happening. They are eating swiftly.

-Srila Prabhupada (Room Conversation with Dr. Theodore Kneupper, November 6, 1976, Vrndavana)

buy unpackaged, unlabelled goods, particularly from small to medium-sized neighborhood stores.

Even liquor is not spared. Adulterated batches of bootleg liquor kill hundreds every year.

Some other examples of adulteration are:

Bitter Gourd and Capsicum: Banned malachite added to make them green and shiny

Tea Dust: Iron filings

Milk: Detergent, dirt, water, flour, urea, caustic soda

Ground Spices: Sawdust and colours

Sugar: Chalk powder

Wheat Flour: Sand, dirt and chalk powder

Honey: cheap Jaggery

Most Milk In India Contaminated With Bleach, Fertilizer, Food Safety Regulator Finds

Times of India, Jan 10, 2012

India's food safety regulator found 68 percent of milk samples from cows and buffalo to be contaminated with additives such as fertilizer, bleach and detergent.

Cows may be sacred in India, but their by-product - milk - evidently is far from it.

During testing by the country's food safety regulator, 68 percent of milk samples from cows and buffalo were found to be contaminated with additives such as fertilizer, bleach and detergent.

The study, conducted by the Food Safety and Standards Authority, found that the milk was also "diluted with water or sweeteners, fat,

---

We have seen in India. Nowadays there is no eatables. The government cannot supply food, failure, the problem which is not even amongst the beasts and birds. The birds and beasts, they have no such problem. They are freely living, jumping from one tree to another, because they know there is no problem of eating. And human society, there is problem of eating. What is the advancement? And there is enough place for producing food. I have seen Africa, Australia. Enough place.

~ Srila Prabhupada, (Room Conversation with Richard Webster, chairman, Societa Filosofica Italiana -- May 24, 1974, Rome)

non-edible solids, glucose and skimmed milk powder to increase volume. "Addition of water not only reduces the nutritional value of milk but contaminated water may also pose health risks," the study says. However, the presence of the bleaching agent hydrogen peroxide and the fertilizer urea "are far more serious," the report notes, and can lead to gastroenteritis and other intestinal ailments.

The regulator blamed a "lack of hygiene and sanitation in the milk handling." Dirty water comes with the increased risk of hepatitis infection. Synthetic milk is also becoming common.

Commonly used adulterants are: caustic soda, urea, detergent, chalk, animal fat, neutralizers, hydrogen peroxide, sugar, starch, glucose, formalin and vegetable fat. Sorbitol is used as a thickening agent.

According to The National, India is one of the world's biggest producers of milk but struggles to meet domestic demand.

A national grid links more than 700 Indian cities and towns to the milk producers in the villagers. The processing and distribution of milk starts with dairy farmers across villages in India, who bring their daily supplies to a local collection center in their village.

The paper quoted one farmer from Binaural in the state of Uttar Pradesh as saying: "We don't even know what we are drinking anymore. The milk the dairy farmers give to the collection centers in their respective villages is fair and good. But it is the greed of manufacturers, and because demand is so high, that they don't care about who drinks the milk and can add all these additives." The states of West Bengal, Orissa, Bihar, Chhattisgarh and Jharkhand fared the worst, The National wrote, with not a single sample passing the tests. In the national capital Delhi, 70% samples failed the test.

Yes. Just like the Germans, they extracted fat from stool. And that was used as butter. This is scientific. They'll have to eat stool even. They have eaten. In the last war, concentration camp, they have eaten their own stool. There was no food. So nature will punish them in that way. They'll eat everything. This godless civilization will lead people to such condition of life. Kadharya bhaksana kare, tara janma adho pate yaya. This life they will eat everything, all nonsense thing, and next life they become pig, cats, dogs. That's all. This will be.

~ Srila Prabhupada

"These are very harmful to the heart, liver and kidneys, and is specifically dangerous for pregnant women and the foetus," says Dr Nutan Desai, a gastroenterologist at Fortis Hospital, Mumbai. The samples were collected randomly and analysed from 33 states totaling a sample size of 1,791. Just 31.5% of the samples tested (565) conformed to the FSSAI standards while the rest1,226 (68.4%) failed the test.

These samples were sent to government laboratories like Department of Food and Drug Testing of Puducherry, Central Food Laboratory in Pune, Food Reasearch and Standardization Laboratory in Ghaziabad, State Public Health Laboratory in Guwahati and Central Food Laboratory, Kolkata, for testing.

Meanwhile, India's second largest state milk federation body, the Karnataka Milk Federation, has been forced to withdraw its full cream milk from the market because it found that vendors were using water to dilute the milk and later adding starch to thicken it.

This shows the trade off between the risk of getting caught and the reward of profits is skewed heavily in favour of the latter. The government must focus on raising the risks to the adulterer. One way of doing this is by hiking the penalty, including making it analogous to attempt to murder in some cases.

These toxic chemicals are particularly harmful to the children. Phenomenal growth of health care sector in India can be attributed, at least in part, to this. It also explains why India has the highest number of malnourished children, even more than Sub-Sahara Africa. Problem is further exacerbated by the government policy of encouraging slaughterhouses and beef export. Now a dead cow fetches more money than a living one. India in 2012 became the world leader in beef export. Also due to lack of draught animals and cow dung manure, agriculture is dying off. Every year, close to 40,000 farmers commit suicide and many are abandoning field work to work as labourers or coolies in cities.

87.

Fat, Sick And Nearly Dead

150 pounds overweight, loaded up on steroids and suffering from a debilitating autoimmune disease, Joe Cross is at the end of his rope and the end of his hope. In the mirror he saw a 310lb man whose gut was bigger than a beach ball and a path laid out before him that wouldn't end well— with one foot already in the grave, the other wasn't far behind. Fat, Sick & Nearly Dead is an inspiring film that chronicles Joe's personal mission to regain his health.

With doctors and conventional medicines unable to help him, Joe turns to the only option left, the body's ability to heal itself. He trades in the junk food and hits the road with juicer and generator in tow, vowing only to drink fresh fruit and vegetable juice for the next 60 days. Across 3,000 miles Joe has one goal in mind: To get off his pills and achieve a balanced lifestyle.

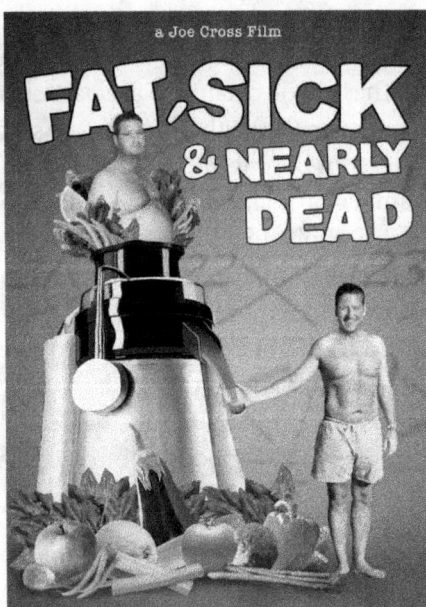

a Joe Cross Film

FAT, SICK & NEARLY DEAD

While talking to more than 500 Americans about food, health and longevity, it's at a truck stop in Arizona where Joe meets a truck driver who suffers from the same condition. Phil Staples is morbidly obese weighing in at 429 lbs; a cheeseburger away from a heart-attack. As Joe is recovering his health, Phil begins his own epic journey to get well.

What emerges is nothing short of amazing – an inspiring tale of healing and human connection.

Part road trip, part self-help manifesto, this movie defies the traditional documentary format to present an unconventional and uplifting story of two men from different worlds who each realize that the only person who can save them is themselves.

This is a 2010 production and Joe Cross follows the juice fast under the care of Dr. Joel Fuhrman, Nutrition Research Foundation's Director of Research. Cross and Robert Mac, co-creators of the film, both serve on the Nutrition Research Foundation's Advisory Board.

Following his fast and the adoption of a plant-based diet, Cross lost 100 pounds and discontinued all medications.

The film has been credited with doubling the sales of Breville juicers since the documentary launched on Netflix in the US in July 2011.

Fat, Sick, and Nearly Dead won the Turning Point Award and shared the Audience Choice Award – Documentary Film, at the 2010 Sonoma International Film Festival.

Full movie can be watched here: http://vimeo.com/45359005

I remember growing up in Arlington, VA in the early '50s, and the word "farmer" was like the worst put-down that a person could call another person, at least among the young.
~ Michael Baker, May 25 2011

88.

Organic Water Is Here

This isn't just a dream. Finally, Organic bottled water without antibiotics, growth hormones, synthetic pesticides or even genetic modification is here.

Safeway is selling bottled water which doesn't even have growth hormones in it! People are queuing up for a healthy sip.

So what if we have made a mess of our food. At least something wholesome to drink is still there.

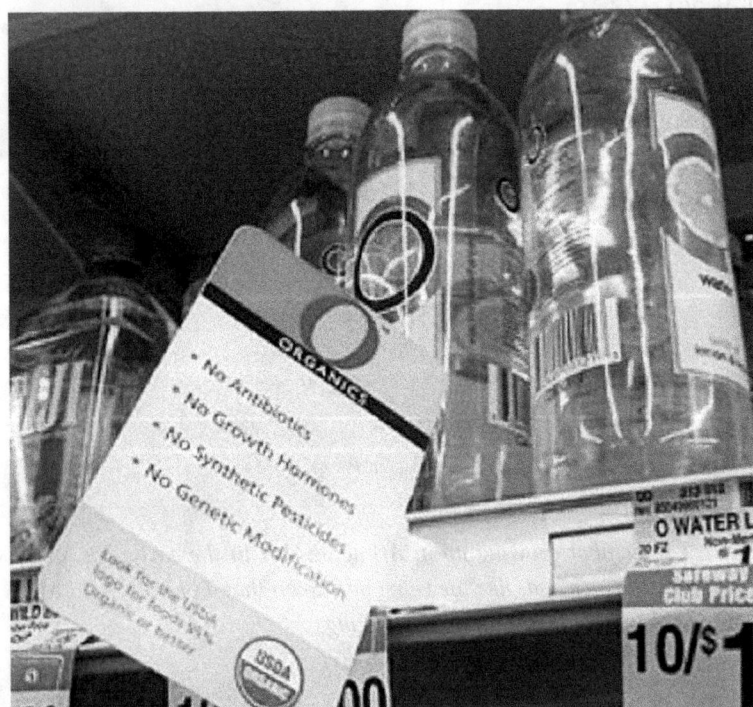

89.

Pesticides

Poisoning The Planet

Dr. Walter Crinnion, The Huffington Post

In my Earth Day blog I mentioned that 1.2 billion pounds of pesticides were sprayed per year in the United States with an annual cost of $11 billion, while the total world pesticide use exceeded 5.0 billion pounds in 2000 and 2001 (for a combined total of $64.5 billion). That should take care of all those nasty bugs! But, less than 0.01 percent of all those billions of pounds that are sprayed actually make it to the intended pest! Oops. Kind of surprising that such an inefficient system is still in use today, isn't it?

It probably wouldn't be so bad if the pesticides were only harmful to a few bugs, but they are not. All pesticides kill bugs by poisoning their nervous systems (think "brain" and "nerves"). Today the bulk of pesticides used are either organophosphates or pyrethroids. Organophosphates came out of nerve gas research in Germany between the first and second world wars. This is also the same class

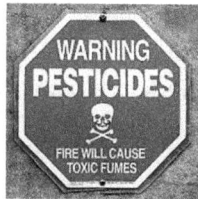

> *"I asked the feedlot manager why they didn't just spray the liquefied manure on neighboring farms. The farmers don't want it, he explained. The nitrogen and phosphorus levels are so high that spraying the crops would kill them. He didn't say that feedlot wastes also contain heavy metals and hormone residues, persistent chemicals that end up in waterways downstream, where scientists have found fish and amphibians exhibiting abnormal sex characteristics."*
>
> *~Michael Pollan, The Omnivore's Dilemma: A Natural History of Four Meals*

of compounds that was released into a Tokyo subway a number of years ago by a cult group. So, if you are concerned at all about your brain, your children's brains and the brains of your elected officials and everyone driving cars on the road around you, then maybe you want to help to start reducing the 99.99 percent of the 1.2 billion pounds of neurotoxic pesticides that are floating around because you decided to save a buck by buying a commercially raised apple.

While no pesticides or herbicides are used to grow crops that are certified organic, the idea that these crops are free of insecticide residue is actually not true. Those that are raised in open fields are open to the air and get contamination from pesticides and heavy metals that are blowing around. And these pesticides have been shown to fly around the globe, travelling thousands of miles. However, it is true that organically raised foods are significantly less contaminated with these chemicals than the same foods grown in non-organic methods (including integrated pest management systems). The levels of pesticide residue on foods in the United States is monitored through the Pesticide Data Program of the US Department of Agriculture. A review that utilized their data, along with data from Consumers Union and the Marketplace Surveillance Program of the California Department

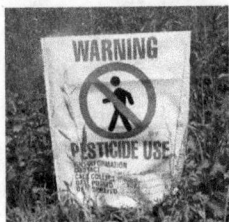

And Prabhupada would add, "They think Vedic culture is primitive, but actually it's most scientific."

Paramananda and Nirmal walk toward an eggplant patch where two bamboo crosses stand like scarecrows. Says Nirmal, "You've heard of Laksmi, the goddess of fortune? She represents everything that comes from the soil -- crops, jewels, raw materials -- all wealth. Anyway, when rats were destroying the crops, I got some zinc phosphate from Bombay. It worked well for a while, but the rats were so intelligent they stopped eating it. Then the Vedas gave me a hint. The sages describe Laksmi as riding on an owl, a nocturnal predator. To give the owls the hint, I put up these bamboo perches, and watched them land at night. One by one, the rats came out of their holes and ended up in the owls' stomachs. Krishna's natural pest control."

~ Suresvara dasa (Simple Living High Thinking)

of Pesticide Regulation reported that organically raised foods had one-third the amount of chemical residues that were found in conventionally raised foods. When compared to those grown with integrated pest management techniques, the organics had half the amount of residues. In addition, organic foods were far less likely (by a factor of 10) to have two or more residues on them than conventional foods were. While only 2.6 percent of all organic foods had multiple residues detected, 26 percent of the conventional did. Data from the Pesticide Data Program revealed that the conventional produce that had the highest percentages of positive (insecticide residue) findings were: celery (96 percent), pears (95 percent), apples (94 percent), peaches (93 percent), strawberries (91 percent), oranges (85 percent), spinach (84 percent), potatoes (81 percent), grapes (78 percent) and cucumbers (74 percent) (45). That study found that an average of 82 percent of all conventional fruits were positive for insecticide residues while only 23 percent of the organics were. When it came to vegetables, 65 percent of the conventional tested positive, compared to only 23 percent for the organics.

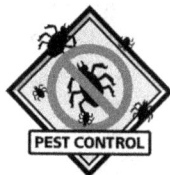

The sufferings of human society are due to a polluted aim of life, namely lording it over the material resources. The more human society engages in the exploitation of undeveloped material resources for sense gratification, the more it will be entrapped by the illusory, material energy of the Lord, and thus the distress of the world will be intensified instead of diminished. The human necessities of life are fully supplied by the Lord in the shape of food grains, milk, fruit, wood, stone, sugar, silk, jewels, cotton, salt, water, vegetables, etc., in sufficient quantity to feed and care for the human race of the world as well as the living beings on each and every planet within the universe. The supply source is complete, and only a little energy by the human being is required to get his necessities into the proper channel. There is no need of machines and tools or huge steel plants for artificially creating comforts of life. Life is never made comfortable by artificial needs, but by plain living and high thinking.
~ Srila Prabhupada (Srimad Bhagavatam 2.2.37)

The fruits and vegetables with the highest and lowest percentages of residues in the USDA study is very similar to the listing of the most and least toxic foods that is available on the web through Environmental Working Group. The current list given by them lists the top 12 most toxic fruits and vegetables as (In order of toxicity):
- Peach
- Apple
- Bell Pepper
- Celery
- Nectarine
- Strawberries
- Cherries
- Kale
- Lettuce
- Grapes (Imported)
- Carrot
- Pear

And the least toxic ones as:
- Onion
- Avocado
- Sweet Corn
- Pineapple
- Mango
- Asparagus
- Sweet Peas
- Kiwi
- Cabbage

You are given a field, a piece of land. You can grow twice, thrice in a year very nice foodstuff, sometimes pulses, sometimes paddy, sometimes the mustard seed. Any land... In India, we have seen that a cultivator produces three, four kind of food grains in a year. That is the system... That is the system that in India every man is producing his food grains independently. Now it is stopped. Formerly, all these men, they used to produce their food grain. So they used to work for three months in a year, and they could stock the whole year's eatable food grains. Life was very simple. After all, you require to eat. So this Vedic civilization was that keep some land and keep some cows. Then your whole economic question is solved.
~ Srila Prabhupada

- Eggplant
- Papaya
- Watermelon
- Broccoli
- Tomato
- Sweet Potato

Not only have repeated studies shown that organic foods have lower levels of insecticides, but there is also now clear evidence showing lower pesticide levels in the actual consumers of the organic foods (i.e. You!). I also talked about these fascinating studies in Seattle (with Dr. Fenske at the University of Washington) in my Earth Day blog. It started with a simple study that looked at the organophosphate pesticide presence in the urine of preschoolers in the Seattle area. The researchers found that all but one child had pesticide residue in their urine (which meant it was in their bloodstream, as well). When they questioned the parents of this one child, they learned that they only fed organic food to their children.

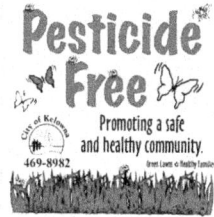

So, the researchers began to plan another study to see if eating organic foods really did lower one's pesticides levels. Well, their

Nature already has an arrangement to feed us. By the order of the Supreme Personality of Godhead, there is an arrangement for eatables for every living entity within the 8,400,000 forms of life. Eko bahunam yo vidadhati kaman. Every living entity has to eat something, and in fact the necessities for his life have already been provided by the Supreme Personality of Godhead. The Lord has provided food for both the elephant and the ant. All living beings are living at the cost of the Supreme Lord, and therefore one who is intelligent should not work very hard for material comforts. Rather, one should save his energy for advancing in Krishna consciousness. All created things in the sky, in the air, on land and in the sea belong to the Supreme Personality of Godhead, and every living being is provided with food. Therefore one should not be very much anxious about economic development and unnecessarily waste time and energy with the risk of falling down in the cycle of birth and death.

~ Srila Prabhupada (Srimad Bhagavatam 7.14.14)

follow-up study with preschoolers proved that it did. They enrolled families into the study by standing outside of the Puget Consumers Co-op (for families buying organic foods) and outside Larry's Market (for families buying conventional foods). When they broke the code on the samples they found that the children whose parents supplied them with mostly conventional foods had six to nine times higher levels of pesticides in their urine than the children who ate mostly organic foods. How nice to be able to take some simple steps that keep neurotoxic compounds from entering the bodies of our children and ourselves.

Section - VI

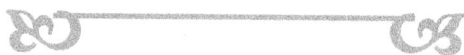

Future Of Humanity

90.

Back To Natural Foods

Dr. Weston A. Price

Simply stated, the practical application of the primitive wisdom for accomplishing this would involve returning to the use of natural foods which provide the entire assortment of bodybuilding and repairing food factors. This means the recognition of the fact that all forms of animal life are the product of the food environments that have produced them. Therefore, we cannot distort and rob the foods without serious injury. Nature has put these foods up in packages containing the combinations of minerals and other factors that are essential for nourishing the various organs. Some of the simpler animal forms are able to synthesize in their bodies some of the food elements which we humans also require, but cannot create ourselves. Our modern process of robbing the natural foods for convenience or gain completely thwarts Nature's inviolable program. I have shown how the robbing of the wheat in the making of white flour reduced the minerals and other chemicals in the grains, so as to make them sources of energy without normal body-building and repairing qualities. Our appetites have been distorted so that hunger

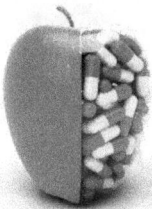

> *The roots of peace and prosperity lie in working the land, protecting the cow, and loving Krishna.*
> ~ Suresvara dasa

appeals only for energy with no conscious need for body-building and repairing chemicals.

One dairy farmer I know sells his own cows' milk for $1 a gallon while his wife pays $1.80 for the man-handled, store-bought stuff. Most vegetable farmers trade their harvest for inedible paper. This paper money buys complex machinery that they hope will save them time and bring in more paper money. But greed never pays. In a recent national study of 130 stressful occupations, the job of farm manager ranked twelfth. Farmers are going out of business at the rate of one thousand per week, because the cost of farming has become greater than the profits. And since the industrialization of agriculture, the number of American families who live on farms has shrunk from 30% in 1920 to 2.5% today.

Nevertheless, Secretary of Agriculture John Block claims the industrialization of agriculture has "enabled the vast majority of Americans to engage in other economic activities that have produced the vast array of necessities and consumer goods which make possible the high standard of living Americans enjoy today."

Is it prosperity to have two locks on the door instead of one, special hot-lines to the police, fire, and riot squads, and a gun in every house? Or motorcycles and cars screeching into the morning hours? Or high-school seniors graduating with their brains 'washed' by fifteen thousand hours of television? And ten thousand Russian megatons inspired by American expertise now aimed at Americans' living rooms? The answer must be a resounding NO! if we are to be honest.

Although Lord Krishna gave us the land and the cows as our natural economic base, we don't find much talk about them in Business Week, Money, or Fortune. We find, instead, the latest bank rates and high-tech investments, bargains in wines and personal computers, and speculation that gold may soar to $4,000 an ounce by 1986.

But others, like financial adviser Howard Ruff and survivalist Sally Harrington, are more down to earth. In a world spinning toward political, economic, and ecological disaster, Ruff explains why grains and beans are at least as good an investment as silver and gold.

"You spend hundreds of dollars every year to insure your cars against the accident you fully expect not to have," says Ruff, "and you can't eat the cancelled checks. Your money is wasted unless you're 'lucky' enough to have an accident. Food storage is the insurance you can eat."

Adds Harrington, "Wheat, if kept dry and protected from rodents and insects, will last for two or three thousand years. Some that was found in King Tut's tomb was still edible, and it even germinated."

~ Sruresvara dasa

535

One of our modern tendencies is to select the foods we like, particularly those that satisfy our hunger without our having to eat much, and, another is to think in terms of the few known vitamins and their effects. The primitive tendency seems to have been to provide an adequate factor of safety for all emergencies by the selection of a sufficient variety and quantity of the various natural foods to prevent entirely most of our modern afflictions. Their success demonstrates that their program is superior to ours.

An important advance in modern international relationships provides for exchange of professorships and, thus, interchanges of wisdom. We have shown a most laudable and sympathetic interest in carrying our culture to the remnants of these primitive races.

Would it not be fortunate to accept in exchange lessons from their inherited knowledge? It may be not only our greatest opportunity, but our best hope for stemming the tide of our progressive breakdown and also for our return to harmony with Nature's laws, since life in its fullness is Nature obeyed.

91.

City Farms

Or Edible Cities

The Future Of Humanity

Cities cover only 2% of the Earth's surface, but consume 75% of its resources. Cities are black holes, they're swallowing our planet. But, there is a faint ray of hope. More and more are joining the Green City or Grow Your Food movements. Millions around the world are producing food in their apartments, balconies, lawns, rooftops and window-sills.

Jac Smit, President of the Urban Agriculture Network and co-author of "Urban Agriculture: Food, Jobs, and Sustainable Cities", paints a vision of what the world would be like if cities were nutritionally self-reliant: "As we consider a dominantly urban Earth early in the next century, in a world with less land and water per-capita, the return of agriculture to where we live presents us with a new paradigm."

What if the urban landscape were edible? What if vacant, waste land in cities were productive and enhancing the environment for living? What if urban areas were increasing biodiversity rather than diminishing it?"

"Ideally we believe that simply by changing from suit to jeans, digging up a bit of lawn, and planting vegetable seeds, the city person will begin asking questions about his environment and about his urban behavior and thinking patterns."

~ Founding director of City Farmer, addressing science teachers at the 20th International Science Education Symposium in 1979.

It's happening. Growing your own food in cities has long been the way in Asia, and it's expanding enormously in Africa, Latin America, and all over the world.

In many places, urban food production is growing more rapidly than urban population -- in spite of urban drift.

In greater Bangkok, 72% of all urban families are engaged in raising food, mostly part-time. In Moscow, the share of families raising food more than tripled between 1972 and 1992. In Dar-es-Salaam in Tanzania the number of households engaged in food production grew from 20% to more than 65% between 1970 and 1990.

In Argentina the number of participants in the community agriculture program grew from 50,000 to 550,000 between 1990 and 1994, and the number of supporting institutions grew from 100 to 1,100. The area devoted to urban agriculture in Harare in Zimbabwe doubled between 1990 and 1994.

Industrialised Nations

City farming is growing just as rapidly in the rich cities of the West, perhaps more because of environmental concerns, but also to feed the hungry: the Urban Agriculture Network was "founded in response to the increase of persistent hunger in urban areas in both poor countries and rich countries".

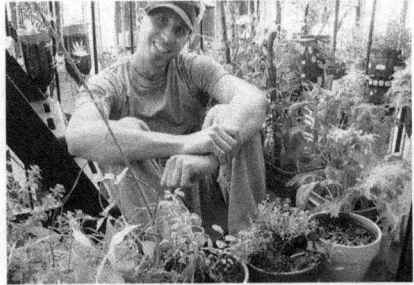

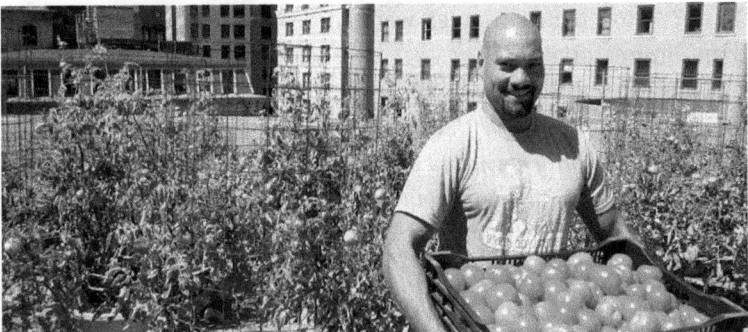

The city farming movements have been intensely studied in the 20 years or so and they has been found to deliver a rich harvest of benefits -- benefits that social workers, community organizations, educators, psychologists, health workers, nutritionists and crime fighters can only dream of where there are no city farms or community gardens.

By 1994, 300,000 households in the US were using a community garden, and 6.7 million more said they'd do so too if there was one nearby (National Gardening Association).

The US government's Urban Gardening program estimates that a $1 investment in food growing projects yields $6 of produce in a single season.

We are Humans. We Grow Food.

By Mike Lieberman

When people ask why they should grow their own food, I don't break out all kinds of reports and studies that tell how it's better for you and the environment. I break it down even simpler and tell them it's because we are human. It's what we do.

It's not until the last 100 or so years that we've stopped growing our own and put that responsibility in the hands of others. Think about it. Humans have grown their own food for hundreds and thousands of years.

Civilizations and societies were built around fertile land and access to water. Communities were built around food. There is so much that goes into it from the planning to the planting, tending to the harvesting and most importantly the preparing and sharing of it. It's what brings people together on so many levels.

We now just skip right to the eating, which is often done on the run too.

Our 'throw away' society doesn't realize that depending upon others to make/grow/package what we eat lends itself to people not knowing what they are eating and what it can (and will) do to their health over time. Like I said before..get rid of the dollar menu and learn to grow/bake/preserve your own! ~ *Edward, Portsmouth*

These days we've come to sit at a desk in front a computer all day or in a large SUV traveling through space. That's not what we are designed to do. That's all relatively new to us.

This is why I keep it simple and say that the reason we should grow our own food is because we are humans. I'm not saying an entire garden, but growing just one thing will make a difference.

Urban Homesteading

According to UC-Davis, "an urban homestead is a household that produces a significant part of the food consumed by its residents. This is typically associated with residents' desire to live in a more environmentally conscious manner.

Aspects of urban homesteading include:

- Resource reduction: using solar/alternative energy sources, harvesting rainwater, using greywater, line drying clothes, using alternative transportation such as bicycles and buses.

- Edible landscaping: growing fruit, vegetables, culinary and medicinal plants, converting lawns into gardens.

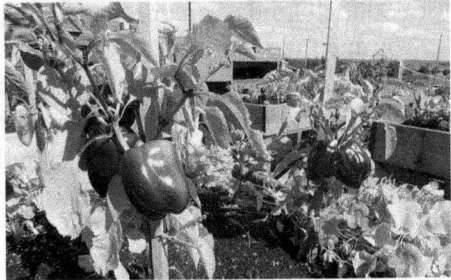

- Self-sufficient living: re-using, repairing, and recycling items; homemade products.

- Food preservation including canning, drying, freezing, cheese-making, and fermenting.

- Community food-sourcing such as foraging, gleaning, and trading.

- Natural building

- Composting

Having an allotment or vegetable garden has been common throughout history. A wealth of urban homesteading books

I think people feel better if the simply interact with any bit of nature. Growing food included. Why else do all little children love to pick flowers?
~ Brianna

(Urban Homestead by Kelly Coyne, Erik Knutzen; The Backyard Homestead by Carleen Madigan; Urban Homesteading by Rachel Kaplan, K. Ruby Blume; Toolbox for Sustainable City Living by Scott Kellog) have been published in the past decade. All over the world, people have found ways of growing their own food in inner-city urban areas.

92.

Joy Of Farming

In One Of The Densest Cities In The World

Mumbai is one of the densest cities in the world, 48,215 persons per km² and 16,082 per km² in suburban areas. There was twelve fold increase in its population in last one century. Greater Mumbai, formed by City Island and Salsette Island, is the largest city in India with a population of 16.4 million, according to 2001 census.

In a scenario like this, urban agriculture seems unlikely since it must compete with real estate developers for vacant lots. Alternative farming methods have emerged as a response to scarcity of land, water, and economic resources.

Dr. R T Doshi's is taking a lead in popularizing terrace/balcony gardens. His methods are revolutionary and do not require big investment or long hours of work. His farming practice is organic and is mainly directed towards domestic consumption. He utilizes locally available materials such as sugarcane waste, polyethylene bags, tires, containers, garbage cans, cylinders, and soil. The containers and bags (open at both ends) are filled with sugarcane stalks, compost, and garden soil.

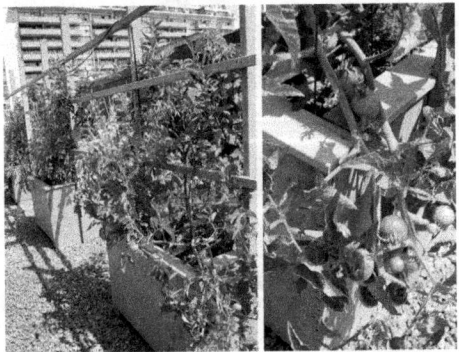

The water requirement is much less compared to conventional field farming.

He has grown different types of fruit such as mangos, figs, guavas, bananas, and sugarcane stalks on his terrace of 1,200 sq ft (110 m2) in Bandra. This concept of city farming consumes the entire household's organic waste. He subsequently makes the household self-sufficient in the provision of food: 5 kilograms (11 lb) of fruits and vegetables are produced daily for 300 days a year. (RUAF Foundation. Handouts on Case Studies)

This idea is being taken up by the local schools. In the Rosary High school, Dockyard Road, a city farm was created on a terrace area of 400 sq ft (37 m2). The main objective of the project was to promote economic support for street children, beautify the city landscape, supply locally produced organic food and to manage organic waste in a sustainable manner. This project had the participation of street children. The farm produced vegetables, fruits, and flowers. There was noticeable change in the behaviour of street children after their participation in the project.

Mumbai Port Trust has developed an organic farm on the terrace of its central kitchen, in an area of approximately 3,000 sq ft (280 m2). This central kitchen serves food to approximately 3,000 employees daily, generating large amounts of organic waste.

This terrace farm was started initially to dispose of the kitchen waste in an eco-friendly way. This project recycles ninety percent of this waste. Staff members, after their duty hours, love to tend the garden which has about 150 plants.

93.

Three Tons Of Food Per Year

From A 1/10 Acre City Lot

Self-sufficient in the city, A Family Of Four With No Jobs

Jules Dervaes is an urban farmer and a proponent of the urban homesteading movement. Dervaes and his three adult children operate an urban market garden in Pasadena, California as well as other websites and online stores related to self-sufficiency and "adapting in place."

Dervaes has a one-tenth acre lot in Pasadena, California, on which he and his family raise three tons of food per year. This provides 75 percent of their annual food needs and helps them sustain an organic produce business. They also raise bees and compost worms.

Dervaes started experimenting with self-sufficiency while he lived in New Zealand and later in Florida, then decided to see how efficient he could make an urban homestead in Pasadena, California, USA. According to Natural Home magazine, *"The Dervaeses' operation is about 60 to 150 times as efficient as their industrial competitors, without relying on chemical fertilizers and pesticides."*

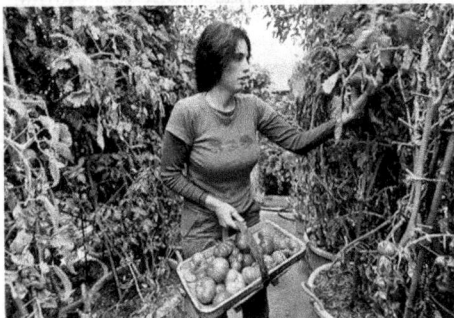

In addition to growing a significant amount of food, the Derveas family attempts to live off-grid as far as possible and have invested significant amounts of money to experiment with other ways of attaining self-sufficiency. They have 12 solar panels on the roof of the house, a biodiesel filling station in the garage, and a solar oven in the backyard; they use a wastewater reclamation system, a dual-flush toilet, a composting toilet, and a number of hand-cranked kitchen appliances (to reduce power consumption). They also use solar drying, and have a cob oven.

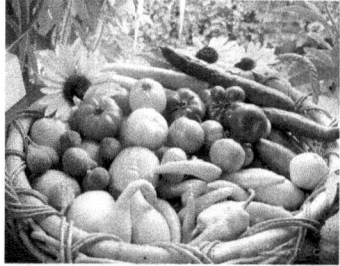

Dervaes owns several websites, including julesdervaes.com, pathtofreedom.com, urbanhomestead.org, urbanhomesteading.com, freedomgardens.org, peddlrswagon.com, backyardchickens.org, barnyardsandbackyards.org, thehiddenyears.org, and dervaesinstitute.org. As of 2008, Path to Freedom got five million hits per month from over 125 different countries.

The Dervaes family was featured on National Geographic Channel's Doomsday Preppers in 2012 and briefly appeared in a trailer for the show.

94.

No Space?

Grow Your Own Food With Vertical Gardens

And Put A Farmer's Market On Your Back Porch

With the growing trends in eating organic foods and local foods, the Vertical Garden may be a perfect fit for people who want to grow their own food without any of the weeding, tilling, fertilizing or other typical chores of gardening. Many restaurant owners in New York are now growing food on the rooftops using their Vertical Gardens.

Vertical Gardens simplifies traditional gardening, using a unique vertical garden system that makes it easy to grow your own fresh fruits and vegetables at home.

It's perfect for rooftops, patios, balconies, terraces—just about any relatively sunny place outside.

The O'Hare airport (Los Angeles) has embraced the concept of vertical gardening in full force and now grows much of the produce for restaurants at the airport in their vertical gardening display.

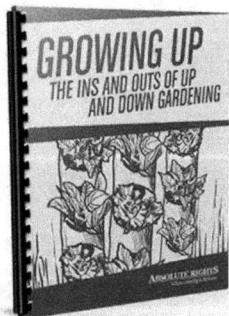

A Do It Yourself Manual

A do it yourself vertical garden can be created with a little imagination and some guidance from the experts. Survival Life and Managing Editor 'Above Average' Joe have produced a Special Report to help people make the most of the space they have, and enjoy the benefits of growing their own food.

Growing Up: The Ins and Outs of Up and Down Gardening is the blueprint for growing all the produce a family could eat in a fraction of the space they think they might need. Vertical gardening is all about constructing practical and inexpensive planting systems that are just as good as a large plot of soil, and sometimes even more so. As little as two square feet of space, up to an average ceiling height, indoors or out, can be enough to grow an entire season's worth of food.

There's no denying the fact that more of the population lives in urban areas, where land is at a premium. With more apartment-style living comes fewer yards, and fewer opportunities to plant gardens. Growing Up will show people how easy it can be to become farmers without any acreage to speak of.

With vertical gardening, farmers actually have better control of their crops. They can extend the life and yield potential of almost everything they plant, giving them fresh food longer than traditional farmers. Manipulating the water, light, and size of vertical garden plants gives far more control over the final outcome.

Any productive garden needs care and attention, but with a vertical garden there's no need for expensive tools, back-breaking work, or protection from nature and the elements. Growing Up

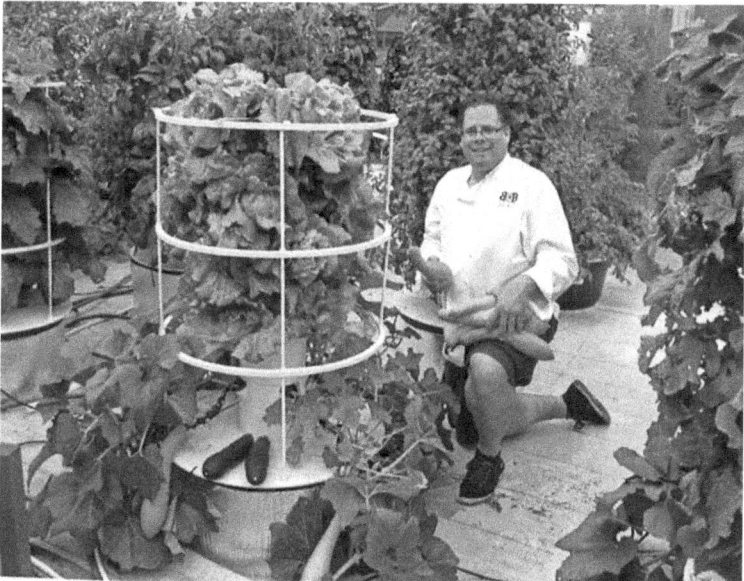

will share the best techniques for creating the most successful yet inexpensive growing systems. Vertical gardens can be set up in an afternoon, with far less time and money spent on a large plot of land.

Ultimately, a food supply grown in a vertical garden could become a life-saving decision. Should a major disaster hit an area, the supply lines of grocery stores and super markets would easily be disrupted. Those who are already growing their own food in a controlled environment won't have to worry about going hungry.

Potential farmers can spend a small fortune trying to make a vertical garden themselves, or they can consult a guide that will talk them through the best ways to do it.

95.

Fast Food, Fast Track To Slow Food, Slow Track Life

A True Story

By L. Kevin & Donna Philippe-Johnson, The Sun, January 2, 2008.

As a middle class American, it's been difficult for me to understand how we are supposed to make a living when there are so many things working against us. How can we go on day after day with the rising cost of food, fuel, utilities, car insurance, taxes and health care, while dealing with the insecurity of unemployment? In the past, whenever I considered these things, I felt a hopeless sense of impending doom in the pit of my stomach. There is so much talk about how to solve these issues, but nothing ever seems to stop the downward spiral of struggle and stress that millions of folks are experiencing.

Like many working people, my life went along fine during the 1980s. I had a good paying job ($42,000 a year) and though I didn't enjoy the kind of work I was doing as an industrial draftsman, receiving a steady paycheck every week kept me going without much complaint.

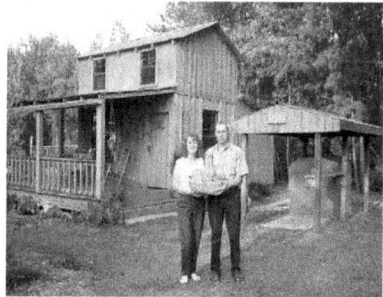

But then came the Gulf War in the 1990s and after that point I faced nine layoffs over the span of 10 years. By the time September 11 happened, I hadn't been able to maintain steady employment in the petrochemical industry for over a decade. I would work about three or four months, then back again to the unemployment line.

It was at this point that I realized that something was wrong. The life strategy I had grown up to believe in was no longer working and there didn't seem to be any answers. Obviously no one was going to get me out of this, so I decided I needed to take matters into my own hands and figure out a way to redefine my basic approach to living.

Lucky for me, I have an adventurous wife. She was on the same page with me and was willing to make some drastic changes in our lifestyle. As a committed team, we decided to figure out another way to survive despite these uncertain, hard economic times. Since we didn't have a lot of money and because it was getting harder to find steady employment, we decided to rethink our basic values in order to create a life for ourselves where we could be independent and free of needing a career or a full-time job.

And for us, that meant first and foremost, moving to the country. If we were going to be poor, we thought, at least it would be better to be poor in the country. That way we could grow our own food and reduce our expenses. Eventually we discovered that there were others who felt the same way we did. Today there is a small, but growing movement in this country towards a lifestyle we call "Voluntary Creative Simplicity."

We decided to start over, to shake loose from all the things holding us down. We got rid of all the stuff we didn't need and worked on paying off debt. Then canceling our credit cards and using cash, we followed an efficient financial plan that taught how to track every penny. By doing this we were able eventually to save a little bit of money.

Also, we wanted to be strong and healthy to do the work required for this basic lifestyle so we changed our eating habits. We broke away from the standard American fast food, pre-packaged supermarket diet in favor of organically grown whole grains, raw fruits and vegetables, fermented dairy, nuts, seeds and sprouts and eliminated all junk foods and prescription drugs. We started exercising regularly by walking, practicing yoga, and gardening. Since we no longer wanted to pay health insurance premiums, we decided to start a special savings account ($1,000) just for emergency first-aid treatment. And of course we got rid of the cell phone, cable television and Internet bills and greatly minimized our use of air conditioning. The beginning of the path to the simple life was a process of elimination in every aspect of our lives.

Eventually we found 2-1/2 acres of land, 35 miles out of the city. Inspired by our new vision, one summer we said goodbye to the city, permanently moved out to our new place and set up a dome tent to live in. We happily lived in our tent that summer while clearing the land and constructing a rustic 10' by 12' room with a sleeping loft. We did this on a "pay-as-you-go" plan, hauling all the materials in the back of our old pickup truck. Never having built anything before, we worked hard and gained the skill of building our own shelter.

As the tiny outbuilding took shape, next came the installation of an underground cistern for collecting rainwater, and finally, the construction of our three-room (500 square foot) cabin. Since we had to borrow $9,000 to purchase the property, I continued to take whatever jobs I could find (drafting, clerk work, courier, dishwasher, bakery assistant, etc.) while Donna (my wife!) stayed busy working on our organic garden, planting fruit trees and composting. She enjoys learning about native plants and healing herbs that she can grow.

Over the next few years, while working toward our goals of self-reliance and independence, we became stronger, healthier and more confident in our ability to rely on our own skills. It was quite an empowering experience. We learned how to build things, grow our own food, take responsibility for our own health, and best of all, we learned how to laugh and have fun again. The simple joys and true pleasures of fresh, home-grown food, watching everything grow and prosper in harmony, working with our own hands and spending quality time together replaced all of the costly false values that had occupied our time before.

Gradually we paid off the land, finished the cabin and succeeded in minimizing our basic utility costs. We began to notice that our expenses were decreasing as the quality of our life was increasing. As long as we stayed home and didn't travel to a steady job we really didn't need very much money. The lifestyle of voluntary creative simplicity was resulting in compounding efficiency and improvement in every area of our lives.

Soon, we saw the proof of the inefficiency of working a full-time job. After figuring in the work-related expenses of one job, I realized that my take home pay was only $3 an hour! At that point I was convinced that it was far more cost effective to stay home, grow our own food, split our own firewood and bake our own bread than it was to travel to a job day after day. Yet we still needed some form of income.

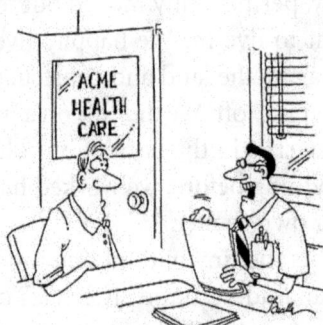

"I'm sorry, but stress caused by trying to figure out your health insurance is not covered by it."

Though we had reduced the amount we needed to around $540 a month (way below the poverty level in America), we still had to find a way to generate that income without relying on full-time employment. Once we had succeeded in drastically reducing the amount of money we needed, I knew it would be easy to earn this income by working odd jobs such as building rustic furniture, playing guitar for tips, simple carpentry, part-time drafting, office work, plumbing, etc. However, there was one thing I really loved to do...bake handmade whole-grain sourdough bread in an outdoor wood-fired clay oven! I had always shared my bread with friends and family, but it never really occurred to me to do it as a way to earn extra money.

We soon discovered that there was no authentic, handmade sourdough bread being produced in our area, and little by little, people began asking if they could trade or buy from us. Within a year we had enough bread customers to generate the supplemental income needed to meet our modest expenses. And now there is even more demand and a waiting list of neighbors and friends who want our bread regularly. They know our bread is special because the organic wheat is freshly hand milled, the loaves are lovingly made entirely by hand and baked in our outdoor clay oven.

While the key to the lifestyle of voluntary simplicity, is "thinking small," many people still believe the opposite is true-"bigger is better." For example, people often tell us we should invest in a commercial bakery and produce more sourdough bread. But in order to expand and make a career out of baking and selling bread, we would have to go into debt to purchase commercial mixers, freezers and large ovens, work longer hours and face the mountain of bureaucratic permits, codes, fees and restrictions. As a result, the simple, authentic handmade artisan bread that our customers love would have to be sacrificed in favor of expanding volume and making more money. Everybody loses but the bankers and the bureaucrats. We would fall right back in the same old trap, getting into debt and sacrificing our freedom and quality of life for a job. This is an example of compounding inefficiency.

The downfall of many people who would like to break the bonds of stress and financial enslavement to the system is their tendency to think too big. But we must realize that this has been programmed into us by the industrial society and loan institutions, all attempting to excite and feed our insatiable desires. Friends, it takes a lot of mindful awareness to break free of all these traps. It also requires an ability to improvise and adapt towards an alternative model. The lifestyle of voluntary simplicity is one option and the resulting benefits are transformational.

The point I'm making is this: many of us can no longer think in terms of

"Those who think they have no time for healthy eating, will sooner or later have to find time for illness"

having a lifetime career anymore. For whatever reason, things are changing in this country. Outsourcing and cheaper labor costs in other countries will continue to eliminate jobs in the United States. And though the opportunity still exists to work, we must understand that it may be only temporary. While continuing to work at a job or career one should be wise and set up a plan to survive without steady employment for certain periods of time if necessary.

This could mean storing some supplies, purchasing a piece of property where a small shelter, tent or tipi can be erected if necessary, or getting out of the city and into the country where

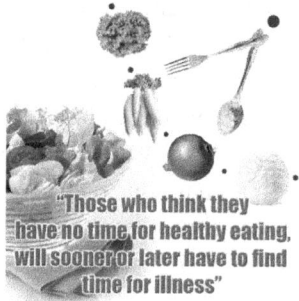

one can provide food for themselves. My old Grandpa used to say, "all the troubles in this country began when people stopped growing their own food." And he was right. The younglings of this modern age don't even know what real food is, much less how to grow or prepare it! This has to change. (That's another reason we promote sourdough bread baking. It is time to start a "slow-food" movement).

Thinking small is one of the most intelligent and powerful things one can do. Consciously reducing one's life down to the simple basics is the secret to happiness. And it is so easy. What is the solution? This is our advice, especially to young people:

"Don't get in debt, don't think in terms of a career (work at a job for one reason only, to get paid so you can buy a place to live and grow some food), live in a small shelter, unload unnecessary stuff, reduce monthly expenses, extract yourself from the enslavement of modern technological materialism, stay healthy by exercising, eat a simple, wholesome diet, develop some practical skills, practice your art or trade and serve your local community. Teach your children to value true pleasures. Real wealth is perishable: food, health, trees, flowers, herbs, healthy soil, clean water, fresh air, friends and art. Learn to value and appreciate these above all else."

Of course we realize that everyone has to creatively work out their own unique plan according to their particular circumstances, especially if there are children to raise. (We have six grown children.) But with "small thinking," so many opportunities open up and the more one can release, the more freedom there is to experience with each passing year.

If someone would have suggested to us ten years ago that there was a way for the two of us to live on much less, build our own little hut, buy our freedom, give up steady employment, work fewer hours, become happy, healthy, debt free, self-reliant, and live fearlessly without health insurance, I would have told them they were crazy. This has been an incredible, radical journey for us, but now we know from first hand experience that with vision, patience, self-discipline and courage, it is possible to create such a reality.

Creative voluntary simplicity expands faster than inflation for those who can do it, rather than waste time and energy thinking too big and chasing after more money to find happiness and security.

96.

Timeless Science

Of Sanctified Eating And Good Health

By Adiraja Dasa

India is the home not only of vegetarian cooking, but also of the science of healthful living. The scripture known as the Ayur-veda, is the oldest known work on biology, hygiene, medicine, and nutrition. This branch of the Vedas was revealed thousands of years ago by Sri Bhagavan Dhanvantari, an incarnation of Krishna. "Old" is not the same as "primitive", however, and some of the instructions of the Ayur-veda will remind today's reader of modern nutritional teachings or just plain common sense. Other instructions may seem less familiar, but they will bear themselves out if given the chance.

We shouldn't be surprised to see bodily health discussed in spiritual writings. The Vedas consider the human body a divine gift, a chance for the imprisoned soul to escape from the cycle of birth and death. The importance of healthful living in spiritual life is also mentioned by Lord Krishna in the Bhagavad-gita (6.16-17), "There is no possibility of becoming a yogi, O Arjuna, if one eats too much or eats too little, sleeps too much or does not sleep enough. One who is temperate in his habits of eating, sleeping, working, and recreation can mitigate all material pains by practicing the yoga system."

Proper eating has a double importance. Besides its role in bodily health-over-eating, eating in a disturbed or anxious state of mind, or eating unclean foods causes indigestion, "the parent of all diseases"-proper eating can help the aspiring transcendentalist attain mastery over his senses. "Of all the senses, the tongue is the most difficult to control," says the Prasada-sevaya, a song composed by Srila Bhaktivinoda Thakura, one of the spiritual predecessors of Srila Prabhupada, "but Krishna has kindly given us this nice prasada to help us control the tongue."

Here are a few guidelines for good eating taken from the Ayurveda and other scriptures.

Spiritualize Your Eating

The Bhagavad-gita (17.8-10) divides foods into three classes: those of the quality of goodness, those of the quality of passion, and those of the quality of ignorance. The most healthful are the foods of goodness. "Foods of the quality of goodness [milk products, grains, fruits, and vegetables] increase the duration of life; purify one's existence; and give strength, health, happiness, and satisfaction. Such foods are sweet, juicy, fatty, and palatable."

Foods that are too bitter, sour, salty, pungent, dry or hot, are of the quality of passion and cause distress. But foods of the quality of ignorance, such as meat, fish, and fowl, described as "putrid, decomposed, and unclean," produce only pain, disease, and bad karma. In other words, what you eat affects the quality of your life.

The purpose of food, however, is not only to increase longevity and bodily strength, but also to purify the mind and consciousness. Therefore the spiritualist offers his food to the Lord before eating. Such offered food clears the way for spiritual progress. There are millions of people in India and around the world who would not consider eating unless their food was offered first to Lord Krishna.

Eat At Fixed Times

As far as possible, take your main meal at the solar midday, when the sun is highest, because that's when your digestive power is strongest. Wait at least three hours after a light meal and five after a heavy meal before eating again. Eating at fixed times without snacking between meals helps make the mind and tongue peaceful.

Eat In A Pleasant Atmosphere

A cheerful mood helps digestion; a spiritual mood, even more. Eat in pleasant surroundings and center the conversation around spiritual topics.

Look upon your food as Krishna's mercy. Food is a divine gift, so cook it, serve it, and eat it in a spirit of joyful reverence.

Combine Foods Wisely

Foods should be combined for taste, and for efficient digestion and assimilation of nutrients. Rice and other grains go well with vegetables. Milk products such as cheese, yogurt, and buttermilk go well with grains and vegetables, but fresh milk does not go well with vegetables.

The typical Vedic lunch of rice, split-lentil soup, vegetables, and chapatis is a perfectly balanced meal.

Avoid combining vegetables with raw fruits. (Fruits are best eaten as a separate meal or with hot milk). Also avoid mixing acidic fruits with alkaline fruits, or milk with fermented milk products.

Share Prasada With Others

Srila Rupa Gosvami explains in the Upadesamrta, a five-hundred year-old classic about devotional service, "One of the ways for devotees to express love is to offer prasada and accept prasada from one another." A gift from God is too good a thing to keep to oneself, so the scriptures recommend sharing prasada with others, be they friends or strangers. In ancient India-and many still follow the practice-the householder would open his door at mealtime and call out, "Prasada! prasada! prasada! If anyone is hungry, let him come and eat!" After welcoming his guests and offering them all the comforts at his disposal, he would feed them to their full satisfaction before taking his own meal. Even if you can't follow this practice, look for occasions to offer prasada to others, and you will appreciate prasada more yourself.

Be Clean

Vedic culture places great emphasis on cleanliness, both internal and external. For internal cleanliness, we can cleanse the mind and heart of material contamination by chanting Vedic mantras, particularly the Hare Krishna mantra. External cleanliness includes keeping a high standard of cleanliness when cooking and eating. Naturally this includes the usual good habits of washing the hands before eating, and the hands and mouth after.

Eat Moderately

Vitality and strength depend not on how much we eat, but on how much we are able to digest and absorb into our system. The stomach needs working space, so instead of filling it completely, fill it just halfway, by eating only half as much as you think you can, and leave a fourth of the space for liquids and the other fourth for air. You'll help your digestion and get more pleasure from eating.

Moderate eating will also give satisfaction to your mind and harmony to your body. Overeating makes the mind agitated or dull and the body heavy and tired.

Don't Pour Water On The Fire Of Digestion

Visible flames and invisible combustion are two aspects of what we call "fire". Digestion certainly involves combustion. We often speak of "burning up" fat or calories, and the word "calorie" itself refers to the heat released when food is burned. The Vedas inform us that our food is digested by a fire called Jatharagni (the Fire in the Belly). Therefore, because we often drink with our meals, the effect of liquid on fire becomes an important consideration in the art of eating.

Drinking before the meal tempers the appetite and, consequently, the urge to overeat. Drinking moderately while eating helps the stomach do its job, but drinking afterwards dilutes the gastric juices and reduces the fire of digestion. Wait at least an hour after eating before drinking again, and, if need be, you can drink every hour after that until the next meal.

Don't Waste Food

The scriptures tell us that for every bit of food wasted in times of plenty, an equal amount will be lacking in times of need. Put on your plate only as much as you can eat, and save any leftovers for the next meal. (To reheat food it is usually necessary to add liquid and simmer in a covered pan. Stir well and frequently).

If for some reason prasada has to be discarded, then feed it to animals, bury it, or put it in a body of water. Prasada is sacred and should never be put in the garbage. Whether cooking or eating, be careful about not wasting food.

Try An Occasional Fast

According to the Ayur-veda, fasting strengthens both will power and bodily health. An occasional fast gives the digestive system a rest and refreshes the senses, mind, and consciousness.

In most cases, the Ayur-veda recommends a water fast. Juice fasting is popular in the West because Western methods encourage long fasts. In Ayur-vedic treatment, however, most fasts are short- one to three days. While fasting, one should not drink more water than needed to quench one's thirst. Jatharagni, the fire of digestion, being freed from the task of digesting food, is busy incinerating the accumulated wastes in the body, and too much water inhibits the process.

Devotees of Krishna observe another kind of fast on Ekadasi, the eleventh day after the full moon and the eleventh day after the new moon, by abstaining from grains, peas, and beans. The Brahma-vaivarta scripture says, "One who observes Ekadasi is freed from all kinds of reactions to sinful activities, and thereby advances in pious life."

Purify Your Existence

In the Bhagavad Gita, one of the main spiritual texts of India, Krishna, or God, offers a very salient point: "If one offers Me with love and devotion a leaf, a flower, fruit or water, I will accept it." The point being made here is that God isn't looking for elaborate and complicated offerings from the devotees. Instead, Krishna is looking for the love and devotion, or the bhakti, behind the offering.

The other very important facet of the offering is that it can't be a product of cruelty. It is a well known fact that animals undergo tremendous emotional and physical suffering when killed. In the classic Hindu text Manusmriti, it is stated, "Having well considered the origin of flesh-foods, and the cruelty of fettering and slaying corporeal beings, let man entirely abstain from eating flesh." Such food items are not only unhealthy for the our bodies, but also unhealthy for our consciousness.

When food is offered to the Divine or God, it becomes sanctified. In the bhakti tradition, food is offered through devotional mantras that focus our intention. It is understood that God then accepts the offering of food and partakes of it. Because the food came in contact with the divine, it also adopts divine qualities. In this way, matter is transformed into spirit.

When an individual consumes this offered or "karma-free" food, one's mind, senses and consciousness get purified of such tendencies as greed, anger, envy and selfishness. One comes simultaneously closer to the divine. This is known as the yoga of eating.

Advancing spiritually and elevating one's consciousness can often involve rigorous practices. However, it's nice to know that just by engaging in simple and creative endeavors, such as cooking and eating, one can move closer to that ultimate spiritual goal.

THE AUTHOR

Dr. Sahadeva dasa (Sanjay Shah) is a monk in vaisnava tradition. Coming from a prominent family of Rajasthan, he graduated in commerce from St.Xaviers College, Kolkata and then went on to complete his CA (Chartered Accountancy) and ICWA (Cost and works Accountancy) with national ranks. Later he received his doctorate.

For close to last two decades, he is leading a monk's life and he has made serving God and humanity as his life's mission. He has been serving as the president of ISKCON Secunderabad center since last twenty years.

His areas of work include research in Vedic and contemporary thought, Corporate and educational training, social work and counselling, travelling in India and aborad, writing books and of course, practicing spiritual life and spreading awareness about the same.

He is also an accomplished musician, composer, singer, instruments player and sound engineer. He has more than a dozen albums to his credit so far. (SoulMelodies.com) His varied interests include alternative holistic living, Vedic studies, social criticism, environment, linguistics, history, art & crafts, nature studies, web technologies etc.

Many of his books have been acclaimed internationally and translated in other languages.

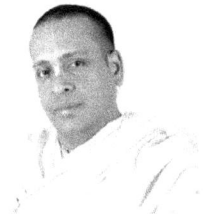

By The Same Author

Oil-Final Countdown To A Global Crisis And Its Solutions

End of Modern Civilization And Alternative Future

To Kill Cow Means To End Human Civilization

Cow And Humanity - Made For Each Other

Cows Are Cool - Love 'Em!

Capitalism Communism And Cowism - A New Economics For The 21st Century

Noble Cow - Munching Grass, Looking Curious And Just Hanging Around

Let's Be Friends - A Curious, Calm Cow

Wondrous Glories of Vraja

We Feel Just Like You Do

(More information on availability at DrDasa.com)